1990
YEAR BOOK OF
SPORTS
MEDICINE®

The 1990 Year Book® Series

Year Book of Anesthesia®: Drs. Miller, Kirby, Ostheimer, Roizen, and Stoelting

Year Book of Cardiology®: Drs. Schlant, Collins, Engle, Frye, Kaplan, and O'Rourke

Year Book of Critical Care Medicine®: Drs. Rogers and Parrillo

Year Book of Dentistry®: Drs. Meskin, Ackerman, Kennedy, Leinfelder, Matukas, and Rovin

Year Book of Dermatology®: Drs. Sober and Fitzpatrick

Year Book of Diagnostic Radiology®: Drs. Bragg, Hendee, Keats, Kirkpatrick, Miller, Osborn, and Thompson

Year Book of Digestive Diseases®: Drs. Greenberger and Moody

Year Book of Drug Therapy®: Drs. Hollister and Lasagna

Year Book of Emergency Medicine®: Dr. Wagner

Year Book of Endocrinology®: Drs. Bagdade, Braverman, Halter, Horton, Kannan, Korenman, Molitch, Morley, Odell, Rogol, Ryan, and Sherwin

Year Book of Family Practice®: Drs. Rakel, Avant, Driscoll, Prichard, and Smith

Year Book of Geriatrics and Gerontology®: Drs. Beck, Abrass, Burton, Cummings, Makinodan, and Small

Year Book of Hand Surgery®: Drs. Dobyns, Chase, and Amadio

Year Book of Hematology®: Drs. Spivak, Bell, Ness, Quesenberry, and Wiernik

Year Book of Infectious Diseases®: Drs. Wolff, Barza, Keusch, Klempner, and Snydman

Year Book of Infertility: Drs. Mishell, Paulsen, and Lobo

Year Book of Medicine®: Drs. Rogers, Des Prez, Cline, Braunwald, Greenberger, Wilson, Epstein, and Malawista

Year Book of Neonatal and Perinatal Medicine: Drs. Klaus and Fanaroff

Year Book of Neurology and Neurosurgery®: Drs. Currier and Crowell

Year Book of Nuclear Medicine®: Drs. Hoffer, Gore, Gottschalk, Sostman, Zaret, and Zubal

Year Book of Obstetrics and Gynecology®: Drs. Mishell, Kirschbaum, and Morrow

Year Book of Occupational and Environmental Medicine: Drs. Emmett, Brooks, Harris, and Schenker

Year Book of Oncology: Drs. Young, Longo, Ozols, Simone, Steele, and Weichselbaum

Year Book of Ophthalmology®: Drs. Laibson, Adams, Augsburger, Benson, Cohen, Eagle, Flanagan, Nelson, Reinecke, Sergott, and Wilson

Year Book of Orthopedics®: Drs. Sledge, Poss, Cofield, Frymoyer, Griffin, Hansen, Johnson, Springfield, and Weiland

Year Book of Otolaryngology–Head and Neck Surgery®: Drs. Bailey and Paparella

Year Book of Pathology and Clinical Pathology®: Drs. Brinkhous, Dalldorf, Grisham, Langdell, and McLendon

Year Book of Pediatrics®: Drs. Oski and Stockman

Year Book of Plastic, Reconstructive, and Aesthetic Surgery: Drs. Miller, Bennett, Haynes, Hoehn, McKinney, and Whitaker

Year Book of Podiatric Medicine and Surgery®: Dr. Jay

Year Book of Psychiatry and Applied Mental Health®: Drs. Talbott, Frances, Frances, Freedman, Meltzer, Schowalter, and Yudofsky

Year Book of Pulmonary Disease®: Drs. Green, Loughlin, Michael, Mulshine, Peters, Terry, Tockman, and Wise

Year Book of Speech, Language, and Hearing: Drs. Bernthal, Hall, and Tomblin

Year Book of Sports Medicine®: Drs. Shephard, Eichner, Sutton, and Torg, Col. Anderson, and Mr. George

Year Book of Surgery®: Drs. Schwartz, Jonasson, Peacock, Shires, Spencer, and Thompson

Year Book of Urology®: Drs. Gillenwater and Howards

Year Book of Vascular Surgery®: Drs. Bergan and Yao

1990

The Year Book of SPORTS MEDICINE®

Editor-in-Chief

Roy J. Shephard, M.D., Ph.D., D.P.E.
Director, School of Physical and Health Education, and Professor of Applied Physiology, Department of Preventive Medicine and Biostatistics, University of Toronto

Editors

Col. James L. Anderson, PE.D.
Director of Physical Education, United States Military Academy, West Point

Edward R. Eichner, M.D.
Professor of Medicine and Chief, Section of Hematology, University of Oklahoma Health Sciences Center, Oklahoma City

Francis J. George, ATC, PT
Head Athletic Trainer, Brown University, Providence

John R. Sutton, M.D.
Acting Deputy Principal, Cumberland College for Health Sciences, Lidcombe, New South Wales, Professor of Medicine and Exercise Physiology, University of Sydney

Joseph S. Torg, M.D.
Professor of Orthopedic Surgery, and Director, Sports Medicine Center, University of Pennsylvania School of Medicine, Philadelphia

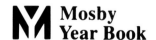

Mosby Year Book

St. Louis   Baltimore   Boston   Chicago   London   Philadelphia   Sydney   Toronto

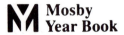

**Mosby
Year Book**

Dedicated to Publishing Excellence

Editor-in-Chief, Year Book Publishing: Nancy Gorham
Sponsoring Editor: Gretchen C. Templeton
Manager, Medical Information Services: Edith M. Podrazik
Senior Medical Information Specialist: Terri Strorigl
Assistant Director, Manuscript Services: Frances M. Perveiler
Associate Managing Editor, Year Book Editing Services: Elizabeth Fitch
Production Coordinator: Max F. Perez
Proofroom Supervisor: Barbara M. Kelly

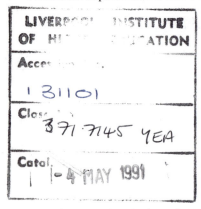

Mosby-Year Book, Inc.
11830 Westline Industrial Drive
St. Louis, MO 63146

Editorial Office:
Mosby-Year Book, Inc.
200 North LaSalle St.
Chicago, IL 60601

International Standard Serial Number: 0162-0908
International Standard Book Number: 0-8151-7738-0

Table of Contents

The material in this volume represents literature reviewed from February 1989 through January 1990.

Journals Represented

Mosby–Year Book subscribes to and surveys nearly 850 U.S. and foreign medical and allied health journals. From these journals, the Editors select the articles to be abstracted. Journals represented in this YEAR BOOK are listed below.

Acta Orthopaedica Scandinavica
American Family Physician
American Heart Journal
American Journal of Cardiology
American Journal of Clinical Nutrition
American Journal of Diseases of Children
American Journal of Obstetrics and Gynecology
American Journal of Occupational Therapy
American Journal of Physical Medicine & Rehabilitation
American Journal of Physiology
American Journal of Roentgenology
American Journal of Sports Medicine
American Review of Respiratory Disease
Angiology
Annales de Chirurgie de la Main
Annals of Emergency Medicine
Annals of Internal Medicine
Archives of Emergency Medicine
Archives of Internal Medicine
Archives of Orthopedic and Traumatic Surgery
Archives of Otolaryngology—Head and Neck Surgery
Archives of Physical Medicine and Rehabilitation
Arteriosclerosis
Arthritis and Rheumatism
Arthroscopy
Athletic Training
Australian Journal of Science and Medicine in Sport
British Heart Journal
British Journal of Family Planning
British Journal of Sports Medicine
British Medical Journal
Canadian Family Physician
Canadian Journal of Sports Sciences
Chest
Circulation
Clinica Chimica Acta
Clinical Endocrinology
Clinical Nephrology
Clinical Orthopaedics and Related Research
Clinical Pediatrics
Clinical Physiology
Clinical and Laboratory Haematology
Ergonomics
European Heart Journal
European Journal of Applied Physiology and Occupational Physiology
Fertility and Sterility
Gastroenterology
Gerontology
Injury

International Journal of Cardiology
International Journal of Sports Medicine
Journal of Applied Physiology
Journal of Applied Sport Science Research
Journal of Biomechanics
Journal of Biomedical Engineering
Journal of Bone and Joint Surgery (American volume)
Journal of Bone and Joint Surgery (British volume)
Journal of Cardiopulmonary Rehabilitation
Journal of Clinical Endocrinology and Metabolism
Journal of Clinical Investigation
Journal of Computer Assisted Tomography
Journal of Gerontology
Journal of Hand Surgery (American)
Journal of Musculoskeletal Medicine
Journal of Neural Transmission
Journal of Neurological Sciences
Journal of Orthopaedic and Sports Physical Therapy
Journal of Pediatrics
Journal of Sports Medicine and Physical Fitness
Journal of Sports Sciences
Journal of Trauma
Journal of Vascular Surgery
Journal of the American College of Cardiology
Journal of the American Medical Association
Lancet
Medecine du Sport
Medicine and Science in Sports and Exercise
Metabolism
Neurology
New England Journal of Medicine
Nursing Research
Orthopaedic Review
Orthopedics
Pace
Pediatrics
Physician and Sportsmedicine
Physiotherapy Canada
Postgraduate Medicine
Quarterly Journal of Experimental Physiology
Quarterly Journal of Medicine
Radiology
Research Quarterly for Exercise and Sport
Scandinavian Journal of Rehabilitation Medicine
Scandinavian Journal of Work Environment and Health
Sports Medicine
Sports Training, Medicine, and Rehabilitation
Stroke

STANDARD ABBREVIATIONS

The following terms are abbreviated in this edition: acquired immunodeficiency syndrome (AIDS), the central nervous system (CNS), cerebrospinal fluid (CSF), computed tomography (CT), electrocardiography (ECG), and human immunodeficiency virus (HIV).

Introduction

The past year has brought to light many interesting new themes in the field of sports medicine, and representative papers covering these topics are included in the present volume.

One of the most exciting findings of the past year has been the strong new proof of the value of exercise in decreasing both cardiac and all-cause mortality in sedentary adults. Moreover, it has become apparent that the amount of exercise required to obtain protection is not at a heroic level that is impracticable to prescribe for the average patient—the greatest advantage is seen in a progression from total inactivity to modest daily energy expenditures.

The growing prevalence of HIV infections continues to cause concern in public health authorities, and the epidemic has sparked a tremendous surge of investigation into immune function. One encouraging feature for those already affected by this disease is that moderate activity boosts various aspects of immune function. Through stimulation of natural killer cell activity, exercise may also have some value in both the prevention of cancer and as secondary treatment after surgical excision or radiotherapy.

There is interesting new work concerning the treatment of hypothermia by radio-energy, and disturbing evidence that repeated exposure to extreme altitudes may cause deterioration of cerebral function.

Despite the disqualification of Olympic participant Ben Johnson, surveys show an alarming prevalence of anabolic steroid abuse in the United States, extending from the high school to the professional level. The search continues for methods of detecting blood doping, and new hazards associated with this abuse are coming to light.

There have finally been major developments in cardiac rehabilitation. The need to restore muscle function as well as oxygen-transporting capacity is finally receiving recognition, and the boundaries of the rehabilitation center are extending beyond the typical myocardial infarction patient to include those with congestive failure and others who have undergone vascular bypass and cardiac transplantation.

These and many other topics important to the practitioner of sports medicine are discussed in this 1990 edition of the YEAR BOOK OF SPORTS MEDICINE.

Roy J. Shephard, M.D. Ph.D., D.P.E.

Exercise After Myocardial Infarction: Translating the Expertise of Sports Medicine Into Clinical Practice

ROY J. SHEPHARD, M.D., PH.D., D.P.E.
School of Physical and Health Education, Department of Preventive Medicine and Biostatistics, Faculty of Medicine, University of Toronto

The Paradox of Knowledge and Practice

The benefits of progressive exercise after myocardial infarction are well known to experts in sports medicine. Recent meta-analyses, based on controlled experiments involving more than 5,000 patients, have provided clear proof of the value of exercise in the secondary and tertiary treatment of ischemic heart disease (1–4). An appropriately graded training program reduces the risk of a fatal recurrence by 17% to 29% in the first few years after myocardial infarction, and although the number of nonfatal reinfarctions changes very little, the proportion of fatal recurrences is reduced by such therapy (4). Moreover, recent studies suggest that the proportion of patients who return to work is increased (5), and the average time for a return to normal employment is shortened (6). Aerobic power is increased by an average of some 20% relative to controls (7). If exercise sessions are continued for 6 to 12 months there are accompanying gains in cardiac stroke volume (8–10), with a lessening of electrocardiographic ST segmental depression (11, 12) and improved myocardial perfusion (13–15). The average gain in oxygen transport is equivalent to a 10-year reduction in functional age (16), and in some patients who have chosen to train particularly vigorously, gains of maximal oxygen intake have exceeded 100% of the initial values (17). Finally, and perhaps most importantly, the quality of life is substantially improved for the exercisers (18).

Few other treatments of myocardial disease (or, indeed, of other chronic clinical conditions) can claim such a catalog of proven therapeutic benefits. Nevertheless, in 1990 one can find clinical articles advising family physicians that "It is not justified to recommend special exercise programs of cardiac rehabilitation as a routine measure in the care of most patients who have had an infarction" (19).

The unwillingness to accept evidence established by many years of careful and costly experimentation plainly has important implications for the practical application of the new knowledge presented in this and other scholarly volumes, and possible reasons for the "communication gap" merit further analysis. The article already cited (19) will be used as a primary text for our discussion of this issue, although there have been other recent dogmatic and doctrinaire condemnations of exercise therapy, both by clinicians (20) and economists (21).

General Factors

Limited knowledge base.—One reason why clinicians tend to be uncomfortable with exercise as a practical form of therapy is that, despite the vigorous educational efforts of groups such as the American College of Sports Medicine, many family practitioners remain unfamiliar with even the basic concepts of exercise testing and exercise prescription. Medical schools still offer far too little training in this important area of instruction.

When writing technical articles it then becomes tempting to rely on secondary opinions, rather than to reach a personal decision after a careful review of the original data. Thus, in dismissing exercise rehabilitation, the paper under detailed discussion (19) admits that it ". . . is based, in large part, on their outline and review. . . ."

Similarly, when the average family physician offers advise to a patient in an office setting, it is easier to opt for the familiar approach of pharmaceutics than to break the new ground of recommending an exercise program. Pseudoscientific justification for such conservatism can be found in claims that the benefits of exercise are still not fully proven.

Loss of clinical control.—If personal knowledge of exercise methodology is limited, one simple option is referral of the patient to a specialized rehabilitation center for a long-term program of treatment. Although this is an effective solution, it means surrender of some control over the patient's treatment and—dare we say this?—a resultant fear that income will be lost for a considerable period.

The quest for control is a potent human motivator and, consciously or subconsciously, the clinician who lacks expertise in sports medicines often wishes to retain control over the patient through adoption of a pharmaceutical approach. This is readily rationalized by hasty dismissal of evidence that favors the exercise alternative.

Commercial influences.—A careful choice between the options of exercise, pharmaceutics, and surgery is hardly helped by strong commercial interests promoting each of the possible alternatives. Physicians are barraged with glossy covered brochures and "free" luncheon-seminars that offer highly selective information on the merits of drug treatment. Cardiac surgery has also become big business in some hospitals, and there are equally persuasive sales agents arguing that the purchase of an office treadmill can be a major money-maker for a family physician.

Evidence on Mortality and Morbidity

Is the benefit of exercise statistically insignificant?—Authors such as Dunn (19) and Godfrey (20) have suggested that the impact of an exercise program on mortality and morbidity is statistically insignificant. But, by focusing exclusively on probability values from selected papers, they conveniently overlook the consistent trend present in a multiplicity of studies that (when considered individually) lack the sample size needed to prove or disprove the exercise hypothesis.

It is true that of at least 16 controlled studies, only two small (22, 23) and one larger (24) exercise trial have in themselves shown a statistically significant reduction in cardiac mortality. However, with one important exception [the Southern Ontario Exercise-Heart Collaborative Trial (25)], almost all reports have accorded a 20% to 30% advantage to the exercised group. The negative findings in southern Ontario apparently reflect a large "crossover" of subjects between control and exercised groups; if attention is confined to subjects for whom there was objective evidence of adherence to the prescribed regimen, we find (as in other laboratories) a statistically insignificant 28% advantage of mortality in the exercised group (26).

TABLE 1.—Meta-Analyses Showing Influence of Exercise-Centered Rehabilitation Programs on Relative Risk of Fatal Recurrence After Myocardial Infarction

Author	Sample Size	Total Exercise	Deaths Control	Relative Exercise/Control	Risk Significance
May et al (1)	2,752	164	201	0.81	—
Bobbio (27)	2,260	131	184	0.71	0.002
Oldridge et al (2)	3,614	233	291	0.80	0.0044
Oldridge et al (28)	5,243	356	440	0.81	0.0013
Shephard (4)	5,325	370	447	0.83	0.0013

Evidence from meta-analyses.—Several authors (1–4, 27–30) have attempted to overcome the technical problem of inadequate sample size by a pooling of data. This approach, sometimes described as meta-analysis (31), is recognized as both useful and valid in epidemiologic investigations in which individual samples are insufficient for conclusive examination of an issue.

Data from individual trials that meet minimum standards of experimental design are combined (Table 1), yielding statistically significant evidence that an exercise-centered rehabilitation program does indeed bring about a substantial and clinically useful reduction of mortality for the postcoronary patient. The article by May et al. (1) further argues that the gains attributable to an exercise program are larger and more clearly established than those reported for alternative forms of therapy.

In contrast, exercise does not seem to change the total number of recurrent infarctions. But the fact that a smaller fraction of recurrences have a fatal outcome is also an important therapeutic gain.

A major shortcoming of the meta-analyses is that there are inevitable differences in the details of rehabilitation programs from one trial to another (31, 32). The clinical criteria of disease and the date of entry relative to the original myocardial infarction, the intensity and duration of exercise, the mortality experience of the control sample, and the nature of associated therapeutic interventions such as the control of diet have all shown intertrial variations (1, 4). Nevertheless, May et al. (1) concluded that the pooled data used to assess exercise programs were much more acceptable than the information available for most types of pharmaceutical intervention with which exercise has been compared.

Trial duration.—Trial duration has favored the outcome of the pharmaceutical and surgical options with which exercise has been compared. The follow-up period for exercise programs has ranged from a few months to a maximum of 3 years, whereas many years have been required to observe the much-publicized benefits from such tactics as aspirin therapy, or the use of β-blocking drugs or lipid-lowering regimens (33).

Do Risk Factors Change?

Benefit does not result from exercise per se.—The next logical line of retreat for critics of exercise is to admit that a graded increase of physical activity has some beneficial impact on mortality statistics, but to argue that exercise is beneficial *merely* because it reduces known risk factors, e.g., an excessive body mass, high systemic blood pressure, an adverse lipid profile, or the habit of cigarette smoking. Given the lack of success in correcting cardiac risk factors by other means, this hardly seems a valid criticism of exercise (34).

In the specific context of myocardial infarction, Dunn (19) makes the potentially more serious charge that there are "no changes in risk factors among those engaging in supervised exercise programs." Careful analysis of the data from controlled trials (33) in fact shows important benefits to the exercised groups, although in the study of Kallio et al. (24) the issue has been clouded by a multifactorial intervention.

Cigarette smoking.—With regard to smoking, no controlled study has claimed any great advantage for exercise (35). The massive World Health Organization (WHO) study (36) found an initial 65% of smokers in the exercised group, and 68% in the control group. Others have noted even higher baseline proportions of smokers, although in some instances there have been substantial subsequent reductions in the number of smokers among both exercised and control groups.

We have certainly been disappointed that the proportion of smokers seen at the Toronto Rehabilitation Centre has not diminished appreciably over several years of involvement in a progressive exercise program. On the other hand, we have been impressed that in a group in which some 80% of participants were heavy smokers, we have held the proportion of smokers at 3 years post infarction to about 35%, below the male population average (37). If participation in the exercise program has done no more, at least it appears to have countered the normal recidivism that is such a major problem in the treatment of severe cigarette addiction.

An uncontrolled study from Bavaria (38) has claimed much more dramatic benefit from participation in a residential rehabilitation program; in that study the proportion of smokers decreased from 69.5% to 25.3%.

Systemic blood pressure.—Several controlled studies have shown reductions in systolic (39), diastolic (35), or both diastolic and systolic pressures (24) with exercise. In our experience (37), involvement in a cardiac rehabilitation program led to a small but clinically useful reduction of 5 mm Hg in the resting systolic blood pressure. Critics who have ignored or dismissed such changes have apparently overlooked the fact that long-term population responses to pharmaceutical treatments are no larger, but are won at the expense of much more serious side effects.

Blood lipids.—Controlled studies of blood lipids have in some instances shown small decreases in the levels of serum cholesterol (40) or triglycerides (35, 41, 42), or both (24). As might be expected, greater changes have been reported from residential programs (38). Nevertheless, the critical feature of the blood lipid profile is the high-density lipoprotein/low-density lipoprotein-cholesterol ratio, rather than the total cholesterol or the triglyceride reading.

The United States National Exercise and Heart Disease Project (35) saw a small increment of high-density lipoprotein-cholesterol in exercised subjects (1.4 mg/dL vs 0.3 mg/dL), and the Toronto Rehabilitation Centre experience has provided unequivocal evidence that involvement of the postcoronary patient in an appropriate exercise program can bring about substantial and clinically important improvements in the lipid profile (43). As Williams and his associates have emphasized (44), this response is not seen unless the exercise prescription progresses to a substantial weekly walking or jogging distance (18−20 km/wk). But the cost to the patient's life-style is still less than the alternative of a major upheaval in domestic cooking patterns and daily treatment with cholestyramine.

Functional Gains

Many critics of exercise have confined their attention to the impact of a rehabilitation program on morbidity and mortality. From a statistical standpoint there are considerable advantages to the use of such hard end points. However, from the patient's perspective, the quality-adjusted lifespan (45) is much more important than its brief prolongation. By increasing the ability of the heart to pump blood and transport oxygen, has the training program allowed the individual concerned an earlier return to work, a greater enjoyment of leisure, or an improved mood state?

Cardiorespiratory function.—Exercise detractors have argued that the heart will recover spontaneously during the first few months after a myocardial infarction. Functional gains as large as 22% have been reported over the period from 3 to 6 weeks post infarction, with a total increment in aerobic power of 46% from 3 weeks to 6 months postinfarction (46, 47). DeBusk (48) has suggested that such early gains largely reflect the willingness of the patient or the supervising physician to carry an exercise test to a higher peak heart rate. But even if there were some more fundamental change of myocardial function, such criticisms would be more relevant to analyses of phase I (hospital-based) rehabilitation programs than to outpatient or community treatment (which typically begins 2 to 6 months after infarction).

In assessing the functional impact of exercise, a recent review of controlled trials (33) noted gains relative to control subjects in all of eight studies (Table 2), including four in which the period of rehabilitation had been only eight weeks. An exercise critic (19) admitted that the differences of the type shown in this table were statistically significant but suggested that an advantage of 20% to 25% was "relatively small." The source of this opinion seems to be Greenland and Chu (33), who suggested that "In the many sedentary patients without complications whose recreational and occupational activities are of low intensity, resumption of premorbid activities can be achieved without participation in a formal exercise program."

The primary basis for the claim can be traced to the report of DeBusk

---

TABLE 2.—Controlled Trials Examining Gains for Functional Capacity After Exercise-Centered Cardiac Rehabilitation

Author	Sample Size	Program Length	Functional Gain	Test Method
DeBusk et al (47)	28/30	8 wk	16.8%	TM $\dot{V}O_2$
Miller et al (49)	61/34	8 wk	21.4%	TM $\dot{V}O_2$
Carson et al (42)	151/152	3 mo	34.6%	TM time
Hung et al (50)	23/30	8 wk	19.8%	Cycle work
Wilhelmsen et al (39)	114/88	9 mo	20%	Cycle time
Paterson et al (8)	37/42	1 yr	15%	Cycle $\dot{V}O_2$
Marra et al (41)	84/83	8–9 wk	31.2%	Cycle work
Roman et al (51)	93/100	4 mo	25.0%	TM $\dot{V}O_2$

et al. (47); their patients achieved an aerobic power of 8.9 METS (i.e., maximal oxygen intake of 31.2 mL/kg · min) without specific exercise therapy. Greenland and Chu (33) further cited a recommendation made in the United States that it was acceptable to use up to 80% of this maximal aerobic power (52) during the performance of occupational tasks. The chain of reasoning seems flawed on at least three counts: (1) an aerobic power of 31.2 mL/kg · min is not typical of the average postcoronary patient [figures of 21–26 mL/kg · min are much more common at entry into a phase III cardiac rehabilitation program (53)]; (2)it is not acceptable to use 80% of aerobic power during the performance of daily work (the normal ceiling of the industrial physiologist is 33% to 50% of aerobic power, depending on the circumstances of the task (54); and (3) account must be taken not only of current function but also of the future needs of the patient relative to the inevitable deterioration of capacity with aging, a functional loss of at least 10% per decade (16).

Another physiologic argument that is sometimes raised is that, at best, exercise training improves peripheral function (55); the performance of the heart cannot be improved after infarction. The basis for this fallacy seems an inadequate period of observation and (in many studies) an inadequate total period of rehabilitation. When studies have continued for an adequate time (6 months to a year or more), gains in cardiac stroke volume have been observed much as those in a healthy adult who undergoes prolonged training (8–10, 46). The long-term response seems to be associated with decreased myocardial ischemia (12, 13) and increased myocardial perfusion (14, 15). A decrease in left atrial and left ventricular dimensions also points to improvements of ventricular compliance and contractility (56).

Socioeconomic adjustment.—The proportion of patients returning to work after myocardial infarction ranges widely from 50% to 96%, depending on the nature of the work and the extent of available social benefits (5, 6, 36, 57). There may also be disruptions of family life after a heart attack (58), at times related to fears revolving around resumption of sexual activity (59).

The view of the exercise critics seems to be that even if exercise induces a gain of aerobic power, this does not have any material impact on psychosocial function (19). Two controlled trials are adduced in support of this view (60, 61). In the first of the two trials (60), the exercised group did demonstrate a statistically significant advantage of sexual function at 6 months; by 18 months the intergroup difference was small, but there was also little difference in exercise patterns between supposedly active and inactive groups. In the second trial both test and control groups were encouraged to exercise, although supervised exercise classes were provided only for the test subjects. Despite the limited nature of the experimental comparison the test subjects fared better on a scale measuring social adequacy.

Some reports offer little other than anecdotal evidence supporting exercise programs as a means of encouraging a return to work. For example, the WHO study (36) suggested that return to work was more common in exercised patients than in controls at 15 of 17 cooperating centers. The majority of program participants at many centers are "white-collar" workers; few physical demands are imposed by either occupation or transportation, so that the lack of hard evidence is not surprising. Considerations such as motivation, skills, experience, financial status, attitudes of relatives, and the presence of associated disease all influence employment prospects (62). Carson et al. (42) also found that whether allocated to exercise or control groups, subjects expected to complete their experimental trial before return to work.

Nevertheless, the most important variable governing return to work is age (63), and we may immediately remark that an increase in aerobic power has a substantial impact on biological age (16). Moreover, the likelihood of a successful return to work is influenced by the physical demands of occupation relative to the individual's aerobic power (64), and a history of vigorous physical activity before infarction can double the chances of a return to full-time work (63).

Mayou (65) found that an exercise program had little influence on the proportion of patients returning to work, but other studies have reported gains ranging from 5% to 30% (66–70).

Mood-state.—Despite patient tendencies to denial, the period immediately following myocardial infarction is often marked by severe reactive anxiety/depression (71–74). Furthermore, a major reason why people exercise is to "feel better," and an early small-scale controlled trial demonstrated a reduction of anxiety in response to participation in an exercise program, the response being greater in cardiac than in matched healthy subjects (75).

Our own experience has shown a substantial correction of both depression (72) and anxiety (74) with participation in an exercise-centered rehabilitation program, these gains being associated with program compliance (72). Hellerstein and Hornsten (73) had similar findings, but Naughton and associates did not observe any change of mood state with exercise (76). Two substantial controlled trials (60, 61) likewise did not observe any striking psychological benefit, in part because they were unable to sustain differences of activity levels between their test and control subjects. In the study of Stern and Cleary (60), there was some decrease in the mean depression score in exercised patients, but the effect was not statistically significant because the initial depression scores were relatively low; this reflects involvement in a 6-week preliminary exercise program and relatively late program entry (up to 36 months after myocardial infarction).

Costs of Exercise

When the cumulative benefits of exercise can no longer be denied, the argument then becomes that such gains are not sufficient to outweigh the costs of a cardiac rehabilitation program, in terms of both economics and clinical risk to the patient.

Program costs.— In some centers the expense of a cardiac rehabilitation program is quite high (77). Depending on the extent of ECG monitoring, the patient costs during the first 3 months of treatment (phase I and phase II programs) can easily amount to between $4,000 and $5,000, and limited reimbursement by insurers discourages patient compliance. Nevertheless, Noakes (78) has pointed out that this expense is small relative to the costs associated with cardiac transplantation or angioplasty.

Many analyses of program costs ignore space. If a gymnasium is used by a single class of cardiac patients, the annual value of this serviced space could amount to $400 to $500 per patient-year. In the United States the full cost of a tapered phase III program has been estimated at $1,200 per patient (77). At the Toronto Rehabilitation Centre, a 4-year tapered phase III program has been costed at $1,565; this figure includes five routine exercise tests, supervised exercise sessions once per week for 1 year and monthly for a further 6 months, telemetry and ambulatory monitoring when required, further exercise tests if required, access to the patient's exercise supervisor, and psychological screening (77).

The patient may accumulate not only program costs of this order but also personal expenses for the purchase of special clothing and equipment (79). Nevertheless, the major cost to the average participant is a substantial commitment of time, both in the exercise program itself and in travel to and from the rehabilitation center (77). If the activity program is enjoyed, the "opportunity cost" of committed time can perhaps be ignored, but if attendance at the exercise classes is seen as a regrettable necessity, then the time thus allocated should be costed at an appropriate figure, for example, an average industrial wage; 2 years of thrice-weekly attendance might demand an investment valued at $9,000.

Economic Benefits.—The immediate economic benefits of exercise, such as the decreased likelihood of a fatal recurrence and the prospect of an earlier return to work, usually outweigh direct program costs (68, 77, 80).

The magnitude of the mortality effect depends on the assumed decrease in fatal recurrences (20% to 30% of an initial 4% annual rate), the exercise compliance rate (25% to 50% of patients adopting an effective training program), the likely lengthening of productive life (5–10 years), and the resultant economic benefit (25% to 100% of salary). Depending on the assumptions that are made, the savings would range from $10 to $120 per patient-year (77).

On optimistic assumptions (50% effective exercise participation, 30% increase in proportion of workers), the economic benefit from a greater likelihood of return to normal employment might amount to $3,000 per year. With more pessimistic figures (25% effective participation, 10% gain in employment), this saving would drop to $500 per patient year. Data from Sweden (80) and Russia (68) suggest figures of $2,300 and $1,300 per patient-year, respectively.

Together, these two items more than offset program costs. If account is taken of the commitment of the participant's time, the ratio of costs to benefits becomes more problematic, although given the increased functional capacity of the exercisers a true weighing of costs and benefits should probably compare the "quality-adjusted" free time of treated and untreated individuals; on such a scale, exercise would certainly remain a beneficial form of therapy.

Clinical risks.—The ghosts of Pheidippides and Jim Fixx are sometimes conjured up when emphasis is turned to clinical risks, particularly the likelihood that exercise will precipitate a recurrence of myocardial infarction or sudden death.

In fact, the immediate risks of a post coronary exercise program are extremely low (81–86), whether considered in themselves or relative to the hazards of alternative surgical forms of treatment (78). The data recently accumulated by Van Camp and Petersen (81) coincide closely with the cumulative Toronto experience (86), showing one cardiac arrest for every 111,996 patient hours, one myocardial infarction per 293, 990 patient-hours, and one fatality per 783,972 patient hours. In essence, the risks of a recurrence are increased only slightly *during* a bout of exercise (87), but this hazard is more than offset by the favorable experience *between* bouts of exercise, as already discussed.

The search for some indicator of patients who are at increased risk during exercise has generally been unrewarding (88). Possible factors include exceeding prescribed heart rates, intercurrent viral infections, and concomitant business and social worries (88). The American College of Cardiology has recommended the provision of continuous ECG monitoring (89) to patients with (1) a history of cardiac arrest, (2) a ventricular ejection fraction of less than 30%, (3) complex resting ventricular arrhythmias, or ventricular arrhythmias exacerbated by exercise, (4) a history of congestive failure or severe shock during the primary episode, (5) ST segmental depression of more than 2 mm during exercise, and (6) inability to monitor the heart rate while exercising. At first inspection these seem to be high-risk categories of individual meriting careful surveillance, although others have regarded continuous monitoring as an unnecessary and unhelpful expense (81). One report has suggested that the risk of cardiovascular complications is increased by adoption of a high-intensity exercise program (82). Given appropriate progression of training, this has not been our experience, even when patients have carried their training programs through to the level of marathon participation (86).

Compliance Rates

The final argument of the exercise sceptics is that of poor compliance. Even if exercise is very beneficial relative to costs, it is reasoned that patients cannot be persuaded to engage in an exercise program on a long-term basis.

There is certainly need for a further study of factors influencing exercise compliance (90, 91). Many multicenter trials have had some difficulty in establishing a difference of exercise behavior between exercised and control groups, although this has been attributable as much to involvement of the control group in activity programs as to a lack of exercise participation by the experimental subjects. Our experience has been that with good leadership, a compliance of 82% can be sustained over a well-organized 3-year rehabilitation program (92). Oldridge (93) has also secured a compliance rate of 90% with appropriate contracting by program participants. There remains scope for further improvement, but such long-term compliance rates compare extremely favorably with the adherence rates usually found for pharmaceutical treatments.

Educating the Skeptics

Given that exercise is an effective form of theapy for the postcoronary patient, is well accepted by most patients, as has the potential for a high compliance rate and a favorable cost-benefit ratio, what further measures can be suggested to educate the skeptics?

As daily work becomes automated and controlled from home-based computer terminals, there is an ever-growing need for physicians to understand the principles of exercise prescription and to be able to recommend appropriate training programs for all of their patients.

Sports medicine is already served by a vast wealth of specialized journals and textbooks such as this volume but, unfortunately, these resources are used mainly by the converted. Professional associations such as the American College of Sports Medicine have shown phenomenal growth over the past two decades, but again phenomenal growth over the past two decades, but again only a small percentage of clinicians profit from the resultant educational opportunities.

The answer for future generations of physicians may lie in a major restructuring of the medical curriculum, so that both physiology and pathology are taught on the active rather than the recumbent patient. But incentives must also be found to upgrade the knowledge and skills of these currently in clinical practice. One welcome development in this regard has been the recent institution of a Clinical Diploma Examination in Sports Medicine by the Canadian Academy of Sports Medicine (94); this examination gives recognition to those who already have expertise in the therapeutic use of exercise and is also helping to shape a demand for postgraduate medical education among others planning to sit the Diploma examination.

Perhaps even more importantly, there is a need for economic change within the medical establishment. Exercise counseling can be quite labor intensive and many physicians tend to avoid such initiatives, not only because they lack the necessary knowledge but also because they recognize that current fee schedules make the offering of detailed exercise advice financially unattractive. Similarly, insuring agencies in both Canada and the United States have failed to encourage exercise as a useful and appropriate form of therapy. Their policies should recognize that exercise programs are more effective than many of the treatments for which reimbursement is currently provided.

Conclusions

Expressed scepticism about the value of exercise therapy for the postcoronary patient frequently masks a lack of knowledge of exercise testing and exercise prescription. Arguments currently advanced against exercise for the postcoronary patient lack substance. Such treatment is better validated than are many common medical practices. Nevertheless, it will take more than scholarly arguments to bring exercise therapy into the mainstream of clinical practice. New long-term educational programs must be introduced, involving both medical students and practitioners already in the field. Specific recognition of the value of exercise treatment should also be accorded through (1) specialist certification in Sports Medicine, (2) more appropriate fee schedules for exercise counseling and prescription, and (3) patient reimbursement of exercise program costs by insuring agencies.

References

1. May GS, Eberlein KA, Furberg CD, et al: Secondary prevention after myocardial infarction. A review of long-term trials. *Prog Cardiovasc Dis* 24:331–352, 1982.
2. Oldridge NB, Guyatt G, Fischer M, et al: Randomized trials of cardiac rehabilitation. Combined experience of randomized clinical trials. *JAMA* 260:945–950, 1988.
3. Shephard RJ: The value of exercise in ischemic heart disease. A cumulative analysis. *J Cardiac Rehabilitation* 3:294–298, 1983.
4. Shephard RJ: Exercise in the tertiary prevention of ischemic heart disease: Experimental proof. *Can J Sport Sci* 14:74–84, 1989.
5. Borer JS, Brandi-Pifano S, Puigbo JJ, et al: Rehabilitation of patients with left ventricular dysfunction and heart failure, in Wenger NK, Almeida-Feo D, Rosenthal J (eds): *Rehabilitation of the Cardiac Patient*. Basel, Karger Publ, 1986.
6. Hedback B, Perk J: Five-year results of a comprehensive rehabilitation programme after myocardial infarction. *Eur Heart J* 8:234–242, 1987.
7. Kavanagh T, Shephard RJ, Chisholm AW, et al: Prognostic indexes for patients with ischemic heart disease enrolled in an exercise-centered rehabilitation program. *Am J Cardiol* 44:1230–1240, 1979.
8. Paterson DH, Shephard RJ, Cunningham DA, et al: Effects of physical training on cardiovascular function following myocardial infarction. *J Appl Physiol* 47:482–489, 1979.
9. Ehsani AA, Biello DR, Schultz J, et al: Improvement of left ventricular contractile function by exercise training in patients with coronary heart disease. *Circulation* 74:350–358, 1986.
10. Hagberg JM, Ehsani AA, Holloszy JO: Effect of 12 months of intense exercise training on stroke volume in patients with coronary artery disease. *Circulation* 67:1194–1199, 1983.
11. Kavanagh T, Shephard RJ, Doney H, et al: Intensive exercise in coronary rehabilitation. *Med Sci Sports*. 5:34–39, 1973.
12. Ehsani AA: Effects of 12 months of intense exercise training on ischemic ST segment depression in patients with coronary artery disease. *Circulation* 64:1116–1124, 1981.
13. Froelicher V, Jensen D, Genter F, et al: A randomized trial of exercise training in patients with coronary heart disease. *JAMA* 252:1291–1297, 1984.
14. Sebrechts CP, Klein JL, Ahnve S, et al: Myocardial perfusion changes following 1 year of exercise training assessed by thallium 201 circumference count profiles. *Am Heart J* 112:1217–1226, 1986.
15. Hammond HK, Kelly TL, Froelicher VF, et al: Use of clinical data in predicting improvement in exercise capacity after cardiac rehabilitation. *J Am Coll Cardiol* 6:19–26, 1985.
16. Shephard RJ: Physical Activity and Aging, ed 2. London, Croom Helm, 1987.
17. Shephard RJ: Cardiac rehabilitation in prospect, in Pollock ML Schmidt DH (eds): *Heart Disease and Rehabilitation*. New York, John Wiley & Sons, 1986.

18. Shephard RJ: Are we asking the right questions? *J Cardiac Rehabil* 2:21–26, 1982.
19. Dunn EV: Exercise after myocardial infarction: Appraisal of the literature, *Can Fam Physician* 35:1909–1912, 1989.
20. Godfrey C: Is exercise a good thing? *Can Fam Physician* 32:135–137, 1986.
21. Russell LB: Is prevention better than cure? Brookings Inst, Washington, DC, 1986 pp. 1–129.
22. de la Vega PF, Ortiz E, Vicente T, et al: The effect of physical training. *Proceedings*, IVth World Congress of Cardiac Rehabilitation, Brisbane, 1988, p 125.
23. Moczurad KW, Dubiel JP, Curylo AM: Long-term physical training and the fate of man after first myocardial infarction. *Proceedings*, IVth World Congress of Cardiac Rehabilitation, Brisbane, 1988, p 124.
24. Kallio V, Hämäläinen H, Hakkila J, et al: Reduction of sudden deaths by a multifactorial intervention program after acute myocardial infarction. *Lancet* 2:1091–1094, 1979.
25. Rechnitzer PA, Cunningham DA, Andrew GM, et al: Relationship of exercise to the recurrence rate of myocardial infarction in men: Ontario Exercise-Heart Collaborative Study. *Am J Cardiol* 51:65–69, 1983.
26. Cunningham DA, Rechnitzer P, Jones NL, et al: The issue of poor compliance in exercise trials. *J Cardiac Rehabil* Submitted for publication, 1990.
27. Bobbio M: Does post-myocardial infarction rehabilitation prolong survival? A meta-analytic survey. *Proceedings,* IVth World Congress of Cardiac Rehabilitation, Brisbane, 1988, p 92.
28. Oldridge NB, Guyatt G, Fischer M, et al: Randomized trials of cardiac rehabilitation: Overview analysis of mortality. *Proceedings,* IVth World Congress of Cardiac Rehabilitation, Brisbane, 1988, p 128.
29. Staniloff HM: Current concepts in cardiac rehabilitation. *Am J Surg* 147:719–724, 1984.
30. O'Connor GT, Buring JE, Goldhaber SZ, et al: An over-view of randomized trials of exercise after myocardial infarction. *Clin Res* 34:379A, 1986.
31. Louis TA, Fineberg HV, Mosteller F: Findings for public health from meta-analyses. *Annu Rev Public Health* 6:1–20, 1985.
32. Goldman L, Feinstein AR: Anticoagulants and myocardial infarction: The problems of pooling, drowning and floating. *Ann Intern Med* 90:92–94, 1979.
33. Greenland P, Chu JS: Efficacy of cardiac rehabilitation services, with emphasis on patients with myocardial infarction. *Ann Intern Med* 109:650–663, 1988.
34. Shephard RJ: Exercise as an agent of lifestyle change. *Br J Sports Med* 23:11–22, 1989.
35. Oberman A, Cleary P, Larosa JC, et al: Changes in risk factors among participants in a long-term exercise rehabilitation program, in Kellerman JJ (ed): *Comprehensive Cardiac Rehabilitation.* Basel, Karger Publ, 1982, pp 168–175.
36. Lamm G, Denolin H, Dorossiev D, et al: Rehabilitation and secondary prevention of patients after acute myocardial infarction, in: Kellerman JJ (ed): *Comprehensive Cardiac Rehabilitation.* Basel, Karger Publ, 1982, pp 168–175.
37. Kavanagh T, Shephard RJ, Chisholm AW, et al: Prognostic indexes for patients with ischemic heart disease enrolled in an exercise-centered rehabilitation program. *Am J Cardiol* 44:1230–1240, 1979.
38. Angster H, Glonner R, Halhuber M: Risk factor modification in the framework of rehabilitation, in Kellerman JJ (ed): *Comprehensive Cardiac Rehabilitation.* Basel, Karger Publ, 1982, pp 176–179.
39. Wilhelmsen L, Sanne H, Elmfeldt D, et al: A controlled trial of physical training after myocardial infarction. Effects of risk factors, nonfatal reinfarction and death. *Prev Med* 4:491–508, 1975.
40. Vermeulen A, Lie KI, Durrer D: Effects of cardiac rehabilitation after myocardial infarction: Changes in coronary risk factors and long-term prognosis. *Am Heart J* 105:798–801, 1983.
41. Marra S, Paolillo V, Spadaccini F, et al: Long-term follow-up after a controlled randomized post-infarction rehabilitation programme: Effects on morbidity and mortality. *Eur Heart J* 6:656–663, 1985.

42. Carson P, Phillips R, Lloyd M, et al: Exercise after myocardial infarction: Controlled trial. *J R Coll Physicians Lond* 16:147–151, 1982.
43. Kavanagh T, Shephard RJ, Lindley LJ, et al: Influence of exercise and lifestyle variables upon high-density lipoprotein cholesterol after myocardial infarction. *Arteriosclerosis* 3:249–259, 1983.
44. Williams PT, Wood PD, Haskell WL, et al: The effects of running mileage and duration on plasma lipoprotein levels. *JAMA* 247:2674–2679, 1982.
45. Kaplan R: Quantification of health outcomes for policy studies in behavioral epidemiology, in Kaplan R, Criqui MH (eds): *Behavioral Epidemiology and Disease Prevention*. New York, Plenum Press, 1985, pp 31–56.
46. Wohl AJ, Lewis HR, Campbell W, et al: Cardiovascular function during early recovery from acute myocardial infarction. *Circulation* 56:931–937, 1977.
47. DeBusk RF, Houston N, Haskell W, et al: Exercise training soon after myocardial infarction. *Am J Cardiol* 44:1223–1229, 1979.
48. DeBusk R: Physical conditioning following myocardial infarction, in Kellerman JJ (ed): *Comprehensive Cardiac Rehabilitation*. Basel, Karger Publ, 1982, pp 156–161.
49. Miller NH, Haskell WL, Berra K, et al: Home versus group exercise training after myocardial infarction. *Circulation* 70:645–649, 1984.
50. Hung J, Gordon EP, Houston N, et al: Change in rest and exercise myocardial perfusion and left ventricular function 3 to 26 weeks after clinically uncomplicated acute myocardial infarction: effects of exercise training. *Am J Cardiol* 54:943–950, 1984.
51. Roman O, Guitierrez M, Luksic I, et al: Cardiac rehabilitation after myocardial infarction. Nine-year controlled follow-up study. *Cardiol* 70:223–231, 1983.
52. American Heart Association Committee on Exercise: *Exercise Testing and Training of Individuals With Heart Disease or at Risk for its Development: A Handbook for Physicians*. Dallas, American Heart Association, 1975.
53. Kavanagh T, Shephard RJ, Kennedy J: Characteristics of post-coronary marathon runners. *Ann NY Acad Sci* 301:656–670, 1977.
54. Shephard RJ: *Endurance Fitness*, ed 2. Toronto, Univ of Toronto Press, 1977.
55. Clausen JP: Physiological response to exercise in health and disease. *Prog Cardiovasc Dis* 18:459–495, 1976.
56. Hoffman A, Duba J, Lengyel M, et al: The effect of training on the physical working capacity of MI patients with left ventricular dysfunction. *Eur Heart J* 8(suppl G):43–49, 1987.
57. Wenger NK, Hellerstein HK, Blackburn H, et al: Physician practice in the management of patients with uncomplicated myocardial infarction: Changes in the past decade. *Circulation* 65:421–427, 1982.
58. Skelton M, Dominian J: Psychological stress in wives of patients with myocardial infarction. *Br Med J* 2:101–103, 1973.
59. Kavanagh T, Shephard RJ: Sexual activity after myocardial infarction. *Can Med Assoc J* 116:1250–1253, 1977.
60. Stern MJ, Cleary P: The National Exercise and Heart Disease Project: Long-term psychological outcome. *Arch Intern Med* 142:1093–1097, 1982.
61. Erdman RA, Duivenvoorden HJ: Psychological evaluation of a cardiac rehabilitation program: A randomized clinical trial in patients with myocardial infarction. *J Cardiac Rehabil* 3:696–704, 1983.
62. Shephard RJ: *Ischemic Heart Disease and Exercise*. London, Croom Helm, 1981.
63. Weinblatt E, Shapiro R, Frank CW, et al: Return to work and work status following first myocardial infarction. *Am J Public Health* 56:169–185, 1966.
64. Groden BM: Return to work after myocardial infarction. *Scott Med J* 12:297–301, 1967.
65. Mayou RA: A controlled trial of early rehabilitation after myocardial infarction. *J Cardiac Rehabil* 3:397–402, 1983.
66. Dwyer T, Rutherford R: Cost and benefit in cardiac rehabilitation—tertiary rehabilitation. *Proceedings, IVth World Congress of Cardiac Rehabilitation*, Brisbane, 1988, p 87.

67. Klarman HE: Socio-economic impact of heart disease, in Andrus EC (ed): *The Heart and Circulation. Second National Conference on Cardiovascular Diseases*, vol 2. Washington, DC, Community Services and Education, USPHS, 1964.
68. Nikolaeva LF, Karpova GD, Rubanovich A, et al: Medical, social and economic effectiveness of the USSR National staged MI patients rehabilitation programme. *Proceedings*, IVth World Congress of Cardiac Rehabilitation, Brisbane, 1988, p 87.
69. Vasilauskas D, Krisciunas A, Lazaravisius A: Rehabilitation of postinfarctional patients: Socio-economic effectiveness. *Proceedings, IVth World Congress of Cardiac Rehabilitation*, Brisbane, 1988, p 144.
70. Estany ER, de Leon OP, Chesa CS, et al: Influence of comprehensive cardiac rehabilitation on return to work after myocardial infarction. *Proceedings, IVth World Congress of Cardiac Rehabilitation*, Brisbane, 1988, p 145.
71. Ruskin HD, Stein LL, Shelsky IM, et al: M.M.P.I. comparison between patients with coronary heart disease and their spouses and other demographic data. *Scand J Rehab Med* 2:99–104, 1970.
72. Kavanagh T, Shephard RJ, Tuck JA: Depression after myocardial infarction. *Can Med Assoc J* 113:23–27, 1975.
73. Hellerstein HK, Hornsten T: Assessing and preparing the patient for return to a meaningful and productive life. *J Rehabil* 32:48–52, 1966.
74. Shephard RJ, Kavanagh T, Klavora P: Mood state during postcoronary cardiac rehabilitation. *J Cardiopulmonary Rehabil* 5:480–484, 1985.
75. McPherson BD, Paivio A, Yuhasz MS: Psychological effects of an exercise program for post-infarct and normal adult men. *J Sports Med* 7:95–102, 1967.
76. Naughton J, Bruhn J, Lategola M: Effects of physical training on physiologic and behavioral characteristics of cardiac patients. *Arch Phys Med Rehabil* 49:131–137, 1968.
77. Shephard RJ: Exercise in secondary and tertiary rehabilitation. Costs and benefits. *J Cardiopulmonary Rehabil* 9:188–194, 1989.
78. Noakes TD: Criticisms of exercise after heart attack—variations on an old theme? *S Afr Med J* 62:238–240, 1982.
79. Shephard RJ: *The Economic Benefits of Enhanced Fitness*. Champaign, Ill, Human Kinetics Publ, 1986.
80. Perk J, Hedback B: Cost-effectiveness of cardiac rehabilitation. *Proceedings* of IVth World Congress of Cardiac Rehabilitation, Brisbane, 1988, p 110.
81. Van Camp SP, Peterson RA: Cardiovascular complications of outpatient cardiac rehabilitation programs. *JAMA* 256:1160–1163, 1986.
82. Hossack KF, Hartwig R: Cardiac arrest associated with supervised cardiac rehabilitation. *J Cardiac Rehabil* 2:402–408, 1982.
83. Mead WF, Pyfer HR, Trombold JG, et al: Successful resuscitation of two near simultaneous cases of cardiac arrest and review of fifteen cases occurring during supervised exercise. *Circulation* 53:187–189, 1976.
84. Fletcher SF, Cantwell JD: Continuous ambulatory monitoring. Use in cardiac exercise programs. *Chest* 71:27–32, 1977.
85. Haskell WL: Cardiovascular complications during exercise training of cardiac patients. *Circulation* 57:920–924, 1978.
86. Shephard RJ, Kavanagh T, Tuck J, et al: Marathon jogging in post-myocardial infarction patients. *J Cardiac Rehabil* 3:321–329, 1983.
87. Shephard RJ: Recurrence of myocardial infarction. Observations on patients participating in the Ontario Multicentre Exercise-Heart Trial. *Eur J Cardiol* 11:147–157, 1980.
88. Shephard RJ, Kavanagh T: Predicting the exercise catastrophe in the post-coronary patient. *Can Fam Physician* 24:614–618, 1978.
89. American College of Cardiology: Position report on cardiac rehabilitation. *J Am Coll Cardiol* 7:451–453, 1986.
90. Andrew GM, Oldridge NB, Parker JO, et al: Reasons for dropout from exercise programs in coronary patients. *Med Sci Sports Exerc* 13:164–168, 1981.
91. Oldridge NB: Compliance of post-myocardial infarction patients to exercise programs. *Med Sci Sports Exerc* 11:373–375, 1979.

92. Shephard RJ, Corey P, Kavanagh T: Exercise compliance and the prevention of a recurrence of myocardial infarction. *Med Sci Sports Exerc* 13:1–5, 1981.
93. Oldridge NB: Compliance with exercise in cardiac rehabilitation, in Dishman RK (ed): *Exercise Adherence—Its Impact on Public Health.* Champaign, Ill, Human Kinetics Publ, 1988.
94. Jean P, Hart I, Pipe A: A systematic approach to developing diploma examination in sports medicine. *Can J Sports Sci* 14:194–196, 1989.

1 Biomechanics

Rotational and Translational Movement Features of the Pelvis and Thorax During Adult Human Locomotion
Stokes VP, Andersson C, Forssberg H (Karolinska Inst; Karolinska Hosp/St Görans Hosp, Stockholm)
J Biomech 22:43–50, 1989   1–1

Trunk movement is an important aspect of human gait as the movement of the pelvis and thorax are closely related to gait efficiency and smoothness of locomotion. Although the kinematics of limb movement have been well studied, few studies have been published on pelvis and thorax interaction patterns. Features of normal gait patterns were identified to be used as a database for future assessments of developmental gait patterns in children and pathologic gait patterns in patients with gait disturbances.

The movements of the pelvis and thorax were recorded by a SELSPOT system interfaced with an HP1,000 minicomputer to obtain 3-dimensional kinematic/temporal data for the pelvis and thorax. Light-emitting diodes attached to triangular plates fitted to the posterior of the pelvis and thorax via a waist belt and shoulder harness were tracked by 2 cameras. Three women and 5 men performed repeated trials of walking and running on a treadmill with randomized ordering of speeds. The first and last trials were static trials during which the individual was instructed to stand motionless in a relaxed postion in the center of the calibration volume.

Analysis of the movement data revealed a set of complex movement patterns for both the pelvis and the thorax during normal treadmill walking. Although the number of persons tested in this study was small, it is assumed that larger studies of normal adult movement patterns of the trunk during walking will show similar features. The data collected will serve as a baseline for future studies aimed at assessing deviations from these normal patterns.

▶ This is excellent biomechanical research. I had never thought that there would be such complex movement patterns of the pelvis and thorax during normal treadmill walking. The methodology used by the authors for recording the movement made it possible to show the movement of both segments in 3 dimensions with high resolution. Some patterns of movement illustrated 6 rotation/translation directional changes, separated by reversal points. Because the number of subjects was small, it will be necessary to collect more data from a larger group to obtain an accurate picture of normal adult movement patterns of the trunk and pelvis while walking.—Col. J.L. Anderson, PE.D.

Joint Use and Misuse

Radin EL, Yang KH, Whittle MW, O'Conner JJ, Rieger C (West Virginia Univ)
Int J Sports Med 10:S85–S86, 1989
1–2

Osteoarthritis may develop in athletes or the elderly as a result of stress concentration or repetitive impulsive loading, or both. During activity, impulsive loading is superimposed on oscillating movement. Why this form of mechanical loading damages some joints but not others, and the way in which muscles protect the joints, were studied in 21 individuals.

When the generation and transmission of skeletal transients from heel-strike during walking was analyzed, only 7 of the 21 had impulsive peak in ground reaction force and acceleration at heelstrike. Just before heel-strike, quadriceps activity was detected by electromyography. When the quadriceps muscle was paralyzed by injection of lidocaine into the femoral nerve, a heelstrike impulse was present in a volunteer who previously had none. The heelstrike impulse was not altered significantly by inertial forces in the lower limb.

Protection of joints from shock loading requires muscular control of limb deceleration. Osteoarthritis probably can be avoided in athletes who have a normal musculoskeletal system. They should maintain muscle endurance, avoid training when tired, and wear protective gear to facilitate active absorption of impact forces.

▶ The 7 subjects who demonstrated an impulsive peak in ground reaction force and acceleration at heelstrike were demonstrating minor incoordination in that they had not learned to use the quadriceps muscles to decelerate the foot before heelstrike, and this impulsively loads the joints. The authors believe that the main shock absorbing mechanisms are eccentric muscle action and deceleration of the limb before contact with a surface. This incoordination is associated with the aging process. Often, as people age they stop walking up or down stairs and the quadriceps weaken, impulsive loading increases, and osteoarthritis develops. Osteoarthritis is not a disease; rather, it is organ failure of the joint as a result of mechanical circumstances.—Col. J.L. Anderson, PE.D.

Influence of Gait Parameters on the Loading of the Lower Limb

Collins JJ, Whittle MW (Nuffield Orthopaedic Ctr, Oxford, England; Univ of Oxford)
J Biomed Eng 11:409–412, September 1989
1–3

The support of the weight of the body and acceleration of the body comprise the ground reaction force that acts on the foot during walking. To investigate the loading rate of the lower limb during load acceptance and to determine its relationship with cadence, stride length, and velocity, studies were made in 13 healthy men aged 18–63 years. Each man walked at 5 different self-selected speeds. Plots of the ground reaction force were used to determine the loading rate of the limb.

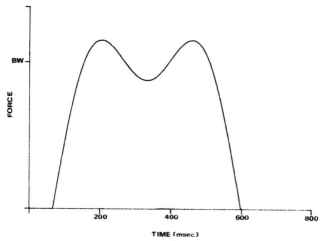

FORCE

BW

TIME (msec)

200   400   600   800

Fig 1–1.—Plot of the vertical component of the ground reaction force in normal walking. (Courtesy of Collins JJ, Whittle MW: *J Biomed Eng* 11:409–412, September 1989.)

Velocity had the highest correlation with loading rate, and stride length had the lowest correlation. Cadence and loading rate had a non-linear relationship (Fig 1–1) The initial loading phase of walking appears to be similar among normal persons. These baseline data can be used in more detailed investigations of the heelstrike transient. A better understanding of the mechanics of walking and a defined normative database are needed for more effective assessment of pathologic gaits and the prevention of joint wear.

▶ Repetitive impulsive loading, such as that experienced during walking, has been linked with the etiology and progression of a variety of pathologic conditions, in particular, osteoarthritis and low back pain. Radin et al. (Abstract 1–2) found that incoordination appears to be responsible for impulsive peak in ground reaction force and acceleration at heelstrike. However, the authors of the present study used a force platform that sampled data only at 50 Hz too low to accurately measure the high-frequency impulsive load at heelstrike; thus their data were not available for use in calculating the loading rate. It would appear that the procedures used in these 2 studies should be combined in order to accurately measure impact forces during walking and effects on the loading rate of the lower limb.—Col. J.L. Anderson, PE.D.

The Axis of Rotation of the Ankle Joint
Lundberg A, Svensson OK, Németh G, Selvik G (Karolinska Hosp, Stockholm; Lund Univ, Lund, Sweden)
J Bone Joint Surg 71-B:94–99, January 1989   1–4

The kinematics of the foot and ankle in normal individuals have not been well studied. The talocrural joint is the only joint to show uniform interindividual kinematic properties, but there is some controversy regarding the axis of this joint during continuous motion. X-ray stereophotography was used to study the axis of the talocrural joint in normal subjects.

Method.—Three or more 0.8-mm tantalum marker beads were introduced into the bones of the lower extremity in 8 healthy volunteers aged 26–38 years. After 2–10 weeks, each subject was placed on a platform that could be tilted by 10-degree increments about a transverse and an anteroposterior axis. Rotation could also be recorded by using a goniometer placed around the lower leg and fixed to the device (Fig 1–2). Simultaneous anteroposterior and lateral radiographs were obtained at 10-degree increments from 30 degrees of plantar-flexion to 30 degrees of dorsiflexion of the foot, from 20 degrees of pronation to 20 degrees of supination, and from 20 degrees of medial rotation to 10 degrees of lateral rotation of the leg.

The axis of the talocrural joint changed continuously throughout the range of movement. In dorsiflexion the axis tended to be oblique downward and laterally; in leg rotation it took varying inclinations between horizontal and vertical. However, all axes were close to the midpoint of a line between the tips of the malleoli.

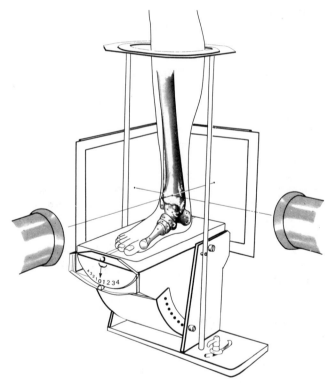

Fig 1–2.—Diagram of apparatus with leg in position and x-ray tubes placed for anteroposterior and lateral exposures. (Courtesy of Lundberg A, Svensson OK, Németh G, et al: *J Bone Joint Surg* 71-B:94–99, January 1989.)

The change between the axes occurred rather abruptly in some subjects and more gradually in others. Special attention should be paid to the position of the center of the talar part of a spherical total ankle prosthesis.

▶ This is an outstanding piece of research using biomechanical techniques. A significant finding is that when dorsiflexion, pronation and supination, and medial and lateral rotational axes for each of the subjects were drawn in the same figure, all axes, irrespective of their inclination, coincided to run very close to one central point in the trochlea of the talar part. This central point seems to constitute a hub, around which the ankle has more freedom of movement than is often assumed. The authors believe that such a center of movement has several implications, one being that attention should be paid to the position of the center of the talar part of a spherical total ankle prosthesis. The wide variation in joint axes calls for care in designing models of the ankle. These authors found the central point to be located at, or slightly lateral to, the midpoint of a line drawn between the tips of the malleoli.—Col. J.L. Anderson, PE.D.

A Stabilometric Technique for Evaluation of Lower Limb Instabilities
Fridén T, Zätterström R, Lindstrand A, Moritz U (Univ Hosp, Lund, Sweden)
Am J Sports Med 17:118–122, January–February 1989   1–5

Detection of functional instability after ligamentous lesions of the ankle occur is difficult and often imprecise. A stabilometry technique was designed to quantify body sway and record the site of the center of pressure in the frontal plane by a strain gauge force plate while the patient stands on 1 leg (Fig 1–3).

Computer analysis of results in 55 healthy, young volunteers and 14 patients who had unilateral injury of the fibulotalar ligament revealed 4 variables that differentiated between the injured and uninjured leg: parameter 2, the standard deviation of the mean distance between the center of pressure and the references line of the foot, which reflects amplitude but not frequency of the sway movement; parameter 4, the mean sway amplitude; and parameters 5 and 6, the number of sway amplitudes that exceed 5 mm and 10 mm. However, most of these variables did not distinguish the injured leg when an ankle brace was worn. The average speed of frontal sway movements, which reflects frequency and amplitude, differentiated the uninjured leg from the reference group, as did parameters 2, 5, and 6.

The stabilometric method is more sensitive than others. Because ligamentous lesions may result from predisposition to impaired postural control, rehabilitation after injury to an ankle ligament should include the contralateral side.

▶ This study has proved to be very timely to us in the Department of Physical Education at West Point. During the fall of 1990 we will begin a 2-year study on the effect of the ankle brace as prophylaxis in the prevention and treatment of ankle injuries. Although we will not be using the stabilometry technique in our

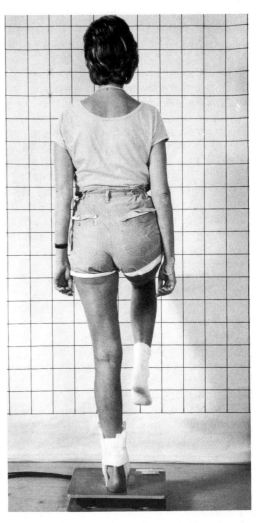

Fig 1–3.—The test person stood on 1 leg during the measurement. (Courtesy of Fridén T, Zätterström R, Lindstrand A, et al: *Am J Sports Med* 17:118–122, January-February 1989.)

study, the information presented here gives us a broader perspective in our study of these injuries.—Col. J.L. Anderson, PE.D.

The Appropriate Use of Regression Equations for the Estimation of Segmental Inertia Parameters

Yeadon MR, Morlock M (Univ of Calgary, Alta)
J Biomech 22:683–689, 1989   1–6

Linear regression equations are often used in conjunction with experimental data to provide linear relationships between dimensionally distinct quantities. However, a close-fitting regression equation may not provide good estimates for data other than that on which the equation is based. A nonlinear scaling procedure that uses only segmental measurements might be more successful. Linear and nonlinear approaches were compared to estimate the segmental moments of inertia from anthropometric measurements determined by Chandler et al. (Fig 1–4). Right-limb data were used to derive equations. Left-limb data were used for cross-validation of inertia estimates calculated from the equations.

Standard error estimates for limb segments averaged 21% for linear equations and 13% for nonlinear equations. When the methods were tested on a boy aged 10 years the mean percentage residuals were 286% for linear equations and 20% for nonlinear equations.

Nonlinear equations are superior to linear equations and can provide reasonable estimates of segmental moments of inertia even when anthro-

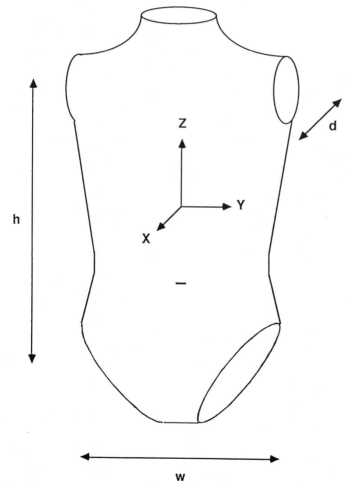

Fig 1–4.—Torso segment of depth *d*, width *w*, and height *h*. (Courtesy of Yeadon MR, Morlock M: *J Biomech* 22:683–689, 1989.)

pometric measurements lie outside the sample range of Chandler et al. The one positive result in this study indicates that it might be worthwhile to test nonlinear equations in a wide range of persons using values calculated from an inertia model as criteria.

▶ Amen! What can one add to this? This outstanding work has determined that nonlinear equations are superior to linear equations. The authors appear to prove that the use of linear equations to express relationships between quantities that are dimensionally distinct may be inappropriate.—Col. J.L. Anderson, PE.D.

The Aging Skeletal Muscle: Effect of Training on Muscle Force and Mass
Klitgaard H, Brunet A, Marc R, Monod H, Mantoni M, Saltin B (Univ of Copenhagen; CNRS, Paris; Rigshospitalet, Copenhagen)
Int J Sports Med 10:S93–S94, 1989   1–7

The decrease in skeletal muscle force and mass that accompanies aging may hinder older athletes in sports performance. Results of attempts to prevent this age-related effect on muscles by strength training as well as by swimming and running were compared in rats and humans.

An increase in plantar flexor force during weight lifting was seen in rats aged 19 to 27 months, after which time it decreased even though training continued. An age-related decline in maximum tetanic tension of plantar and soleus muscles was counteracted by strength training up until 24 months of age, when it started to decline. Swim training did not increase maximum tetanic tension in either muscle. Strength training, unlike swim training, counteracted an age-related decrease in wet weight of plantar and soleus muscles but did not neutralize it.

In physically active men 69–70 years of age, strength training counteracted the age-related decline in maximal isometric torque of elbow flexion and knee extension, whereas swimming had no effect and running had little. An age-related decline in cross-sectional area of elbow flexors and quadriceps muscle of the thigh was counteracted by strength training but not by swimming or running.

Brief, intense strength training allows human skeletal muscle to maintain force and mass during the process of aging but perhaps only up to a certain age-related threshold. Endurance exercise has no such effect.

▶ This study demonstrates what common sense tells most of us who have been involved in physical fitness training. That is, an exercise program should be balanced and should include muscular strength and endurance activities as well as aerobic activities. Many people will say that as we age it is only important to concentrate on cardiovascular fitness. My response to that is that it is important to have a healthy heart and lungs, but it is also important to have a healthy structure in order to carry the healthy cardiovascular system around. None of us would put a new Cadillac engine in a model T Ford with the frame rusted out.—Col. J.L. Anderson, PE.D.

Relationship Between Plasma Somatomedin C and Muscle Performance in a Geriatric Male Population

Capuano-Pucci D, Rheault W, Rudman D (Chicago Med School, North Chicago)
Am J Phys Med 66:364–370, December 1988   1–8

Muscle strength decreases with age. Reportedly, by the seventh decade of life the average maximal voluntary contraction is 20% lower than that in the young adult. This decline increases to 50% by the eighth decade. Growth hormone (GH) secretion also declines with age. The normal plasma somatomedin C (SmC) level at age 20 years averages 1.0 units per mL, but by age 70 years, this decreases to 0.45 units per mL. Declining Gh secretion may be responsible for many of the age-related muscle changes. The plasma concentration of SmC can be used to estimate pituitary GH secretion. The relationship between plasma SmC levels and muscle function was assessed in 18 healthy men aged 55–80 years (mean, 65.8 years). Body weights ranged between 90% and 115% of ideal. After an overnight fast, blood was drawn and plasma SmC levels were measured by radioimmunoassay. Isokinetic muscle strength, power, and endurance were measured on elbow flexors and extensors and on knee flexors and extensors, using the Cybex II dynamometer.

The mean plasma SmC concentration in this group of elderly men was 0.42 units per mL. Only 4 men had plasma SmC levels less than 0.35 units per mL. No relationship was found between SmC levels and muscle function.

▶ This study presents a good lesson in cause and effect. Look at the study immediately preceding this one (Abstract 1–7). Here, the authors report on the average decline in muscular strength in an aging male population. However, the present study shows that the decrease can be reversed by using a strength development program of lifting weights, at least into the early 70s. Animal data show that after a certain age the decline in strength may not be reversed. We do not know that is true for *Homo sapiens*.—Col. J.L. Anderson, PE.D.

Local Bone Mineral Response to Brief Exercise That Stresses the Skeleton

Beverly MC, Rider TA, Evans MJ, Smith R (Nuffield Orthopaedic Ctr, Oxford; Northamptom Gen Hosp, Northampton; Hammersmith Hosp, London, England)
Br Med J 229:233–235, July 22, 1989   1–9

Physical activity is thought to have a role in the prevention and treatment of osteoporosis. Grip strength and bone mineral content were assessed in the forearms of 99 women, and the effects of short periods of exercise that stressed the skeleton on bone mineral content were tested.

There were 69 healthy women whose mean age was 62 years and 30 women with a fractured forearm whose mean age was 53 years. The control women were randomly assigned to exercising either the left or right

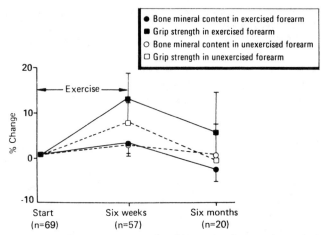

Fig 1–5.—Percentage changes in grip strength and bone mineral content in exercised and unexercised forearms of 69 women. Bars are 95% confidence intervals. (Courtesy of Beverly MC, Rider TA, Evans MJ, et al: Br Med J 299:233–235, July 22, 1989.)

forearm by squeezing a tennis ball as hard as possible 3 times consecutively, morning and evening, every day, for a total of 6 weeks. The unexercised other arm served as a control. The patients similarly exercised their uninjured arm. Bone mineral content of the forearm was measured with a densitometer. Grip strength was measured with a semi-inflated bag connected to an anaeroid barometer. Grip strength and bone mineral content of both wrists were measured at baseline, at 3 weeks and 6 weeks in the patients and at 6 weeks in the controls. All women were asked to return for follow-up 6 months later.

In the 99 women examined before exercising, both bone mineral content in the forearm and grip strength decreased with age. Before exercising, the 2 variables correlated closely, irrespective of age. Fifty-seven volunteers and 20 patients attended the 6-week follow-up examination. There were significant differences in bone mineral content and grip strength between the dominant and nondominant arms of the volunteers. In the exercised forearm a mean gain in grip strength of 12.5% and a mean increase in bone mineral content of 3.1% (Fig. 1–5) were observed.

Twenty volunteers and 13 patients attended the 6-month follow-up evaluation. The volunteers had lost most of their gains in grip strength and bone mineral content, whereas the women who had had a fracture continued to gain strength and bone mineral content in their uninjured arm.

A few seconds of grip exercise daily may stress the forearm skeleton sufficiently to stimulate a local gain in bone mineral content. However, it remains to be determined whether this principle can be applied to the entire skeleton. Moreover, the best method for regularly stressing the entire skeleton of aging and reluctant women remains to be determined.

▶ These authors found support for their hypothesis that a forearm's bone mineral content is closely related to the physical demands made on it by activities that require grip strength. They found a small but significant difference in both the bone mineral content and grip strength of the dominant arm over the non-dominant arm when the measures were made before the exercise treatment was applied. It is important to note that both bone mineral content and grip strength increased after 6 weeks of squeezing a tennis ball 3 times daily. It is equally important to note that those gains were lost after 6 months when the subjects stopped squeezing the tennis ball. Of course, this demonstrates the concept of atrophy and means that exercise must be a lifetime activity if we are to maintain our health in our aging years. It would be interesting to replicate this study using men as the subjects.—Col. J.L. Anderson, PE.D.

The Electromyographic DC Potential as a Correlate of Muscular Activity
Trimmel M, Streicher F, Groll-Knapp E, Haider M (Univ of Vienna)
Eur J Appl Physiol 58:459–465, 1989   1–10

Determining the physiologic significance and origin of slow potential changes is difficult because muscle is both a conducting and a contracting tissue. To demonstrate the effect of muscular force and the duration of muscular work on electromyographic (EMG) DC potential, 30 women lifted different weights by flexing the right forearm within a defined and constant setting.

The weights were held for 20 seconds, followed by a pause of 45 seconds. Weights were lifted 5 times in consecutive order, and the sequence of lifting was crossed over subjects. Weights of 0.5, 1, 2, and 3 kg were used. The EMG recordings were made from the brachii muscle of the right biceps and split into an integrated AC channel (IEMG) and a DC channel (DC-EMG).

There was a positive relationship for weight and time with the IEMG. The average shape of the DC-EMG showed a negative initiation potential, a monotonically increasing negative potential during contraction, a positively peaking off potential, and a slow return to baseline after potential. There was a significant relationship between weight and magnitudes of initiation and termination potentials. Regression analysis demonstrated an inverse relationship between time to termination and time to the resolution potential. The DC-EMG showed higher peaks for heavier weights. A control condition, isometric contraction, suggested that initiation, contraction, and termination potentials of the DC-EMG might also be related to features of the movement.

The DC-EMG appears to be a more complex measure of muscular activity than the IEMG. The DC-EMG is associated with different stages of a voluntary contraction, as well as metabolic processes, particularly after contraction. Because the DC-EMG reflects actual force and the stage of fatigue, it may be a useful measure of muscular activity.

▶ This study includes an interesting discussion of the history of DC-EMG studies of the DC potential of muscle that goes back to the first and second decades of this century. The existence of the DC potential of muscle was first observed back then when studies with the string galvanometer showed the DC electrical activity of muscle. These authors appear to believe that there is still much fruitful research to be done in using DC-EMG to study the DC potential of muscle, which may be an important source of other DC potentials. Another point of interest in this study included the comparison of isotonic and isometric conditions using IEMG and DC-EMG. No differences were found between the 2 conditions using the AC channel IEMG. However, smaller amplitudes were found for initiation, contraction, and the termination potential of the DC-EMG. The authors think that these data suggest that certain aspects of Hurley's sliding filament theory and spatial organization of the muscular filaments may play a part in the DC-EMG generation. If we are going to continue to use the electrical potential of muscle to study muscle action, it appears that DC-EMG may have an important role.— Col. J.L. Anderson, PE.D.

The Fatigability of Two Agonistic Muscles in Human Isometric Voluntary Submaximal Contraction: An EMG Study. II. Motor Unit Firing Rate and Recruitment
Maton B, Gamet D (UA CNRS, Paris)
Eur J Appl Physiol 58:369–374, 1989   1–11

The recruitment and firing rates of motor units (MUs) during fatiguing exercise have been studied principally in maximal isometric contractions. Because it cannot be assumed that findings would be the same with submaximal contractions, the recruitment and firing rate of biceps brachii (BB) and brachioradialis (BR) MUs were studied during the course of fatiguing isometric contractions performed at 20% to 30% of maximum voluntary contraction. To record MU activity, a selective bipolar electrode was inserted into each muscle through a hypodermic needle, which was then removed.

Both continuous discharge of the motoneuron and bursting activity were obseved in both BB and BR recordings. Newly recruited MUs began to discharge in bursts, which gradually lengthened to become a continuous rhythmic firing. Within each burst the first interval between consecutive discharges was the shortest. The MU threshold was reduced immediately after the limit time of the maintained contraction. Regardless of the muscle, the discharge frequency of MUs either remained stable or increased slightly, at least to 60% to 70% of the limit time.

During fatiguing isometric contractions at 20% to 30% of maximum voluntary contraction, contractile failure is compensated for by MU recruitment and a lowered MU threshold. Differences between previously reported BB and BR surface EMG changes cannot be explained on the basis of MU firing rate and recruitment.

▶ This is another excellent study of EMG except that, unlike the previous one (Abstract 1–10), only the IEMG or AC potential was measured. I am not an expert on EMG, but it would appear that we need to use both IEMG and DC-EMG in our studies to achieve a better understanding of how EMG can help us to understand muscular functions.—Col. J.L. Anderson, PE.D.

Influence of Contractile Force on Properties of Motor Unit Action Potentials: ADEMG Analysis
Dorfman LJ, Howard JE, McGill KC (Stanford Univ; VA Med Ctr, Palo Alto)
J Neurol Sci 86:125–136, September 1988   1–12

Quantification of the configurational and firing properties of motor unit action potentials (MUAPs) during electromyographic evaluation is possible only for low-force electromyographic (EMG) recordings. During stronger contractions, MUAPs can only be evaluated qualitatively and subjectively from the appearance and sound of interference patterns. Automatic decomposition EMG (ADEMG) is a computer-based technique for studying the properties of higher-threshold MUAPs. Evaluations were made in 30 normal individuals using this technique.

The study population consisted of 1 woman and 9 men aged 20–40 years, 2 women and 8 men aged 41–60 years, and 5 women and 5 men aged 61–76 years. The average age of the entire group was 48.6 years. All study participants were free of neurologic and neuromuscular disorders. Brachial biceps, brachial triceps, and anterior tibial muscles were studied. Each individual pulled against a strain gauge attached by cable to a cuff encircling the distal forearm or the foot. Ten sites were sampled in each muscle at each of 3 isometric contractile forces: threshold, 10% of maximal voluntary contraction (MVC), and 30% of MVC.

In all, 13,206 different MUAPs were recorded from 2,700 person-muscle-force sites, or an average of 4.9 simultaneously active MUAPs per site. In all muscles the increment in contractile force from threshold to 10% MVC was associated with a significant increase in mean MUAP firing rate and number of turns per MUAP. The increment from 10% to 30% MVC led to a highly significant increase in mean MUAP firing rate, number of turns, amplitude, and rise rate. Each force increment was associated with an increase in the number of simultaneously active MUAPs per recording site and with a significant decrease in mean MUAP duration in all muscles because of noise dependency of the duration measurement. Changes in MUAP properties with force were comparable to or exceeded the effects of age, gender differences, or intermuscular variability.

Automatic decomposition electromyography analysis of threshold MUAPs yielded results similar to those obtained by traditional manual or computer-aided MUAP measurements. The shape and firing properties of MUAPs obtained with ADEMG were strongly influenced by the level of isometric contractile force, at least from zero to 30% MVC. Thus force should be incoporated as an independent stratification variable in databases containing information on MUAP properties.

▶ This study is for people who are or will be using EMG in research. This is excellent work, and the entire paper should be read and studied.—Col. J.L. Anderson, PE.D.

Viscosity of the Flexor Muscles of the Elbow Joint Under Maximum Contraction Condition

Niku S, Henderson JM (California Polytechnic State Univ, San Luis Obispo; Univ of California, Davis)
J Biomech 22:523–527, 1989
1–13

The ability of muscles to develop contractile force decreases as the rate of shortening increases. The mechanism, which is related to the way crossbridges react at higher velocities, may be described as a viscous element having a variable damping coefficient. The damping coefficient of the viscous element of a muscle model was estimated under isometric conditions. A link-segment approach (Fig 1–6) was used to model an arm with its normal and involuntary motions. All of the arm flexors were assumed to constitute a single muscle, providing elbow flexion. The model consisted of a contractile element in parallel with a viscous element, both in series with an elastic element.

The damping coefficient was estimated by measuring maximal isometric tension at different lengths, or elbow angles, and the maximum tension at different shortening speeds at the same lengths. Eleven persons participated in the study, in which a Cybex was used (Fig 1–7). In a typical experiment the maximum torque of 31.5 ft-lb, the isometric contraction, decreased to 13.3 ft-lb as shortening velocity increased to 105 degrees per second. Damping coefficients varied from 44,800 N/sec/m at 15 degrees per second at an angle of 30 degrees to 2,285 N/sec/m at 105 degrees per second at an angle of 120 degrees.

The variation in damping coefficients in this study accords with the pattern of change in force generation expected from the way muscles behave. The coefficient decreases as velocity increases, and it generally is higher at lower upper-lower arm angles than at higher angles. This is a simple, readily repeatable method; however, it has the disadvantage of using a measuring scale with limited accuracy.

▶ These authors have shown a way to demonstrate and measure the damping coefficient of the arm flexor muscles using the Cybex machine. Because there

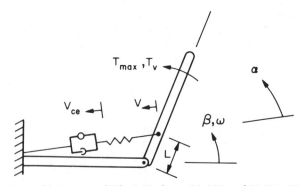

Fig 1–6.—Arm model. (Courtesy of Niku S, Henderson JM: *J Biomech* 22:523–527, 1989.)

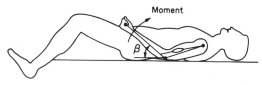

Fig 1–7.—Experimental setup. (Courtesy of Niku S, Henderson JM: *J Biomech* 22:523–527, 1989.)

is no agreement among researchers as to which method is the standard for measuring the damping coefficient, however, different methods are used by different researchers and significantly different values are reported in the literature. These authors spent considerable time explaining the reason for the difference between their values and those reported by Cavagna in 1970. The reasons for the differences were the different research designs and equipment used to make the measurements. This should not surprise anyone. Perhaps if we could get some agreement on a standard for measuring the damping coefficient, we will find more agreement in our values.—Col. J.L. Anderson, PE.D.

Wrist Flexor Muscles of Elite Rowers Measured With Magnetic Resonance Spectroscopy
McCully KK, Boden BP, Tuchler M, Fountain MR, Chance B (Univ of Pennsylvania)
J Appl Physiol 67:926–932, September 1989   1–14

Increasing the metabolic capacity of skeletal muscles is one of the major goals of training programs for endurance sports. Increased endurance performance is associated with increased concentrations and activities of oxidative enzymes. Measurement of the relative values of inorganic phos-

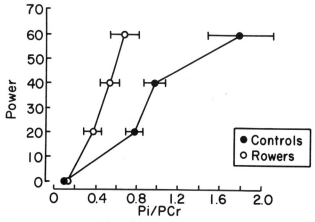

Fig 1–8.—Power vs. P_i/PCr of wrist flexor muscles at rest and during steady-state exercise in 4 rowers and 4 controls. Exercise consisted of 12 contractions of .5-sec duration per minute for 6 minutes at each level. Data are means ± 1 SE for the last 3 minutes of each power level. Each contraction was normalized to maximum voluntary contraction. (Courtesy of McCully KK, Boden BP, Tuchler M, et al: *J Appl Physiol* 67:926–932, September 1989.)

phate (P_i) and phosphocreatine (PCr) has been used as a marker of muscle oxidative capacity. The values of P_i/PCr can be measured by phosphorus magnetic resonance spectroscopy. This procedure was used to assess the metabolic capacity of wrist flexor muscles in trained and nontrained individuals during rest and exercise.

Ten highly trained rowers and 10 nontrained controls of average fitness were matched for age, sex, height, and weight. In vivo muscle metabolism of wrist flexor muscles was measured using a 1.9-T magnet. The study participants performed a series of steady-state and ramp exercise protocols, which involved depressing a handle attached to an isokinetic ergometer. Measured values included P_i/PCr, adenosine triphosphate, and the intracellular pH. Measurements were made at rest, during exercise, and during recovery from exercise.

At rest, rowers and controls had similar P_i/PCr. At each power level during exercise the rowers had lower P_i/PCr values and steeper slopes of the power vs. P_i/PCr at lower power levels (Fig 1–8) when compared with controls. Rowers also had shorter half-time of PCr recovery values than controls. Although the initial linear portion of the recovery curve was difficult to determine (Fig 1–9), rowers had a faster rate of recovery during the first 30 seconds than did controls. They also had smaller changes in pH at the highest power level. At the end of the ramp test the same degree of muscle fatigue was associated with much lower phosphate levels in rowers when compared with controls.

Measurements with magnetic resonance spectroscopy can be used to

Pi/PCr RECOVERY FROM ARM EXERCISE

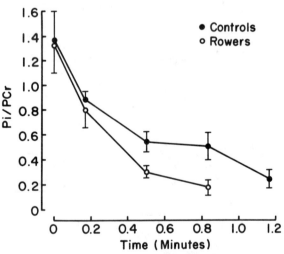

Fig 1–9.—Recovery of P_i/PCr with time for controls and highly trained rowers. Data are means ± 1 SE; 4 persons in each group. Rowers required substantially greater power to reach the same level of PCr/P_i. (Courtesy of McCully KK, Boden BP, Tuchler M, et al: *J Appl Physiol* 67:926–932, September 1989.)

detect differences between trained and untrained human muscle. The muscle fatigue noted in this study did not correlate with phosphate concentrations.

▶ The authors of this excellent study reported that the wrist flexor muscles in highly trained rowers performed considerably better during exercise and recovery from exercise than muscles in control subjects matched for age, sex, height, and weight. They suggest that muscles in the rowers have greater blood flow and/or greater oxidative capacity. However, there was no relationship among the rowers in terms of magnetic resonance spectroscopy results and rowing ability. The amount of fatigue that occurred in the ramp test in the rowers and controls did not correlate with the levels of H_2PO_4, suggesting that muscle fatigue can be related to factors other than H_2PO_4.—Col. J.L. Anderson, PE.D.

Changes in Segment Inertia Proportions Between 4 and 20 Years
Jensen RK (Laurentian Univ, Sudbury, Ont)
J Biomech 22:529–536, 1989   1–15

Growth between the ages of 4 and 20 years produces a redistribution of and an increase in body mass. A model was used to examine changes in whole body and segment shape, volume, mass, mass radius, and moments of inertia.

Data were collected annually over a 9-year period from a sample of males aged 4–20 years. Elliptical zones 2 cm wide were used to model the 16 segments of the body (Fig 1–10). Moments of inertia, mass, and the coordinates of the mass center were determined from these data and

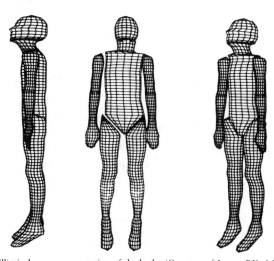

Fig 1–10.—Elliptical zone representation of the body. (Courtesy of Jensen RK: *J Biomech* 22:529–536, 1989.)

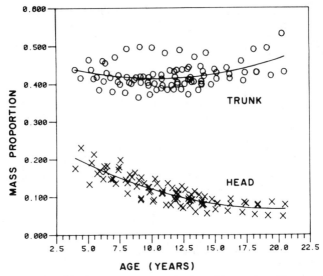

Fig 1–11.—Trunk and head mass proportions and polynomial regressions. (Courtesy of Jensen RK: *J Biomech* 22:529–536, 1989.)

reported segment densities. Reported parameters are inertia parameters useful for a sagittal planar analysis considering the head and neck as a single element, with values given for other fused segments (Figs 1–11 and 1–12 The accuracy of the method was judged against total body mass; other accuracy methods were also assessed. Parameters were presented as proportions of total body mass or segment length.

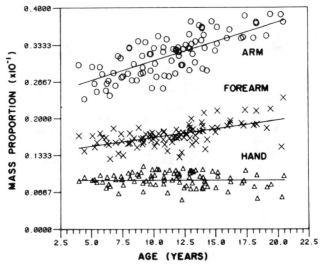

Fig 1–12.—Arm, forearm, and hand mass proportions and polynomial regressions. (Courtesy of Jensen RK: *J Biomech* 22:529–536, 1989.)

Polynomial regressions showed substantial redistribution of the mass between segments over time. This finding is consistent with the principles of cephalocaudal and distal-to-proximal development. The proportions for radius and radius of gyration indicated that mass distribution within segments is relatively small. When the parameters for a 6-year-old child were compared with those expected at ages 18, 24, and 54 years, significant differences were noted. These parameters were then substituted in an analysis of the jump of the 6-year-old child. The changes in joint torque and estimated ground-reaction curves indicated potential development and showed the error that could result if inappropriate parameters are used.

▶ Outstanding work such as this cannot but help biomechanists to do better and more accurate work now and in the future. The concept of body modeling has greatly improved in the past 10 years. Work such as this will help to keep it moving forward.— Col. J.L. Anderson, PE.D.

Reconstruction of the Anterior Cruciate Ligament in Athletes, Using a Fascia Lata Graft: A Review With Preliminary Results of a New Concept
Ekstrand J (Univ Hosp, Linöping, Sweden)
Int J Sports Med 10:225–232, August 1989   1–16

Reconstruction of the anterior cruciate ligament is a challenging procedure. Success depends on appropriate selection of patients, correct choice of graft, careful operative technique, and early, aggressive rehabilitation.

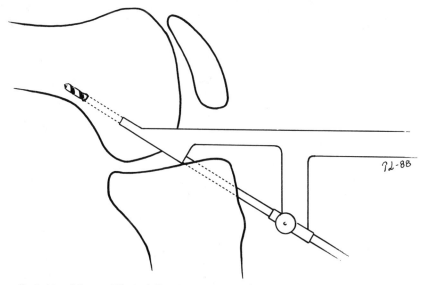

Fig 1–13.—Odensten-Gillquist drill guide is used for anatomical, isometric positioning of drill holes through tibia and femur. (Courtesy of Ekstrand J: *Int J Sports Med* 10:225–232, August 1989.)

Reconstruction is usually recommended only for the young athlete. A modification of the Hey-Groves technique was developed.

Technique.—A fascia lata graft, 4.5 cm wide, is left attached distally. A knee retractor fitting around the lateral femoral condyle provides adequate exposure of the knee without disturbing the patella or extensor apparatus. Notchplasty is performed with removal of osteophytes to restore space for the graft. A drill guide (Fig 1–13) is used to place the drill holes so that the graft can be positioned isometrically. The graft is placed through drill channels in both the tibia and femur (Fig 1–14). The operative procedure lasts for less than 1 hour. Continuous epi-

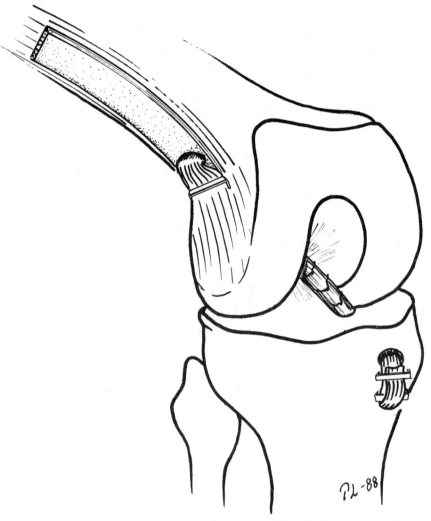

Fig 1–14.—The strip is secured by 1 staple to the femoral condyle and by 2 staples to the tibia in a wrap-back double configuration. (Courtesy of Ekstrand J: *Int J Sports Med* 10:225–232, August 1989.)

dural analgesia for the first postoperative day allows rehabilitation to start immediately. This involves passive motion initially with maximum graft protection, followed by gradually increasing stress on the graft. A gradual return to sports activity follows.

Of 45 patients observed for at least 1 year, 76% returned to games or competition at preinjury levels. After a mean of 6.5 months (range, 5–12 months), no ruptures had occurred. The long-term results require longer follow-up, however.

▶ This operative procedure for reconstruction of the anterior cruciate ligament using a fascia lata graft is quite impressive from the standpoint of when athletes can return to competition. This author reports that, preoperatively, the athletes could perform moderately heavy labor and engage in recreational sports such as cycling or jogging but not in competitive sports. Six months after surgery they could perform heavy labor and participate in competitive sports not involving cutting and contact. At 10 months they could participate in competitive sports such as track and field, gymnastics, or badminton, and at 12 months they could participate in all competitive sports. Of the 45 patients reported on here, 37 (82%) returned to practice in their own sport after a mean of 6.1 months (range, 4–10 months) postoperatively. Four patients decided not to return to their sports, although they had good knee function, and 4 patients were not able to return to sporting activity because of complications such as synovitis or degenerative lesions of the femoral condyle or patella. Although we do not know what long-term follow-up will show, the return to competition figures are impressive.—Col. J.L. Anderson, PE.D.

Is the KT1000 Knee Ligament Arthrometer Reliable?
Forster IW, Warren-Smith CD, Tew M (Univ Hosp, Nottingham, England)
J Bone Joint Surg 71-B:843–847, November 1989   1–17

Results of previous trials with the KT1000 arthrometer have indicated that the difference in laxity between injured and uninjured knees in the same patients was greater than the side-to-side differences in normal persons. If these findings are representative it should be possible to confirm the clinical diagnosis of anterior cruciate ligament (ACL) disruption before surgery. The reliability of the arthrometer is key to such a diagnosis. To determine whether the KT1000 arthrometer would give consistent measurements of anteroposterior laxity, measurements were made by 4 surgeons on the knees of the same persons on the same day at both 15 lb and 20 lb of force (Fig 1–15). Examiners were blinded to results by other examiners. All 4 examiners examined 10 individuals once in turn and then repeated the process in the same order.

There was considerable variation among the 8 measurements of the same knee at each force. Of 40 sets of data (10 right and 10 left knees at 2 forces), only 20% had as many as 4 of 8 like measurements. Of the sets, 40% had at least 7 of 8 measurements within a cluster of 3 mm. In

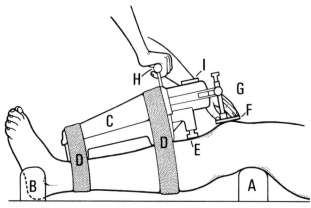

Fig 1–15.—Diagram of the KT1000 arthrometer in use to measure anteroposterior laxity. Adapted from Malcom LL, et al: *Clin Orthop* 196:35–41, 1985. (Courtesy of Forster IW, Warren-Smith CD, Tew M: *J Bone Joint Surg* 71-B:843–847, November 1989.)

70% of sets, the highest of 8 measurements was more than 3 mm greater than the lowest. This finding was more common in injured knees than in normal ones, but there was no tendency for recorded displacement to increase with repeated measuring in either injured or uninjured knees. There were substantial inter- and intraexaminer variations in measurements of side-to-side differences between pairs of knees, as well as in absolute displacement in single knees.

There may have been subjective causes for variation in patients and/or examiners; whatever the reason, the KT1000 arthrometer was not capable of providing a reliable, objective, reproducible measure of ACL laxity. These findings suggest that the KT1000 arthrometer may not be as valuable as thought previously in assessing the relative improvements achieved by different ACL reconstruction techniques.

▶ This study calls into question the reliability of measurements of knee laxity using the KT1000 Knee Ligament Arthrometer. The authors seem to have taken all prudent precautions in designing the study, even taking into consideration the requirements for proper relaxation of the subjects by doing some of the measurements while the subjects were anesthetized. This type of study needs to be replicated by other independent researchers, because we now have valid questions concerning the measurement reliability of this instrument.—Col. J.L. Anderson, PE.D.

Effect of Electro-Motor Stimulation on the Power Production of a Maximally Stretched Muscle
Tachino K, Susaki T, Yamazaki T (Univ of Kanazawa, Kanazawa, Japan)
Scand J Rehab Med 21:147–150, 1989   1–18

Electromotor stimulation (EMS) is a passive method to strengthen muscles. The effects of EMS on the increase in power production of the tibialis anterior muscle (TA) were compared in both the maximally stretched and the maximally shortened positions in 20 healthy female college students.

The students were divided into 2 groups. In 1 group each woman was seated with the left ankle immobilized pain free in a fully plantar-flexed position (ST); in the other group, the ankle was immobilized in a fully dorsiflexed position (SH). The TA was stimulated electrically with a frequency of 50 Hz for a duration of 0.2 ms; a rectangular wave was applied for 10 seconds with a 10-second interval, repeated 10 times daily for 6 weeks.

The ST group had significant gains of 9.4% after 2 weeks, 15.5% after 4 weeks, and 16.4% after 6 weeks. The SH group also had significant, but less pronounced, gains: 5.1%, 8.3%, and 3.0% in the same time periods. At the end of 6 weeks the ST group had significantly greater gains. The increase in power production of the unstimulated TA in the ST group was 5.5%, 8.0%, and 4.3%, which was significant at the ends of the second and fourth weeks of stimulation. The SH group had a nonsignificant increase in torque of −2.7%, 1.8%, and −1.5%. Comparison between the groups showed a significant increase in the power production of the unstimulated TA in the ST group beginning in the second week. To increase muscle strength in the TA, EMS should be performed with the muscle in the maximally stretched position. There may be a cross-educational effect with the muscle in this position.

▶ This study of the effect of EMS is quite interesting. This technique has been used for some time in eastern European countries, including Russia, to train their athletes. The authors of this study chose to allow the subject to control the intensity of the electrical stimuli by using the maximum intensity that could be tolerated. When Larry Butler from our physical education staff visited the Soviet Union several years ago, he allowed them to demonstrate their EMS techniques on him. He reported that there was nothing comfortable or tolerable about the electrical stimuli he received during the demontration, and he was not eager to repeat it. As impressive as the strength gains were with the TA in a fully stretched position and allowing the subjects to determine the amount of electrical stimuli applied, I still wonder what the strength gains would be if the Soviet protocol were used.—Col. J.L. Anderson, PE.D.

2 Women in Sports

Physiological Parameters Related to Distance Running Performance in Female Athletes
Fay L, Londeree BR, LaFontaine TP, Volek MR (Univ of Missouri)
Med Sci Sports Exerc 21:319–324, June 1989   2–1

Many factors influence performance in distance running. The relationships between maximal oxygen uptake, pace at 2 predetermined plasma lactate points, and running economy and performance at distances of 5 km, 10 km, and 10 miles were investigated. Linear regression equations were also developed to predict a runner's race pace for each of these distances.

Thirteen female runners aged 18–33 years underwent a series of submaximal treadmill tests to determine oxygen uptake (running economy), a maximal oxygen uptake test, and another series of 10-minute treadmill runs to identify pace and oxygen uptakes that elicited plasma lactate levels of 2.0 mmol/L and 4.0 mmol/L. Competitive time trials were also conducted for distances of 5 km, 10 km, and 10 miles, and the times for each event and paces in meters per minute were recorded.

The correlation coefficients between each race pace and maximal oxygen uptake ranged between 0.84 and 0.94. The oxygen costs of running at each of 3 submaximal paces correlated moderately with each race pace. With hierarchal stepwise multiple regression, equations with 2 independent variables that explained 94% to 97% of the variability in race performance were developed. The accuracy of these equations should be verified by other studies.

▶ Unless I missed something in the reading of this research, I find it incredible that regression equations with 2 independent variables can explain 94% to 97% of the variability in race performance with no psychological variables being tested. Or, maybe the psychological variables are there but are not identified.— Col. J.L. Anderson, PE.D.

Percentages of Maximal Heart Rate, Heart Rate Reserve, and $\dot{V}O_2$peak for Determining Endurance Training Intensity in Sedentary Women
Weltman A, Weltman J, Rutt R, Seip R, Levine S, Snead D, Kaiser D, Rogol A (Univ of Virginia, Charlottesville)
Int J Sports Med 10:212–216, June 1989   2–2

The use of 60% to 95% of maximal heart rate, heart rate reserve, and maximal oxygen consumption ($\dot{V}O_2$peak) as exercise training intensity measures was evaluated in 33 sedentary women whose mean age was

32.5 years. The $\dot{V}O_2$peak was determined using a continuous horizontal treadmill running protocol; the fixed blood lactate concentrations and lactate threshold were estimated.

The minimal exercise intensity required for most women to achieve values above the lactate threshold was 75% of maximal heart rate. Most required 90% of peak heart rate in order to exceed lactate concentrations of 2 mmol and 2.5 mmol. At 95% of peak heart rate, 12 women exceeded 4 mmol. For most of them to exceed the lactate threshold, 55% of heart rate reserve was necessary. The exercise intensities in percent $\dot{V}O_2$peak for the majority of subjects to exceed the lactate threshold, 2 mmol, 2.5 mmol, and 4 mmol were 55%, 75%, 80%, and 95%, respectively.

If lactate threshold or fixed blood lactate concentrations of 2, 2.5, or 4 mmol are used as criterion training intensities for sedentary women, alternative exercise prescription methods may be necessary.

▶ The purpose of this study was to examine the utility of the percent of maximum concept for exercise prescription in sedentary women when the lactate threshold and fixed blood lactate concentrations of 2.0 mmol, 2.5 mmol, and 4.0 mmol are used as criterion values for exercise intensity. Previous data indicate that use of the standard heart rate intensity guidelines results in differing levels of metabolic stress across subjects.. The authors of this study confirm that sedentary women have widely varying metabolic responses to exercise at intensities of specified percentages of maximum heart rate, heart rate reserve, and maximum oxygen uptake. They have found that if the lactate threshold is used as the exercise intensity, sedentary women would need to incorporate at a minimum of 75% maximum heart rate, 55% of heart rate reserve or 55% of $\dot{V}O_2$ maximum as part of their training routines on their heavy workout days. That is a quantum increase in exercise intensity from the 60% to 75% target heart rate that we have been using in these past years.—Col. J.L. Anderson, PE.D.

Predicting Maximal Oxygen Uptake From Treadmill Testing in Trained and Untrained Women
Martin AD, Notelovitz M, Fields C, O'kroy J (Univ of Florida, Gainesville)
Am J Obstet Gynecol 161:1127–1132, November 1989   2–3

Maximal treadmill exercise testing is often used to establish exercise prescriptions and to assess aerobic exercise training programs. To develop an equation for predicting maximal oxygen uptake from test results in women before and after aerobic training, 181 women aged 29–75 years underwent maximal treadmill exercise testing.

The maximal oxygen uptake in mL/kg/min was equated with 10.34 + 1.29 (exercise time). The correlation coefficient was 0.88 and the standard error of the estimate was 2.1. When 33 women were retested after 6 months and 12 months of aerobic exercise training, the predicted and

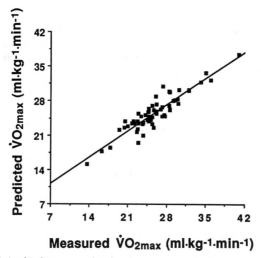

Measured V̇O₂ₘₐₓ (ml·kg⁻¹·min⁻¹)

Fig 2–1.—Relationship between predicted and measured maximal oxygen uptake (V̇O₂max) for cross-validation group. The difference between the 2 measures was not significant ($P = .52$); however, the correlation between measured and predicted V̇O₂max was significant, $r = .89$, SE of the estimate = 1.7; $P < .0001$. (Courtesy of Martin AD, Notelovitz M, Fields C, et al: *Am J Obstet Gynecol* 161:1127–1132, November 1989.)

measured posttraining peak oxygen uptake values did not differ significantly (Fig 2–1).

A strong predictive relationship exists between treadmill exercise time and peak oxygen uptake in trained and untrained women. It is possible to predict peak oxygen uptake with clinically acceptable accuracy using a treadmill and ECG.

▶ The mean age of the subjects for this study was between 54 and 55 years, and their aerobic fitness was quite modest, with a mean maximum oxygen uptake of about 26 mL . kg⁻¹ . min⁻¹. The authors rightfully caution against using this regression equation for predicting the V̇O₂ max outside an exercise time range of 7–20 minutes. Those exercise times equate to 19.37 and 36.14 mL . kg⁻¹ . min⁻¹, respectively. Because the young women who come to West Point arrive here with a mean V̇O₂ max of about 44 mL . kg⁻¹ . min⁻¹, I would be reluctant to use this equation for them. It would be helpful if we could expand the range of this equation, especially at the higher levels.— Col. J.L. Anderson, PE.D.

Differences in Training Responses on Cycle and Rowing Ergometers in Collegiate Women Rowers
Mahler DA, Ward JL, Lentine T, Baron JA (Dartmouth Univ)
Sports Train Med Rehabil 1:197–201, 1989   2–4

Endurance training involving large muscle groups may lead to cardiovascular adaptations as well as crossover muscular adaptations, whereas training for a specific sport (e.g., cycling) leads to cardiovascular adaptations but is specific only for the muscles of the particular sport. The assumption that training on the cycle ergometer would predominantly result in adaptations in the cardiovascular system whereas training on the rowing ergometer would result in combined cardiovascular and muscular adaptations, was evaluated in 7 collegiate women in training for the competitive rowing season.

The women were tested on both the cycle and rowing ergometers at the start and on completion of the 6-month winter training program. Incremental exercise testing was performed on successive days in random order on the cycle and rowing ergometers. The testing protocols consisted of 5 minutes of submaximal, steady-state exercise before increments in power each minute until exhaustion.

With 6 months of training, the maximal oxygen consumption increased by 6% on cycling and by 12% on rowing; the oxygen consumption at the ventilatory threshold increased by 5% for cycling and by 23% for rowing. Comparison of the absolute changes in maximal oxygen consumption and oxygen consumption at the ventilatory threshold showed that the increases were significantly greater for rowing than for cycling. These greater physiologic improvements presumably represent training-induced changes in the specific muscles used in rowing. Muscle biopsies to evaluate muscular structure and function directly were not performed. The importance of specific training for rowing, rather than alternative modes of exercise in preparation for competitive rowing, is supported.

▶ This study should not surprise any of us. The concept is called specificity of training. Naturally, athletes who are rowers will get better conditioning by practicing rowing than by practicing cycling. We should also not be surprised that the increase in the $\dot{V}O_2$ max will be greater after rowing, because more large-muscle groups are working when rowing than when cycling. I would image that the reason coaches would have rowers cycle during the off-season would be to break the monotony and add variability to the training routine while maintaining cardiovascular fitness until time to get back into the rowing routine.— Col. J.L. Anderson, PE.D.

The Effect of Low Impact Dance Training on Aerobic Capacity, Submaximal Heart Rates and Body Composition of College-Aged Females
McCord P, Nichols J, Patterson P (San Diego State Univ)
J Sports Med Phys Fitness 29:184–188, June 1989   2–5

A modified form of low-impact aerobic dancing is used today in which 1 foot remains in contact with the floor at all times, eliminating the suspension phase. The effects of 12 weeks of low-impact aerobic dance conditioning were studied in 16 females aged 17–29 years who had not exercised regularly and had peak oxygen uptake values of less than 43 mL/kg/min. The women exercised 3 times a week for 45 minutes, including 20–35 minutes of low-impact exercise.

Peak oxygen uptake increased by 7.6% during the study period. Submaximal heart rates decreased significantly. The percent body fat decreased from 25% to 21%, as lean body mass increased from 44 kg to 47 kg (6.8%). Body weight did not change significantly.

These data indicate that 12 weeks of low-impact aerobic dance exercise produces a small but significant increase in peak oxygen uptake. Given proper supervision, this appears to be a form of endurance training that is both safe and pleasurable.

▶ Low-impact aerobic dance or exercise training is especially effective for training people who begin with below-average fitness levels. The sedentary population must begin training at a reasonable intensity level that will neither drive them away nor cause unnecessary injuries. Low-impact aerobic exercise can also be used by better-conditioned athletes as part of an "easy day" workout and can add variety to the exercise regimen. However, low-impact aerobic exercise is not the panacea for everyone's exercise needs.—Col. J.L. Anderson, PE.D.

Peripheral Effects of Endurance Training in Young and Old Subjects
Meredith CN, Frontera WR, Fisher EC, Hughes VA, Herland JC, Edwards J, Evans WJ (Tufts Univ)
J Appl Physiol 66:2844–2849, June 1989   2–6

Individuals who have maintained regular exercise into old age are leaner, less likely to have cardiovascular disease or diabetes, and more likely to live longer than sedentary persons. The effects of endurance training on the health of previously sedentary elderly persons were investigated in 10 sedentary elderly men and women and 10 sedentary young healthy men and women. Participants were studied at rest and during maximal exercise, before and after a 12-week training program. The program consisted of 45-minute sessions on a cycle ergometer 3 times per week.

Training did not affect weight or body composition in either group. Elderly subjects had more adipose tissue and less muscle mass than did the younger group. Although the initial peak oxygen capacity was lower in the elderly, absolute increases after training were similar in both groups. Before training, muscle biopsy specimens obtained at rest showed that muscle glycogen stores were 61% higher in the young. Before training, glycogen utilization during submaximal exercise was higher in the elderly. Glycogen stores and muscle oxygen consumption increased significantly in the elderly after training but not in the young. After training the proportion of energy derived from whole-body carbohydrate oxidation during submaximal exercise declined in the young but not in the elderly.

Absolute changes in oxygen capacity were similar in both groups with training, but the elderly had a 128% increase in muscle oxidative capacity. Peripheral adaptations are apparently important factors in the response to aerobic exercise training in the elderly, allowing them to achieve a relative improvement in aerobic capacity equal to or greater than that in young subjects.

▶ This study is extremely valuable. Although it included only 10 elderly subjects, we need all of the information we can get concerning ways to keep our elderly fit. The Center for the Study of Aging in Albany, New York, along with other organizations, is attempting to keep our aging population healthy through exercise, and they need the assistance of university researchers. We are all certain that we can greatly reduce health care costs if we can learn more about how to keep our population physically active as we age.—Col. J.L. Anderson, PE.D.

Aerobic Fitness and Running Performance of Male and Female Recreational Runners
Ramsbottom R, Williams C, Boobis L, Freeman W (Univ of Technology, Loughborough; Leicester Royal Infirmary, Leicester; East Birmingham Hosp, Birmingham, England)
J Sports Sci 7:9–20, Spring 1989   2–7

The reasons why running performance fails to correlate closely with peak oxygen uptake are not clear. The running performance of 18 male and 13 female recreational runners was examined in relation to maximal oxygen uptake and the findings on vastus lateralis muscle biopsy. The mean age of the men was 26 years and of the women, 24 years.

Maximal oxygen uptake correlated well with treadmill running speeds equivalent to blood lactate level of 2 or 4 mmol/L, running economy, and 5-km running times. Muscle fiber composition correlated only modestly with running performance. Submaximal exercise testing indicated that the female runners were as well trained as the male runners, but men nevertheless had faster 5-km times (19.2 vs. 21 minutes).

Although women may use a higher proportion of peak oxygen uptake at a given reference lactate level on submaximal exercise, male recreational runners take less time to complete a 5-km run. The faster running times for men are best explained by a higher maximal oxygen uptake, not a higher training status per se.

▶ I doubt that we can be certain that the faster 5-km running times for men can best be explained by the higher maximal oxygen uptake or any other purely physiologic factor. Psychological factors must be considered, even though we are not certain how to accurately measure them.—Col. J.L. Anderson, PE.D.

Gender-Related Differences in Cardiac Response to Supine Exercise Assessed by Radionuclide Angiography
Hanley PC, Zinsmeister AR, Clements IP, Bove AA, Brown ML, Gibbons RJ (Mayo Clinic and Found, Rochester, Minn)
J Am Coll Cardiol 13:624–629, March 1, 1989   2–8

There is evidence that more women than men with chest pain but normal coronary arteries fail to have an ejection fraction (EF) response to exercise. Gender differences during supine exercise were studied in 192 men and 67 women who had a low probability of coronary artery disease. All were younger than age 50 years, had no anginal or other chest pain, had a nonischemic exercise ECG response, and had a peak exercise heart rate above 120 beats per minute.

Men had a lower resting heart rate and a higher peak exercise systolic blood pressure and rate-pressure product. The median workload reached by men was nearly twice that achieved by women. The median resting EF was 0.63 in men and 0.66 in women. However, the change in EF and the peak value were significantly less in women than in men. The EF decreased on exercise in 30% of women and 16% of men. The end-diastolic volume index increased slightly in women and decreased slightly in men.

There are gender differences in the responses of EF and end-diastolic volume index to both upright and supine exercise. However, gender differences in exercise capacity do not appear to explain the observed differences in these responses.

▶ The authors of this study also found that the men had significantly higher values for exercise workload and exercise intensity than women. These subjects were judged by their obesity and exercise intensity levels to be sedentary in their life-styles. However, at West Point we find similar gender differences in exercise workload and exercise intensity when the subjects are well conditioned. What we do not know is whether these differences are the result of physiologic gender differences or societal-cultural life-style differences from birth. We must continue our studies to answer these questions.—Col. J.L. Anderson, PE.D.

Flexibility Characteristics of Elite Female and Male Volleyball Players
Lee EJ, Etnyre BR, Poindexter HBW, Sokol DL, Toon TJ (Rice Univ, Houston)
J Sports Med 29:49–51, March 1989   2–9

Increased range of motion is commonly assumed to be related to a high level of performance. However, because of the many variables contributing to skilled performance, it is hard to provide conclusive evidence for this assumption. Shoulder and hip flexibility was compared with jumping height among members of the men's and women's United States Olympic Festival volleyball teams.

Twenty-two women and 24 men were measured for standing vertical jump, approach vertical jump, range of shoulder extension, and hip flexion. Among the men approach vertical jump was significantly positively correlated with hip flexion. Among the women there was a significant negative correlation between standing vertical jump and hip flexion and between approach vertical jump and hip flexion. The women with the highest vertical jumps had the least amount of hip flexibility.

The positive correlation between hip flexion and approach vertical jump in the men supports the notion that greater flexibility is related to more skilled jumping performance. However, the opposite was true for the women. Greater hip flexibility may be more advantageous for men than women in jumping ability.

▶ In this study the authors have presented us with an interesting problem: Why do men with greater hip flexibility jump higher than men with lesser hip flexibility, whereas the reverse is true for women? Maybe it is more the result of anatomical differences between men and women. Maybe it is because hip flexibility accounts for such a small percentage of the variance and other variables are much more important. I feel that there is room for both of these possibilities, and more studies need to be done using more variables to account for the excellence in jumping height.—Col. J.L. Anderson, PE.D.

Sex Difference in Muscle Cross-Sectional Area of Athletes and Non-Athletes
Bishop P, Cureton K, Conerly M, Collins M (Univ of Alabama, Tuscaloosa; Univ of Georgia, Athens)
J Sports Sci 7:31–39, Spring 1989   2–10

That sex difference in arm strength is larger than sex difference in leg strength is thought to be related to a sex difference in habitual physical activity. Alternatively, a sex difference in upper body/lower body muscle cross-sectional area could account for the difference in upper body/lower body strength independent of sex differences in physical activity.

Limb fat-free cross-sectional areas (FFCSAs) were calculated from circumferences corrected for subcutaneous fat thickness in 24 male and 25 female swimmers and 23 male and 25 female nonathletes. Fat-free weight was estimated from body density measured under water. Participants were 15–28 years of age.

Male swimmers had 32% greater fat-free weights and 49% larger upper arm, similar forearm, and 23% larger thigh FFCSAs than female swimmers. Male nonathletes had 34% greater fat-free weights and 61% larger upper arm, 54% larger forearm, and 35% larger thigh FFCSAs than female nonathletes. When adjusted for variance in body size, there were no significant differences in FFCSAs for swimmers; however, for nonathletes, men had significantly larger adjusted upper arm and forearm FFCSAs than women, but thigh FFCSAs were not significantly different.

Sex differences in muscle area of the arms may be partially attributable to habitual activity differences between the sexes. When comparing functional or performance measures between sexes, possible long-term differences in activities between sexes should be considered.

▶ This study suggests that apparent biologic sex differences may be more the result of sociocultural differences, and possibly sample selection, than real differences. Although this is interesting information from research that was well done, I wonder whether it addresses the most important question. Today, more and more women are moving into nontraditional jobs, the more important question has to do with functional performance differences and how they are affected by physiologic differences between the sexes. Here at West Point we study the performance differences between men and women and attempt to relate those differences to physiology or culture; we cannot be too concerned with relative measures of strength or endurance compared to body size. The 75-lb pack weighs the same for everyone, and the distance and speed of travel are also the same for everyone in the organization. I have not been able to determine the practical importance of these relative measures.—Col. J.L. Anderson, PE.D.

Contrasts in Muscle and Myofibers of Elite Male and Female Bodybuilders
Alway SE, Grumbt WH, Gonyea WJ, Stray-Gundersen J (Univ of Texas, Dallas)
J Appl Physiol 67:24–31, July 1989   2–11

Muscle adaptation to heavy resistance training has been studied in men but not often in women. Researchers hypothesized that potential adaptations of fiber area and fiber number could be determined in muscles of elite bodybuilders and that these findings could be compared in male and female bodies. Biopsy specimens were obtained from the biceps brachii of 8 elite male bodybuilders and 5 elite female bodybuilders with similar training characteristics. The biopsy samples were examined for muscle cross-sectional area (CSA), fiber area, and fiber numbers.

Biceps CSA was twice as large in male bodybuilders as in female bodybuilders, and it was strongly correlated with lean body mass (Fig 2–2).

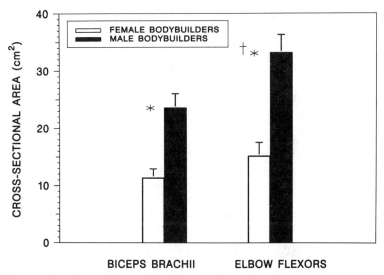

Fig 2–2.—Biceps brachii and total elbow flexor cross-sectional area (means ± 1 SE) in female and male bodybuilders. *$P < .05$, males vs. females; †$P < .05$, male biceps vs. elbow flexors. (Courtesy of Alway SE, Grumbt WH, Gonyea WJ, et al: *J Appl Physiol* 67:24–31, July 1989.)

Per kilogram of lean body mass or per centimeter of height, biceps CSA was 35% greater in men than in women. Most of the gender difference in muscle CSA was the result of greater absolute mean fiber areas in men; however, men also had a significantly greater proportion of small type II fibers than women. Type I fiber areas were similar between the groups. Biceps CSA correlated positively with fiber CSA and fiber number.

Because muscle characteristics before training were unknown, these data suggest that either apparent training adaptations are genetically determined attributes, or that adaptations to resistance training are complex and may involve fiber hypertrophy and fiber number.

▶ This excellent study indicates that women are capable of substantial increases in muscle cross-sectional area, fiber number, and hypertrophy of both fiber types compared with data from untrained women. Limitations in the magnitude of lean body mass and muscle cross-sectional area in women may reflect an inability to achieve the same degree of hypertrophy in type II fibers per kilogram body mass or per centimeter of body height, compared with male bodybuilders. A point of interest to me, which was not mentioned by these investigators, is whether these male and female bodybuilders were taking steroids.—Col. J.L. Anderson, PE.D.

Influence of Dietary Iron Source on Measures of Iron Status Among Female Runners
Snyder AC, Dvorak LL, Roepke JB (Ball State Univ, Muncie, Ind)
Med Sci Sports Exerc 21:7–10, February 1989 ˙   2–12

Female athletes have various degrees of iron deficiency, but not iron-deficiency anemia. These differences have been variously attributed to inadequate dietary intake, low bioavailability of iron, or high rates of iron loss. Running endurance time is significantly related to serum iron variables. Many female athletes are modified vegetarians. Whether runners who consume a modified vegetarian diet are predisposed to iron deficiency was determined in 9 women (median age, 37.8 years) who consumed a diet based on the 4 basic food groups, including red meat, and 9 women (median age, 39.2 years) who consumed a modified vegetarian diet that included very little or no red meat.

All women had adhered to the same dietary pattern for at least 1 year. Both groups were closely matched for body weight, number of pregnancies, years since last pregnancy, aerobic capacity, and miles run per week. Each woman performed an incremental, maximal exercise test on a treadmill to determine aerobic capacity. Serum iron and total iron-binding capacity were measured at the midpoint of the menstrual cycle.

Women in the modified vegetarian group had significantly lower serum ferritin levels and significantly higher serum total iron-binding capacity than women in the red-meat group. The mean dietary iron intake of the vegetarian was similar to that of the red-meat group, but the former had significantly lower bioavailability of dietary iron, probably reflecting the difference in the amount of heme iron consumed. These findings support previous studies, which found that athletes have various degrees of iron deficiency but not of iron-deficiency anemia.

▶ This study agrees with other studies showing that athletes may have various degrees of iron deficiency but not iron-deficiency anemia. Iron deficiency without anemia reduces endurance capacity and leads to excess lactate production. The 2 groups of women in this study differed only in their nutritional intake. One group followed a modified vegetarian diet and the other followed a balanced diet of the 4 basic food groups. Intake averaged less than 1,800 kcal/day, with about 8 mg of iron available per 1,000 kcal, in both groups. Neither group ingested enough iron to meet the Recommended Daily Allowance. The modified vegetarian group consumed almost all of their iron from nonheme sources, however, which is probably why, even though the 2 groups ingested basically the same amount of iron daily, the blood iron in the vegetarian group was less than in the balanced food group eating meat, poultry, and fish. This is because the bioavailability of nonheme iron is influenced by the composition of the diet, with increased bioavailability occurring in the meat-poultry-fish diet. What is the solution for vegetarian runners? Should they be administered supplemental iron? Because we don't know whether that is helpful, iron supplements should not be given to athletes routinely until further documentation is available.—Col. J.L. Anderson, PE.D.

Zinc Status of Highly Trained Women Runners and Untrained Women
Deuster PA, Day BA, Singh A, Douglass L, Moser-Veillon PB (Uniformed Services Univ of the Health Sciences, Bethesda; Univ of Maryland, College Park)
Am J Clin Nutr 49:1295–1301, June 1989   2–13

The trace mineral zinc, one of the most widely distributed metals in the human body, plays important roles in metabolism, endocrine function, and immune integrity. Highly trained female runners may be at risk for zinc deficiency. Endurance training effects on zinc status were assessed in 13 highly trained and 10 untrained women; all received a 25-mg oral zinc load. Blood and 24-hour urine samples were obtained before and after the dose, and 3-day dietary records were kept.

In both groups mean daily zinc intakes were below the Recommended Daily Allowance. Fasting concentrations of plasma zinc, serum albumin, α_2-macroglobulin, and erythrocyte zinc content also were similar in trained and untrained women. However, the highly trained women had significantly greater urinary zinc excretion and reduced response to the oral dose of zinc (Fig 2–3). This may reflect a higher rate of skeletal muscle turnover. Trained women had a decreased response to 25 mg of zinc in terms of the maximal response observed, the area under the curve, and the slope estimating the rate of zinc appearance in plasma. Whether these findings reflect differences in absorption, differences in entry or removal of zinc from plasma, or differences in plasma volume remain unresolved.

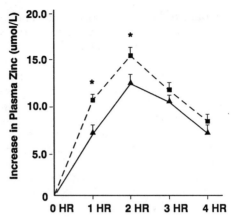

Fig 2–3.—Mean ± SEM increases in plasma zinc for highly trained *(triangles)* and untrained *(squares)* women in response to ingesting 25 mg of zinc. *Significantly different from highly trained (*P* < .01). (Courtesy of Deuster PA, Day BA, Singh A, et al: *Am J Clin Nutr* 49:1295–1301, June 1989.)

▶ The authors have surfaced a problem but were not able to find a solution. We need to continue studying this problem to better determine the consequences of zinc excretion by highly trained women. Also, perhaps zinc taken as part of a well-balanced diet, rather than as a supplement, will be better absorbed and not as easily excreted.—Col. J.L. Anderson, PE.D.

Effect of a Season of Competition and Training on Hematological Status of Women Field Hockey and Soccer Players
Douglas PD (Univ of Connecticut, Storrs)
J Sports Med Phys Fitness 29:179–183, June 1989   2–14

A so-called sports anemia has been noted in the early course of physical training that may adversely affect sports performance and lower resistance to fatigue. Because female athletes may be low in dietary iron, the effects of training and competition on hematologic status were examined in 30 collegiate soccer and field hockey players. The athletes, whose mean age was 19 years, were compared with 30 female college students who did not participate regularly in strenuous activity.

Hemoglobin levels did not differ significantly in the athletes and controls, but the increase over time was more marked in the nonathletes. Nonathletes had much higher hematocrit levels, whereas red blood cell counts increased comparably in both groups over the 14-week study period. Athletes had lower mean corpuscular volumes than nonathletes. The mean iron intake did not differ significantly from the daily recommended intake of 18 mg.

Further studies are needed of female athletes participating in longer seasons and in sports in which the intensity of training may differ. The present study failed to demonstrate conclusive evidence of "sports anemia" in female soccer and field hockey players.

► "Sports anemia" is the same as iron-deficiency anemia, i.e., a condition characterized by a reduced number of erythrocytes and a smaller than normal erythrocyte mass, or a reduced concentration of hemoglobin in the peripheral blood.

This study appears to support the contention that an adequate nutritional diet prevents "sports anemia"—at least for college-aged field hockey and soccer players. These female athletes were not dieting and were consuming the Recommended Daily Allowance of iron. However, those who are dancers, gymnasts, or runners may experience sports anemia because it is more likely that they will be dieting and will not consume the recommended amount of iron daily.—Col. J.L. Anderson, PE.D.

Some Medical Problems Related to Women's Sports (A Review)
Graevskaya ND, Petrov IB, Belyaeva NI (State Inst of Physical Culture of the Moscow Region)
Sports Training Med Rehabil 1:77–83, 1989   2–15

Women compete internationally in most sports. In the Union of Soviet Socialist Republics they account for up to 30% of master athletes, and the proportion of women participating in sports activities worldwide continues to increase. Clearly, regular activity is important for optimal health in women as in men. Women who exercise regularly are better developed physically and have greater functional reserves and general resistance than others. They are better able to adapt to adverse environmental factors. They also have less eventful pregnancies and give birth to healthier children than women who are not athletic.

Whereas the morphological, functional, and mental characteristics of women allow them to excel in some sports, they make high levels of achievement in others problematic. Participation by women in super distance running, sport walking, judo, and football, among others, may not be possible. The achievements of women in sports that depend largely on endurance are notable.

Sport activities have no negative effect on reproductive function, given proper regimens and training techniques. Dysmenorrhea and premenstrual syndrome are no more frequent than in nonathletic women, and there actually are fewer problems during pregnancy and parturition. Data on the time of sexual maturation are conflicting; delayed menarche is most frequent in gymnasts and skaters. Comprehensive studies and combining the experience gained by trainers and physicians working with female sports teams will help female athletes to achieve more while remaining healthy.

► This is an excellent review from the perceptions of USSR sports medicine personalities after studying the research from around the world. I believe that most Western sports medicine experts, certainly in the United States, can learn a great deal from our Soviet counterparts. They have years more experience in the high-level training of elite female athletes, and they recognize the necessity to organize comprehensive studies, to collect data from every nation, and to share these data.—Col. J.L. Anderson, PE.D.

An Epidemiologic Investigation of Injuries Affecting Young Competitive Female Gymnasts

Caine D, Cochrane B, Caine C, Zemper E (Univ of Oregon; Internatl Inst for Sport and Human Performance, Eugene, Ore)

Am J Sports Med 17:811–820, November–December 1989   2–16

Female gymnasts participate in the sport and train more rigorously at an increasingly younger age, but the long-term consequences of pediatric sports injuries are uncertain. Fifty highly competitive female gymnasts whose mean age was 12.6 years were studied for 1 year. At baseline, investigators determined injury status, maturity level, and selected anthropometric indices. Athletes were visited once every 2 weeks to determine injury status.

During the surveillance year 50 gymnasts trained for 40,127 hours. There were 147 injuries distributed among 43 gymnasts, for an overall injury rate of 3.66 injuries per 1,000 hours of participation. The injury rate was particularly high during the first few months of the season. The largest number of injuries involved the lower extremities, especially the knee and ankle. The wrist was the most frequently injured part of the upper extremity and the lower back the most commonly injured area of the spine and trunk. Nonspecific pain accounted for 40% of the complaints, followed by sprains and strains. The overall reinjury rate of 32.7% was even higher for specific body parts; the reinjury rate in the lower back was 72.2%, for example. Most reinjuries were characterized by gradual onset, suggesting a chronic condition. Only 29 gymnasts were still training by the end of the year; 11 of 21 girls who ceased training were injured at the time they withdrew.

The high reinjury rate among these young athletes suggests the need for complete rehabilitation before the child returns to full participation. Rapid periods of growth and advanced levels of competition are also related to risk of injury. Reduced training loads are recommended for athletes experiencing growth spurts.

▶ Injury prediction is a very inexact science. However, the authors of this study have done a great job in alerting health care professionals and those of us involved with sports medicine to the real problems and concerns involved in the training of young female gymnasts. None of us knows the total price in terms of injuries to all of the young women in the United States who have dreams of becoming Olympic champions. I wonder how many are left on the side lines with injuries in order to train the few who ultimately make the national teams? It is important to note that the most injury-prone gymnasts were the class I and elite athletes, who were characterized by a rapid period of growth. One interpretation of this finding is that the risk of injury increases because the skills are more difficult and hazardous. Another possible explanation is that higher degrees of skill require more sound and healthy bodies. Health care professionals must be more proactive in protecting these young women athletes from overzealous coaches, parents, and themselves by developing a better understanding of the injury phenomenon.—Col. J.L. Anderson, PE.D.

The Incidence of Female Hockey Injuries on Grass and Synthetic Playing Surfaces

Jamison S, Lee C (Univ of Newcastle, New South Wales, Australia)
Aust J Sci Med Sport 21:15–17, June 1989   2–17

The use of artificial playing surfaces for competitive sports is increasing. Studies of injury rates on synthetic surfaces have mainly investigated men who play contact sports. However, women who play contact sports may have different injury patterns. Possible differences were examined in rates of injuries incurred on natural grass and on Astroturf in the sport of women's field hockey.

The Australian National Women's Hockey Championships were played on grass in 1984 and on Astroturf in 1985. Players were first asked to complete a questionnaire before the tournament to provide baseline data on injury status. A follow-up questionnaire was completed during the tournament by those players who sustained any type of injury.

Baseline data were completed by 110 women playing on grass and 95 women playing on Astroturf. The 110 women who played on grass reported 86 injuries, or an average of 0.78 injuries per player. The 95 women who played on Astroturf reported 92 injuries, or an average of 0.97 injuries per player. There was a trend for a higher proportion of injuries to the head, body, and upper limbs when playing on Astroturf, but the difference did not reach statistical significance. Injuries to the lower limbs were the most common in both groups. When lower limb injuries were subdivided into injuries of the major joints and soft tissue injuries, 53% of lower limb injuries incurred on grass and 37% of those incurred on Astroturf were of the major joints. The difference was statistically significant.

The reason for the increased injury rate on Astroturf may be attributed in part to the changes in playing style and in part to the faster and less absorptive qualities of the playing surface. Coaches and trainers should ensure that players are adequately prepared physically for the particular demands of their playing positions and that they wear adequate protective gear.

► Having studied athletic injuries for 21 years, I can say that a single study such as this does not really show anything we can consider conclusive. The results of this study comparing injuries occurring on grass with those occurring on artificial surfaces are similar to many I have seen. The numbers of injuries are about the same, but the types are somewhat different. One of the most important problems in doing athletic injury research is to first identify what is an injury.—Col. J.L. Anderson, PE.D.

Women's Soccer Injuries in Relation to the Menstrual Cycle and Oral Contraceptive Use

Möller-Nielsen J, Hammar M (Linköping Univ Hosp, Linköping, Sweden)
Med Sci Sports Exerc 21:126–129, April 1989   2–18

The effect of menstruation on athletic performance is variable among women, with some reporting better and others reporting decreased performance. Whether more traumatic injuries occur during premenstruation and menstruation, and whether the use of oral contraceptives influences the rate of injury during any portion of the menstrual cycle, were determined in 86 female soccer players who responded to a questionnaire. The women also noted their menstrual periods and any alteration in contraceptive status for a 1-year period. The duration of exercise sessions and matches and the number of traumatic injuries also were noted.

In general, women were more susceptible to traumatic injuries during premenstrual and menstrual periods than during the rest of the menstrual cycle. This was particularly true of women who had premenstrual symptoms, such as swelling and discomfort in the breasts, irritability, and swelling and congestion in the abdomen. Women using contraceptive pills had a lower rate of traumatic injury than those not using contraceptive pills.

Oral contraceptives apparently ameliorate some premenstrual/menstrual symptoms that might affect coordination and thus reduce the risk of injury. Further study of the preventive effects of contraceptive pills on traumatic injury are necessary before recommendations can be made.

▶ This is an excellent study done in Sweden. I recognize that the findings may seem strange, but the authors seem to have reviewed all logical reasons why their results are what they are, and their conclusions seem sound. They do not ascribe any cause and effect to their findings, but we all must wonder why these women were more susceptible to traumatic injuries during premenstrual and menstrual periods than during the rest of the menstrual cycle. Also, why did it appear that women using contraceptive pills had a lower rate of traumatic injury than those women not using contraceptive pills? This study must be replicated to test these findings.—Col. J.L. Anderson, PE.D.

Influence of Transcutaneous Electrical Nerve Stimulation on Pain, Range of Motion, and Serum Cortisol Concentration in Females Experiencing Delayed Onset Muscle Soreness
Denegar CR, Perrin DH, Rogol AD, Rutt R (Slippery Rock Univ, Slippery Rock, Pa; Univ of Virginia, Charlottesville; Univ of Oklahoma)
J Orthop Sports Phys Ther 11:100–103, September 1989   2–19

Identification of endogenous opioids and the isolation of β-endorphin led to new models of stimulation-induced analgesia. Current theory proposes that stimulation-induced breakdown of the prohormone proopiomelanocortin, a component of β-endorphin produced by the anterior pituitary gland, results in elevation of blood cortisol levels. Serum cortisol concentrations in response to a 30-minute transcutaneous electrical nerve stimulation (TENS) treatment were measured to determine the potential application of TENS as an anti-inflammatory procedure.

Eight women received low-frequency, 300-μsec pulse-width TENS at 4 sites to control pain in the upper arm induced through repeated eccentric muscle contractions. Patients received TENS treatments before pain was induced and while experiencing induced delayed-onset muscle soreness of the elbow flexor muscle group. Blood samples were withdrawn 15 minutes before and immediately before treatment and at 1, 20, and 40 minutes afterward.

The TENS treatment did not elevate serum cortisol concentrations. Nevertheless, subjects perceived a significant reduction in pain and improvement in range of elbow extension after treatment for induced muscle soreness.

Apparently, the anterior pituitary is not a source of β-endorphin in TENS-induced pain relief. If β-endorphin is active in TENS-induced analgesia, the source may be within the blood-brain barrier.

▶ Although these authors believe that the decreased pain and increased elbow extension after TENS done while the subjects were experiencing delayed-onset muscle soreness were the result primarily of the treatment, the results also suggest that the effects were not caused by release of β-endorphin from the anterior pituitary. The authors did agree that, although their results do not rule out β-endorphin as an active agent in TENS-induced analgesia, the source is probably within the brain, as β-endorphin does not easily cross the blood-brain barrier. The data also do not support TENS as an anti-inflammatory agent.— Col. J.L. Anderson, PE.D.

Generalized Equation for Predicting Body Density of Women From Girth Measurements
Tran ZV, Weltman A (Arizona State Univ, Tempe)
Med Sci Sports Exerc 21:101–104, February 1989   2–20

Most laboratory methods for measuring body density are impractical in field settings. Equations that use only girth are somewhat less accurate than those using skinfold-fat measures, but measurements are easy to obtain and there is less possibility for measurement error. A generalized regression equation using girth measurements, age, height, and weight was developed that provides valid body-density estimates for women over a wide range of ages and weights.

Researchers weighed 482 white women in air on a beam scale and under water and recorded girth for thigh, hips, iliac, and abdomen. They also recorded age, weight, and height and computed residual volume to determine percent of body fat. Stepwise multiple regression was used to select the best set of predictors of body density.

The use of 3 girth measurements—average abdomen, average abdomen^2 (mean of abdomen 1 and abdomen 2), and hips—in combination with body weight, height, and age resulted in a multiple correlation *(R)* of 0.89. The correlation between hydrostatically determined body density and predicted body density using the equation was slightly higher than the *R* value.

An equation using 3 girth measures and body weight, height, and age can predict body density in women with a wide range of ages and body composition. This equation is comparable in accuracy to those previously published using skinfold thickness.

▶ The Army presently uses a generalized equation for predicting percent of body fat for the women in the Army. This equation was developed at Natick Laboratories and is applicable to both black women and Caucasian women. I am not certain that our equation is any more accurate than the one presented in this research. The Army equation was developed to give us a method to be used in field settings and is easy to use, yet accurate.—Col. J.L. Anderson, PE.D.

Impact of Total Body Water Fluctuations on Estimation of Body Fat From Body Density

Bunt JC, Lohman TG, Boileau RA (Univ of Illinois, Urbana)
Med Sci Sports Exerc 21:96–100, February 1989   2–21

The calculation of body fat content on the basis of body density assumes that the density of the fat-free body remains constant. However, women often experience significant fluctuations in body weight as a result of temporary water retention associated with the menstrual cycle. Because water content represents approximately 73% of the fat-free body, fluctuations in body water content could significantly alter estimates of body fat content. To determine whether variability in body weight caused by water retention leads to variability in body density values as determined by hydrostatic weighing, studies were made in 7 men and 7 women aged 19–24 years.

The women had regular menstrual cycles ranging between 25 days and 35 days in length, and all reported experiencing considerable weight fluctuations. None of the women was taking oral contraceptives. During an initial 4-week period fluctuations in weight were monitored by daily weigh-ins early in the morning after an overnight fast. Each woman was tested at 2 different times in the menstrual cycle, corresponding to her low and high body weight. Hydrostatic weighing was done simultaneously with measurement of residual lung volume. Total body water was determined by deuterium oxide dilution. The men were randomly tested approximately 3 weeks apart.

There were significant mean differences in these women for body weight, body density, and percent body fat as determined by the hydrostatic weighing method. Some women, particularly those who experience noticeable fluctuations in body weight, may have significantly different estimates in percent body fat when the hydrostatic weighing method is used.

▶ This study shows us that when measuring women for body fat percentage using body density, we must be alert to the total body water content, which can change significantly for many women depending on their menstrual cycle.

An increase in total body water would cause an overestimation of percent body fat.—Col. J.L. Anderson, PE.D.

The Menstrual Cycle's Effect on the Reliability of Bioimpedance Measurements for Assessing Body Composition
Gleichauf CN, Roe DA (Cornell Univ, Ithaca, NY)
Am J Clin Nutr 50:903–907, November 1989   2–22

Repeated estimates of bioimpedance and body weight were obtained for 25 apparently healthy women aged 20–41 years who had regular menses for the past year. Bioimpedance was measured daily over a single cycle, and sodium intake was determined at the same time.

Most of the error in bioelectrical impedance analysis (BIA) measures came from the undependability of the measures or the error associated with the effect of non-nutritional factors. Sodium intake varied significantly over the cycle, but overall intake averaged 2,937 mg per day. After controlling for intersubject variation, body weight contributed significantly to variation in resistance measures. After controlling for weight change as well, sodium intake did not explain variation in resistance measures but was associated with weight changes during the cycle.

The bioimpedance method is a valid approach to determining body composition in a community setting. When large weight fluctuations occur in relation to the menstrual cycle, the average of several bioimpedance measurements should be obtained, rather than relying on a single measurement.

▶ The validity of bioimpedance analysis for measuring body composition must be questioned because it relies on the assumptions of cylindrical body geometry, a constant and uniform distribution of body water and electrolytes, and constant body temperature. The authors of this study, who found what they believe to be a systematic overestimation of body fat as they used the bioimpedance analysis method, compared their results to measurements using anthropometric measurements with the Durnin and Womersley equation. These authors do not confirm the validity of the bioimpedance analysis techniques for assessing body composition. They believe that the results of this study suggest that the effect on resistance and fat-free mass estimates obtained during the menstrual cycle are related to changes in body weight, presumably caused by changes in water retention. However, they think that the bioimpedance analysis method does appear to be accurate enough to be used when a high degree of sensitivity and specificity is not required, such as in a community setting.—Col. J.L. Anderson, PE.D.

Menstrual Irregularities in Athletic Women May Be Predictable Based on Pre-Training Menses
Cavanaugh DJ, Kanonchoff AD, Bartels RL (Ohio State Univ)
J Sports Med Phys Fitness 29:163–169, June 1989   2–23

Factors predictive of menstrual irregularity were sought in 161 highly competitive female athletes and 65 age-matched nonathletic women. Professional dancers, basketball players, gymnasts, swimmers, and fencers were among the athletes evaluated. The age range was 17–24 years. Those using oral contraceptives were excluded.

Thirteen of 63 athletes who had begun training before menarche (21%) reported current menstrual irregularity. In all, 22% of the athletes and 8% of controls had current irregular cycles. Women who currently had irregular cycles were significantly older at menarche than those with regular cycles. Mean body weights were comparable in the athletes and control women. Athletes with the highest anxiety scores and lowest anger scores on the Spielberger State-Trait Personality Inventory tended to have irregular menstrual cycles.

Female athletes may have factors that predispose them to menstrual disorder. Nevertheless, exercise training alone does not lead to delayed menarche or menstrual irregularity.

▶ After following the discussion of causes of menstrual dysfunction of women athletes for 14 years, it pleases me to see the direction that the research has taken in the past few years. These authors stated that they were aware ahead of time that no single factor in the human physiologic system worked alone to cause menstrual dysfunction. This knowledge has not always been accepted. Our experience here at West Point led us to accept in 1976 that no single identifiable factor was working alone to cause the menstrual dysfunction. It is helpful that psychological factors as well as physiologic factors are now being studied.— Col. J.L. Anderson, PE.D.

The Immune State of Female Athletes and Its Correlation With Menstrual Function and Conditions of Sports Activities
Surkina ID, Gotovtseva EP (Central Research Inst of Medical and Biological Problems Related to Sports)
Sports Training Med Rehab 1:85–88, 1989   2–24

Elevated morbidity during intense athletic activity is related to the so-called state of sports-related immunodeficiency. The correlation between immune status and menstrual function was investigated during a sports season in adult female skaters aged 18–20 years and junior athletes aged 16–17 years. Most had pursued sports activity for 6–10 years.

Only 4 of 20 speed skaters reported no menstrual changes during training and competition. The others described both prolongation and shortening of the cycle, lower abdominal and lumbar pain, and greater blood loss associated with intense exercise during menses. Six women had had menstrual delays for 18–24 months. Training with maximal workloads was associated with a decline in T lymphocyte functional activity, but no relationship with the menstrual pattern was evident.

Female athletes with menstrual dysfunction may be less resistant to emotional stress than those with normal reproductive function. Immune depression in women with irregular menses is a risk factor for infectious disease. It may be appropriate to stimulate immune reactivity in this setting.

▶ This is another example where these authors from the USSR recognize that there appears to be a relationship between menstrual dysfunction of athletes and the psychological stress they experience in training and completion. They also recognize that physiology also plays a part. It is hoped that during this next decade we can work with the Eastern Europeans and share data both sides have in order to solve some of these puzzles we have been studying for years.—Col. J.L. Anderson, PE.D.

Menstrual Status and Plasma Vasopressin, Renin Activity, and Aldosterone Exercise Response
DeSouza MJ, Maresh CM, Maguire MS, Kraemer WJ, Flora-Ginter G, Goetz KL (Univ of Connecticut, Storrs; St Luke's Hosp and Found, Kansas City, Mo)
J Appl Physiol 67:736–743, August 1989   2–25

Vigorous exercise causes increases in plasma vasopressin, renin activity, and aldosterone in women as well as in men. However, no data are available on the relationship between these hormonal factors and ovarian steroids in athletic women as various phases of the menstrual cycle.

Researchers studied 8 amenorrheic women and 8 eumenorrheic women aged 18–37 years who had been running a minimum of 35 miles per week for at least 1 year. Eumenorrheic runners were studied before and after 40 minutes of running at 80% of maximal oxygen uptake during the early follicular and midluteal phases of the menstrual cycle. Amenorrheic runners were studied once using the same protocol.

Menstrual phase had no significant effect on preexercise plasma vasopressin or renin activity, but aldosterone levels were significantly higher during the midluteal phase than during the early follicular phase. At 4 minutes after the 40-minute run, plasma vasopressin and renin activity were significantly elevated in the eumenorrheic runners regardless of the menstrual phase. By 40 minutes after exercise, these values had returned to preexercise levels. During the midluteal phase plasma aldosterone levels at 4 minutes and 40 minutes after exercise were higher than during the early follicular phase. In amenorrheic runners menstrual status was not associated with significant differences in preexercise plasma vasopressin or renin activity. Plasma aldosterone levels were significantly higher in amenorrheic runners, however. Responses in amenorrheic runners after exercise were comparable with responses of eumenorrheic runners in the early follicular phase.

Submaximal exercise induces significant increases in plasma vasopressin and renin activity regardless of menstrual status or phase. Plasma aldosterone levels, however, are significantly elevated during the midluteal phase and rise even higher with exercise during this phase. In addition, amenorrheic runners have elevated resting levels of aldosterone.

▶ This study demonstrates that female athletes have plasma arginine vasopressin, renin activity, and aldosterone responses to submaximal exercise similar to that previously observed in men. The authors believe that these changes may act to conserve body fluids while exercising. The authors have also noted that it appears the elevated level of aldosterone is consistent with the enhanced adrenal cortical phenomenon previously observed in amenorrheic runners and supports the hypothesis that an alteration in the hypothalamic-pituitary-adrenal axis is an integral component of menstrual alterations in some athletic women.—Col. J.L. Anderson, PE.D.

Changes in the Special Working Capacity and Mental Stability of Well-Trained Woman Skiers at Various Phases of the Biological Cycle
Fomin SK, Pivovarova VI, Voronova VI (Kiev State Inst of Physical Culture, Russia)
Sports Train Med Rehabil 1:89–92, 1989   2–26

The biologic cycle in women is divided into 5 phases, including the menstrual, postmenstrual, ovulatory, postovulatory, and premenstrual phases. There is evidence to suggest that the capacity for volume and intensity of workloads during athletic training is affected by the different phases of the menstrual cycle. The biologic pattern of special working capacity and mental stability were investigated in well-trained female cross-country skiers who were preparing for competition.

One hundred sixty-four cross-country skiers aged 18–22 years participated in 115 training sessions. The mean total training load volume was 1,095 km, and the duration of individual sessions was 90–180 minutes. The main goal of the training sessions was to develop special stamina. The working capacity of the women skiers was assessed during a 5-km test race on the standard track and during a 12.5-km test race on ski rollers. Personality and reactive anxiety were assessed at different phases of the menstrual cycle during training and again immediately before the contest.

Analysis of the data confirmed that phasic changes throughout the biologic cycle affect not only working capacity and functional parameters, but also personality and reactive anxiety levels in female athletes. The best test results were achieved by women who were in the postovulatory and postmenstrual phases. Higher anxiety levels were observed during relatively elevated working capacity whereas moderately high levels of anxiety were seen during phases of relatively decreased working capacity.

The training and mental preparation of female athletes for competitive events should take into consideration their biologic characteristics and their mental condition. In phases of relatively low working capacity, physical loads should be selected with special attention to volume and intensity, and psychological loads should be selected with an eye on the nature and specific orientation of the exercises.

▶ These authors from Russia believe that the successful solution of the task of psychological preparation of women athletes for contests is directly correlated with how completely the coaches have taken into consideration all personality characteristics of female athletes and different phases of their biologic cycle in the process of their training. I don't know of any coaches of women athletes in the United States who pay much attention to the personalities of their athletes and try to develop a correlation with their biologic cycles. There are many things we can learn about sports training from our Soviet colleagues.— Col. J.L. Anderson, PE.D.

Exercise During Pregnancy: Guidelines and Controversies
Leaf DA (Univ of California, Irvine)
Postgrad Med 85:233–238, January 1989   2–27

There are conflicting opinions as to whether exercise is beneficial or harmful during pregnancy. Many concerns reflect the complex physiologic adaptations required during pregnancy. Concerns include the possibility of biomechanical damage to the pregnant woman and/or the fetus and altered hemodynamic responses to exercise that might compromise homeostasis.

Increased caloric expenditure during exercise need not adversely affect fetal nutrition if the pregnant woman compensates for exercise by increasing her caloric intake. Balance and coordination can be affected by pregnancy, so a pregnant woman should limit her mode of exercise to activities that do not require sudden changes in body position. Joint laxity increases during pregnancy, putting the pregnant woman at greater risk of sports-induced injury. To avoid injury pregnant women should warm up thoroughly before exercise and should not load excessive weight on their joints. Exercises that do not put the fetus in position to compromise venous blood return are recommended; for example, cycling is preferable to supine exercise. Changes in fetal heart rate during maternal exercise are transient and do not interfere with normal fetal growth and development.

One study noted that women who exercised throughout pregnancy had infants of lower birth-weights than women who stopped exercising at 28 weeks, but it is not known whether this represents a deleterious affect. Another study found that the outcome of labor and delivery was better in a high-level exercise group than in either a no-exercise or low-exercise group.

Healthy pregnant women with no contraindications should be encouraged to participate in aerobic exercise, but they should avoid exercises that might cause orthopedic injuries. Exercising pregnant women also need to augment nutrition to compensate for increased needs for themselves and their fetuses as a result of caloric expenditure during exercise.

▶ It is generally accepted that women who were physically active before pregnancy can continue to exercise, possibly in a modified form, during pregnancy. In 1985 the American College of Obstetricians and Gynecologists approved recommendations for exercise during pregnancy, although without total scientific basis addressing the clinic issues related directly to the outcomes of labor and delivery. Later studies have supported the approved recommendations by showing that the outcome of labor and delivery in a high-level exercise group involved in both aerobic and weight training exercises was better than lower-level and nonexercise groups. Apgar scores and fetal birth weights were higher, cesarean section rates were lower and hospital stays were shorter. A confounding factor, however, was that the high-level exercise group had a younger mean age than the lower level and nonexercise groups. Other studies have shown that aerobic exercise during pregnancy did not increase obstetric complications or neonatal morbidity. It is generally agreed that pregnant women should avoid high-impact injuries that may cause orthopedic injury. See the next study (Abstract 2–28) concerning exercising while immersed in water.—Col. J.L. Anderson, PE.D.

Exercise During Pregnancy
Paisley JE, Mellion MB (Univ of Nebraska, Omaha)
Am Fam Physician 38:143–150, November 1988   2–28

Fifty percent of all women of reproductive age residing in Vermont exercise regularly. Many physically active women want to continue exercising during pregnancy. There are several important benefits of this activity. In addition to maintenance or improvement of maternal fitness and control of excess weight gain, women often have an increased sense of control, improved appearance and posture, increased energy, less backache, and less water retention.

Concerns about the effects of exercise during pregnancy include the possible occurrence of fetal hypoxia, hyperthermia, miscarriage or premature delivery, decreased fetal weight, and maternal musculoskeletal injuries. However, many of these concerns originated with data obtained from animal studies that used untrained pregnant animals and exercised them to exhaustion. Subsequent studies with healthy physically fit pregnant women who exercised at more moderate levels have refuted many of the concerns raised by animals studies.

The American College of Obstetricians and Gynecologists has published a set of guidelines, contraindications, and relative contraindications for exercising during pregnancy and the postpartum period. Some examples of these recommendations are that during pregnancy the maternal heart rate should not exceed 140 beats per minute, strenuous activities should not exceed 15 minutes, and exercise in the supine position after the fourth month of gestation should be avoided. Examples of general contraindications are the presence of hemodynamically significant heart disease or anemia, uncontrolled hypertension, diabetes mellitus, or hypertension, and recurrent cervical incompetence. The presence of essential hypertension, excessive obesity, or multiple gestations are examples of relative contraindications. Although it was recommended previously that bouncing movements be avoided during pregnancy, there is no scientific evidence for this prohibition. Pregnant women should stop exercising if breathlessness, dizziness, nausea, back pain, uterine contractions, vaginal bleeding, or amniotic fluid leakage occur.

Three to 5 exercise sessions per week during pregnancy is a reasonable frequency as long as the woman continues to gain weight adequately and increases her caloric intake to compensate for the extra calories used during exercise.

▶ This paper covers about as well and completely as any all of the up-to-date information on exercising during pregnancy. It advises on specific exercises such as jogging, cycling, aerobics, swimming, weight lifting, contact sports, racquet sports, water skiing, scuba diving, and alpine and nordic skiing. All of the advice appears sound and not overly conservative.— Col. J.L. Anderson, PE.D.

Intense Exercise During the First Two Trimesters of Unapparent Pregnancy
Cohen GC, Prior JC, Vigna Y, Pride SM (Vancouver, BC; Univ of British Columbia)
Physician Sportsmed 17:87–94, January 1989   2–29

Both maternal and fetal responses to activity must be considered in evaluating exercise during pregnancy. Two pregnant runners, not knowing they were pregnant, exercised intensely during their first 2 trimesters.

Woman, 34, gravida 1, para 0, reached menarche at age 13 years and had regular menses during her teens. Her last menstrual period began on July 17, 1982. During the latter part of June and early July, she had decreased running because of relocation. A home pregnancy test in late November was positive, and pregnancy was confirmed on December 3 at approximately 20 weeks' gestation. Before pregnancy she ran an average of 35 miles per week. In 1 race her pace was 8:11 per mile; during pregnancy her pace improved to 7:11 per mile. She ran an average of 42 miles, 28 miles, and 12 miles during the first, second, and third trimesters, respectively. The patient gained a total of 8.1 kg during pregnancy. She went into labor after spontaneous rupture of membranes. After 28 hours of desultory labor, she received oxytocin augmentation and epidural anesthesia. She had a spontaneous vaginal delivery of a normal infant girl 11 hours later. The infant weighed 3,400 g and was determined to be 40 weeks' gestation. Apgar scores were 7 at 1 minute and 10 at 5 minutes. At 10.5 months the infant was in the 90th and 97th percentiles for length and weight, respectively.

Pregnancy should be considered before ascribing amenorrhea to exercise. In this case and in the second patient, the course of pregnancy was not altered by intense exercise. Intense maternal exercise in the first and second trimesters may not harm a normal fetus, but more research in this area is needed.

▶ This study presented 2 case studies of female runners who unknowingly were pregnant and continued intense exercising during their first 2 trimesters.

Upon delivery there was no observable harm to the fetuses. This shows only that women who are involved in intense exercising before pregnancy can probably continue to exercise without danger to themselves or the fetus at least for the first 2 trimesters. This kind of exercise program is not recommended for less well-trained women.—Col. J.L. Anderson, PE.D.

Pulmonary and Ventilatory Responses to Pregnancy, Immersion, and Exercise
Berry MJ, McMurray RG, Katz VL (Univ of North Carolina)
J Appl Physiol 66:857–862, February 1989   2–30

Both pregnancy and immersion affect pulmonary function and ventilation. Swimming has been suggested as the ideal exercise for the pregnant woman, but the combined effects of pregnancy and immersion are unknown. Whether pregnancy and immersion would result in diminished ventilatory capacity for exercise was investigated in 12 pregnant women at 15, 25, and 35 weeks of pregnancy and at 8–10 weeks after delivery. Pulmonary function and ventilation were measured after 20 minutes of rest on land, after 20 minutes of rest during immersion to the level of the xiphoid (IR), and after 20 minutes of exercise at 60% of predicted maximal capacity during immersion (IE).

Except for a decrease at 15 weeks the forced vital capacity remained relatively constant during pregnancy despite the fact that the expiratory reserve volume decreased as pregnancy progressed. The forced vital capacity was maintained by an increase in inspiratory capacity during pregnancy. The forced expiratory volume did not differ significantly between stages or as a result of the pregnancy itself. The forced vital capacity was lowest during the IR trial, and the expiratory reserve volume also decreased. Inspiratory capacity increased during IR and IE trials, but not enough to offset the decrease in expiratory reserve volume. Both resting immersion and pregnancy resulted in a significant decrease in maximal voluntary ventilation. Pregnancy resulted in significant increases in minute ventilation associated with increases in oxygen consumption. Because respiratory frequency remained constant, increased minute ventilation during pregnancy was associated with an increase in tidal volume. Immersion also significantly increased minute ventilation resulting from increased respiratory frequency.

Although pulmonary function and ventilation are altered as a result of immersion and pregnancy, the effects of pregnancy on pulmonary function and ventilation are not compounded by immersion or exercise during immersion. Therefore, exercise in water seems to be a viable alternative for the pregnant woman.

▶ This study appears to show that swimming, or at least exercising while immersed, is an ideal way to exercise while pregnant. However, the authors did not tell us how "at home" with the water were the subjects of this study. This is an important consideration, because we have found here at West Point that people who are not comfortable in the water will have significantly increased respiratory frequency because of the stress they feel. We use a relaxation technique to teach them how to relax when they are immersed in water. The same technique could be used with pregnant women who are exercising while immersed. Another important factor is the water temperature. In this study the temperature of the water was reported to be 30° C, which is 86° F. We have found that the water temperature should be at least 82° F for nonswimmers with the air temperature at least 2° warmer to help them to relax while in the water. Exactly what the water temperature should be for pregnant women should be studied further. Not many swimming pools will keep their water temperatures as warm as 82° F or 86°.—Col. J.L. Anderson, PE.D.

Estrogen 2-Hydroxylase Oxidation and Menstrual Function Among Elite Oarswomen
Snow RC, Barbieri RL, Frisch RE (Harvard School of Public Health; Brigham and Women's Hosp, Boston)
J Clin Endocrinol Metab 69:369–376, August 1989   2–31

To investigate the effects of athletic training on estrogen metabolism and menstrual dysfunction, 10 elite oarswomen aged 22–26 years were monitored for menstrual function by pregnanediol glucuronide assay in overnight 12-hour urine samples collected twice weekly as they progressed from low-intensity training to high-intensity training and then back to low-intensity training. Each training phase lasted for 3 months. Radiometric analysis was used to measure the extent to which the estradiol that was administered was metabolized by oxidation of 2-hydroxylase. Four nonathletic controls matched for age and age of menarche also were studied.

Five women reported no menstrual abnormalities during the previous training year, and 5 reported no disruption of cycles during low-intensity training but did experience disruption of cycles during high-intensity training. The menstrual patterns of the 10 oarswomen were consistent with those reported for the previous training year. All 10 lost weight during high-intensity training and regained it during the third phase.

The 5 women with menstrual dysfunction during high-intensity training metabolized a significantly greater fraction of labeled estradiol by oxidation of 2-hydroxylase. There was no significant difference in oxidation of 2-hydroxylase between the 5 women who had normal menses and the 4 normal controls. There was a positive correlation between the extent of leanness and the extent of estradiol metabolized by oxidation of 2-hydroxylase.

An association between increased oxidation of estradiol 2-hydroxylase and menstrual dysfunction during periods of high-intensity training accompanied by increased relative leanness is suggested. The increased oxidation of estradiol 2-hydroxylase during high-intensity training suggests that a greater fraction of endogenous estrogen may be devoid of peripheral activity.

▶ The study makes another positive contribution to the understanding of the cause of menstrual dysfunction in some female athletes. Although the small sample size did not produce data sets large enough that we can be comfortable with the statistical analyses, the authors made an interesting observation that went beyond the purpose of their research. They noted that differences in estrogen metabolism are associated with several known risk factors for breast cancer, and that elevated 2-hydroxylase oxidation may be protective against that disease. Therefore, the increased 2-hydroxylase oxidation of estrogen in the 10 oarswomen studied may contribute to the lower lifetime occurrence of sex hormone-sensitive cancers observed among former college athletes. Again, an interesting observation that needs further investigation.—Col. J.L. Anderson, PE.D.

Menstrual Disturbances and the Pill on an Expedition in the Western Himalayas, 1988
Cohen J, Morley C, Bass C (Univ College and Middlesex School of Medicine, London; Univ of Cambridge; British Schools' Exploring Society)
Br J Fam Plann 15:44–46, July 1989   2–32

The British Schools' Exploring Society sponsors expeditions for young persons aged 16.5 to 19.5 years into wilderness areas all over the world. In 1988, a group that included 110 young persons from Britain, 12 young persons from India, and 25 adult leaders, scientists, mountaineers, and others went on a 6-week expedition to the Western Himalayas. During the expedition 30 young expeditioners and 5 leaders complained of menstrual problems. Upon their return, questionnaires were sent to these 35 individuals to assess the nature of their problems. Thirty-three questionnaires were returned.

In all, 24 of the 35 women (73%) had some form of menstrual disturbance during the 6-week expedition. Problems included missed periods (16 women), unexplained bleeding (4), prolonged bleeding (6), and more frequent periods (2). Sixteen women had no history of such problems, including 7 who had taken a combination oral contraceptive specifically to control their menstruation during the expedition. Seven women with menstrual disturbances but no history of such disturbances had not taken oral contraceptives. Thirty-one of the 33 responders had taken acetazolamide for a mean of 15 days, 29 women had climbed above 15,000 ft, and 30 women had experienced diarrhea for a mean of 10 days.

Because taking estrogen-containing oral contraceptives at high altitude is associated with an increased risk of thromboembolism, women traveling to high mountain areas should be made aware of these risks before the expedition and should be advised to switch to a progestogen-only oral contraceptive.

▶ The authors of this study have performed a useful service to women who may want to climb, trek, or walk at high altitude in the mountainous regions of the world. They can probably expect some menstrual problems and experience some diarrhea. There is at least a theoretical risk from taking the estrogen part of the combined contraceptive pill above 14,000 ft because of the increased risk of the thromboembolism. Women should transfer to the progestogen-only pill several months before leaving on a mountain-climbing expedition.—Col. J.L. Anderson, PE.D.

Lower Prevalence of Non-Reproductive System Cancers Among Female Former College Athletes

Frisch RE, Wyshak G, Albright NL, Albright TE, Schiff I (Harvard School of Public Health; Harvard Med School; Advanced Med Research Found, Boston; Massachusetts Gen Hosp, Boston)
Med Sci Sports Exerc 21:250–253, June 1989   2–33

A lower risk of breast cancer and cancers of the reproductive system has been reported among women who have undergone long-term athletic training. Whether athletes and nonathletes also differ in the prevalence of cancers of nonreproductive organs and tissues was investigated by means of a detailed questionnaire that was sent to women alumnae of 8 colleges and 2 universities.

Of the 5,398 respondents, 2,622 were former athletes and 2,776 were nonathletes. Nonreproductive system cancers were classified as class I, which included cancers of the digestive system, thyroid, bladder, lung, and other sites, and hematopoietic cancers—lymphoma, leukemia, myeloma, and Hodgkin's disease. Class II included skin cancers and cutaneous melanoma. Former college athletes had a significantly lower prevalence of class I cancers than did nonathletes, with an age-adjusted relative risk of 3.34. Prevalence rates of class II cancers did not differ between athletes and nonathletes.

Women who participate in college athletics apparently are at a significantly lower risk for the development of nonreproductive system cancers, except for skin cancers and cutaneous melanomas, compared with nonathletic women. It might be worthwhile to investigate the prevalence of both reproductive system and other cancers in physically active women and in sedentary women in the general population.

▶ These authors previously reported on the apparent lower prevalence of breast cancer and cancers of the reproductive system among former college athletes compared to nonathletes. This study reports similar findings for nonreproductive system cancers, except for skin cancers and cutaneous melanomas. I agree with the authors that we need to continue to investigate the prevalence of both reproductive system and nonreproductive system cancers among physically active women. It will be important also to consider the age when physical activity became habitual, and how long the active women were in training and at what intensity levels. Can we find similar results of physical activity for men?—Col. J.L. Anderson, PE.D.

3 Exercise Physiology and Biochemistry in Male and Female Patients

---

Cerebral Blood Flow During Submaximal and Maximal Dynamic Exercise in Humans
Thomas SN, Schroeder T, Secher NH, Mitchell JH (Univ of Copenhagen)
J Appl Physiol 67:744–748, August 1989   3–1

Previous studies of changes in cerebral blood flow (CBF) in human beings during dynamic exercise have shown wide variations, some of which have resulted from methodologic differences. Assuming that some of the previous studies were carried out at a low and often undefined work intensity, the changes in CBF during grades of submaximal dynamic exercise were reevaluated in 16 healthy men and women (median age, 28 years).

During exercise sessions the participants were placed behind a Krogh cycle ergometer in a semirecumbent position to keep the head immobile. Two baseline CBF measurements were obtained in this position and additional measurements were obtained during pedaling. Workloads were increased progressively in 10 persons, the last being the maximal effort. The effect of scalp cooling on CBF was assessed in 6 persons both at rest and during exercise. The mean arterial pressure (MAP) was calculated in 10 persons and central venous pressure was calculated in 6.

The major finding was that CBF increased by 31% when calculated as the initial slope index, but by 58% when calculated as the first compartment flow. When both legs were used during cycling, no differences were noted in CBF in the 2 hemispheres. Scalp cooling to a level at which skin flow is decreased or eliminated did not significantly influence CBF measurements. A moderate level of exercise did not significantly change arterial carbon dioxide pressure or central venous pressure; CBF increases duing exercise were associated with increases in MAP.

▶ Cerebral blood flow measurements during exercise are of particular interest but up until recently have presented considerable technical and analytical difficulties. The advent of the ^{133}Xe washout technique has allowed both hemispheric and regional cortical blood flow to be quantified (1). Nevertheless studies of CBF during exercise have yielded variable results. Using graded exercise these authors have demonstrated an increase in CBF, but the magnitude of the increase depended on the analytical technique. Of interest is a similar magnitude of change in cerebral blood velocity on exercise using Doppler ultrasound (2).—J.R. Sutton, M.D.

References

1. Lassen NA: Measurement of regional cerebral blood flow in humans with single-photo-emitting radioisotopes, in Sokoloff L (ed): *Brain Imaging and Brain Function*. New York, Raven Press, 1985, pp 9–20.
2. Huang SY, Bender RR, Groves BM, et al: Cerebral blood flow during exercise at sea level and at high altitude, in Sutton JR, Coates G, Remmers JE (eds): *Hypoxia: The Adaptations*. Toronto, B C Decker Inc, 1990, pp 196–199.

Accuracy of Cardiac Output Measured by Continuous Wave Doppler Echocardiography During Dynamic Exercise Testing in the Supine Position in Patients With Coronary Artery Disease
Maeda M, Yokota M, Iwase M, Miyahara T, Hayashi H, Sotabata I (Nagoya Univ; Fujita-Gakuen Healthy Univ, Hisai, Japan)
J Am Coll Cardiol 13:76–83, January 1989   3–2

Accurate assessment of cardiac output during exercise is important in evaluating pataints with cardiovascular disease. Doppler echocardiography is an accurate noninvasive method for measuring cardiac output instantaneously. It has been compared with invasive methods in patients at rest. However, similar validation has not often been performed during dynamic exercise in patients with coronary artery disease.

Simultaneous thermodilution and Doppler echocardiography were carried out in 25 patients with coronary artery disease at rest and during multistage cycle ergometer exercise testing in the supine position. Pulmonary artery wedge pressure and arterial pressure were recorded each moment during exercise. Selective coronary angiography was also performed. Patients were divided into 2 groups according to pulmonary artery wedge pressure. At peak exercise 11 patients in group 1 had wedge pressures of 20 mm Hg or greater; 14 patients in group 2 had wedge pressures of less than 20 mm Hg; 7 other patients were evaluated only at rest.

The correlation coefficient for thermodilution and echocardiography was .85 at rest and .84 during exercise (Fig 3–1). At rest, differences between the methods were not significant, but thermodilution gave significantly higher values during exercise. There were significant differences in the change in cardiac index and peak aortic velocity between groups 1 and 2. There was a significant linear correlation between the percentage of change in peak aortic velocity and in pulmonary artery wedge pressure from rest to peak exercise.

Continuous-wave Doppler echocardiography is a reliable noninvasive method of measuring cardiac output during dynamic exercise testing in the supine position. Underestimation by the Doppler method may be re-

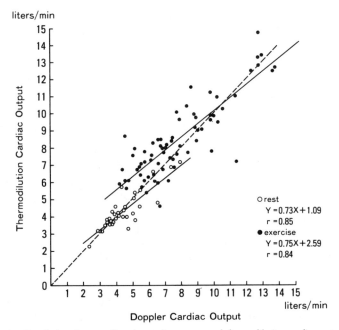

Fig 3–1.—Correlations between Doppler cardiac output and thermodilution cardiac output during supine position ergometer exercise testing. *Open circles* represent cardiac output results at rest (n = 34); *filled circles*, cardiac output results at various stages during exercise (n = 25). (Courtesy of Maeda M, Yokota M, Iwase M, et al: *J Am Coll Cardiol* 13:76–83, January 1989.)

lated to technical problems and/or changes in aortic diameter during exercise. The percentage of change in peak aortic velocity from rest to peak exercise may be helpful in identifying patients with increased pulmonary artery wedge pressures during exercise testing.

▶ The search continues for an ideal noninvasive method of measuring cardiac output during exercise. Here, the technique evaluated is Doppler echocardiography. Unfortunately, this yields a measure of flow velocity rather than cardiac output. It is thus necessary to integrate flow and then to relate this figure to aortic area. Even if the technical problems of chest wall motion and hyperexpansion of the lungs can be overcome, a comparison of changes from rest to exercise can still be invalidated by an alteration of aortic dimensions, such as is likely to occur with an increase of both blood flow and aortic pressure.

The other problem with any new method is to find an appropriate "gold standard" for validation of the data. The authors admit that most clinical measurements of cardiac output have an error of between 15% and 20%. The technique used as a reference here (thermodilution) suffers from technical problems during exercise, particularly inadequate mixing of the injected fluid. Although a close correlation is claimed, the authors' graph shows some data points that depart by more than 100% from the line of identity between the 2 methods of measurement. One final, small point: The correlations seem to have been calculated backward, with the Doppler data as the independent variable!—R.J. Shephard, M.D., Ph.D.

Head-Up Tilt Table Evaluation in a Trained Athlete With Recurrent Vaso-Vagal Syncope

Rechavia E, Strasberg B, Agmon J (Beilinson Med Ctr, Petahtikva, Israel; Tel Aviv Univ)
Chest 95:689–691, March 1989   3–3

The head-up tilt-table test was used to reproduce symptoms of vasovagal syncope and to evaluate various treatments that could prevent the recurrence of symptoms in a professional athlete.

Man, 27, a professional basketball player, had recurrent syncope of at least 15 years' duration and had experienced 3 episodes in the preceding year. Results of physical examination were normal, but ECG revealed prolongation of the PR interval up to .46 second. Holter monitoring showed episodes of bradycardia as low as 30 beats per minute (bpm) during the night in conjunction with escape junctional rhythm. On echocardiography a mildly dilated left ventricle and atrium with normal left ventricular contraction were revealed. Exercise testing showed good functional capacity with a maximal sinus rate of 160 bpm. Results of neurologic testing were normal. The patient underwent a baseline tilt-table test on 2 consecutive days. Forty-five minutes after assuming the upright position, the patient became dizzy. Blood pressure was 80/50 mm Hg and the sinus rate was 60 bpm. When the patient lost consciousness, cardiac monitoring showed an escape nodal rhythm of 35 bpm. Within 15 seconds there was an asystolic pause that lasted for 20 seconds. The patient was evaluated on successive days while receiving transdermal scopolamine and theophylline. On both days syncope recurred. An electrophysiologic study revealed sinus and atrioventricular (AV) nodal dysfunction. The tilt-table test was then repeated on 2 successive days during AV sequential pacing alone and with simultaneous administration of transdermal scopolamine. Syncope related to hypotension occurred on both occasions, despite adequate pacing. The patient was then given ephedrine, 25 mg 4 times a day, and tested in conjunction with sequential pacing. He remained free of symptoms. At discharge ephedrine, 12.5 mg 4 times a day, was prescribed, and the patient was advised to cease athletic activity. At 12-month follow-up he remained asymptomatic.

Upright posture causes a shift of approximately 300–800 mL of blood from the thorax to the lower extremities. Arterial pressure is maintained in the upright posture by an increase in total peripheral resistance. The prime determinant for circulatory failure is a diminution in the volume of blood available to the heart as a result of venous pooling in the legs. In vasovagal syncope the autonomic compensatory reflex may be overpowered and unable to maintain arterial pressure. Several therapeutic measures can theoretically benefit patients with vasovagal symptoms. In this case ephedrine was an effective option.

▶ Syncope or near-syncope is a problem for some distance runners and other endurance athletes. Syncope at the "finish line" after a marathon seems to result from the large decline in total peripheral resistance that develops during exercise, perhaps compounded by volume depletion. Near-syncope on arising from the supine position seems in part related to extreme athletic bradycardia. This detailed case report illustrates how to evaluate and manage disabling vasovagal syncope in athletes. One should note, however, that in healthy persons, active vs. passive changes in posture evoke different cardiovascular responses. Passive head-up tilt causes a gradual increase in the heart rate and diastolic pressure, with little change in systolic pressure. In contrast, active standing causes, within 3–7 seconds, a fall in systolic pressure and a compensatory jump in heart rate, often by 25–30 bpm. This is when dizziness can occur, especially if the subject stands abruptly after a period of supine rest. Normally, systolic pressure recovers fast; within 20 seconds of standing, it exceeds the resting value. Standing up slowly, not abruptly, minimizes postural hypotension and dizziness in athletes and nonathletes alike.—E.R. Eichner, M.D.

Left Ventricular Hypertrophy in Men With Normal Blood Pressure: Relation to Exaggerated Blood Pressure Response to Exercise
Gottdiener JS, Brown J, Zoltick J, Fletcher RD (Walter Reed Army Med Ctr, Washington, DC; Univ of Maryland)
Ann Intern Med 112:161–166, Feb 1, 1990   3–4

Whether nonhypertensive, normally active persons with an abnormal rise in systolic blood pressure may have left ventricular hypertrophy (LVH) was investigated in 25 participants in a health fitness screening program and in 14 normal men with atypical chest pain. Twenty-two men had a systolic pressure of 210 mm Hg or higher during peak treadmill exercise and 17 did not. Left ventricular mass was estimated by echocardiography.

Left ventricular hypertrophy was diagnosed in 14 of the men with an abnormal blood pressure response to exercise and in 1 of those with a normal response. Left ventricular mass correlated linearly with peak exercise systolic blood pressure (Fig 3–2) as well as with resting systolic pressure. The LV mass index was not linearly related to maximal oxygen consumption.

An enhanced pressor response to exercise may indicate increased integrated blood pressure during daily activity that is sufficient to produce a hypertrophic LV response. Alternatively, the presence of LVH and an exaggerated pressor response to exercise may result from a primary pathophysiologic factor—possibly enhanced sympathoadrenal activation. Because LVH is an independent predictor of cardiovascular risk, it may be

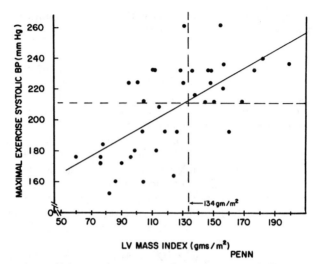

Fig 3-2.—Relation of left ventricular (LV) mass index to maximum systolic blood pressure achieved with exercise. The *vertical dashed line* represents the partition value (134 g/m²) for the diagnosis of LVH. The *horizontal dashed line* indicates partition value (210 mm Hg) for determination of exaggerated systolic blood pressure response to exercise. The linear relationship between maximal systolic blood pressures *(y)* and LV mass index *(x)* is expressed by the equation *y* = .58*x* + 134. The coefficient of correlation *(r)* is .65 (*P* < .0001). (Courtesy of Gottdiener JS, Brown J, Zoltick J, et al: *Ann Intern Med* 112:161–166, Feb 1, 1990.)

important to measure the blood pressure during exercise in evaluating apparently healthy persons.

▶ In most exercise laboratories a small number of patients who are normotensive at rest will have an exaggerated blood pressure response to exercise. There has been speculation that such an observation may be the harbinger of sustained hypertension (1). The present case comparison study used echocardiography to quantify LV mass and to diagnose LV hypertrophy. The authors established a relationship between both systolic blood pressure on exercise and LV mass and concluded that such elevations are significant and can produce end organ effects.—J.R. Sutton, M.D.

Reference

1. Jackson AG, et al: *J Cardiac Rehabil* 3:263, 1983.

Exercise-Induced Alterations of Signal-Averaged Electrocardiograms in Marathon Runners
Smith GS, Vacek JL, Wilson DB, Hawkins JW, Boyer TA, Weatherspoon BG, Mallorca LG (Univ of Kansas)
Am Heart J 118:1198–1202, December 1989   3–5

Sudden cardiac death (SCD) has occurred in distance runners presumably as a result of malignant ventricular arrhythmias. The underlying

	Signal-Averaged Data		
Parameter	*Before race*	*After race*	*Recovery*
QRS (msec)	97.3 ± 10.1	94.4 ± 10.0*	97.8 ± 11.3
RMS (msec)	60.4 ± 35.6	71.0 ± 41.7†	61.6 ± 43.1
LAS (μV)	22.8 ± 8.0	21.8 ± 7.7	23.2 ± 8.5

Abbreviations: LAS, low-amplitude signal duration: *QRS,* duration of filtered QRS; *RMS,* root mean square voltage of last 40 msec of filtered QRS.
*P < .005 vs. both of the other values.
†P < .05 vs. both of the other values.
(Courtesy of Smith GS, Vacek JL, Wilson DB, et al: *Am Heart J* 118:1198–1202, December 1989.)

pathologic condition is usually hypertrophic cardiomyopathy in younger runners and coronary artery disease in those older than 35 years. Noninvasive screening to identify a risk for SCD is not practical with current tests; however, patients with known coronary disease can be evaluated for the risk of SCD and ventricular tachycardia by means of signal-averaged ECG (SAECG). A study was conducted to determine whether late potentials, areas of electrical instability, could be detected by SAECG in 30 asymptomatic runners who completed the 1988 Kansas City Marathon. A baseline SAECG was obtained on the day before the race. Additional tests were administered at an average of 16.7 minutes post race and 7–14 days afterward.

The group baseline results were within the normal range. Only 1 runner had an abnormal SAECG. The SAECGs of all runners were normal immediately after the race, with all 3 parameters showing improvement. The runner who had an abnormal SAECG at baseline and 1 other runner had abnormal measurements during the recovery period. At 1-week follow-up, all parameters were close to those observed at baseline (table). Doppler data did not indicate cardiac fatigue in these runners; 28 runners had some degree of valvular regurgitation, generally of a slight or mild degree.

There was no evidence of the development of late potentials, with their possible effects on the myocardium and conduction system of the heart; however, prolonged exercise changed signal-averaged parameters in these seemingly healthy marathon runners. These changes were most likely caused by exercise, although their significance is uncertain. The risk for SCD appears slight in adult runners without organic heart disease.

▶ There have been reports of cardiac fatigue after ultra-marathon events such as the Hawaii Ironman triathlon (1), with a diminution of myocardial contractility following the race. The starting point of the present investigation was that such fatigue might give rise to electrical instability and thus sudden death.

The subjects were 37-year-old participants in a marathon run in Kansas City at an unspecified environmental temperature. No evidence of cardiac fatigue was seen, and the age of the subjects was relatively young, so that coronary atherosclerosis would have been less advanced than in some long-distance

Masters' competitors. Also, the sample size was only 30, which is small when looking for such a rare event as a precursor of death in a marathon run. Although the concept is an interesting one, there is a need to repeat this study with a larger sample of older runners, preferably those competing in an ultramarathon rather than a marathon event.—R.J. Shephard, M.D., Ph.D.

Reference

1. Douglas PS, et al: *Circulation* 76:1206, 1987.

Impaired Pulmonary and Cardiac Function After Maximal Exercise
Rasmussen BS, Elkjaer P, Juhl B (Central Hosp, Holstebro, Denmark; Univ of Aarhus, Denmark)
J Sports Sci 6:219–228, Winter 1988   3–6

Competitive rowers sometimes experience symptoms of severe cough with expectoration and dyspnea in the supine position after a race. To determine whether oarsmen's symptoms might result from interstitial lung edema and to investigate the duration of pulmonary changes and evaluate the circulatory changes that might provoke the symptoms, 6 healthy well-trained oarsmen underwent testing on a rowing ergometer. Participants warmed up for 15 minutes with a load of 2 kg before rowing hard for 4 minutes with a load of 3 kg.

Each participant was totally exhausted after the test and had intense cough with copious expectoration. Total impedance was monitored as an expression of fluid accumulation in the chest. Participants were also monitored by ECG. Resting values were obtained 1 hour before testing; after exercise measurements were made at 30 minutes and at 2, 4, 8, and 24 hours. Lung diffusing capacity was also measured for carbon monoxide, vital capacity, residual volume, and peak expiratory flow rate.

The lung diffusing capacity for carbon monoxide was significantly decreased below baseline for 2.5 days after exercise. There was a significant increase in residual volume at 30 minutes of recovery but no change in total lung capacity. There was no significant change in total impedance after exercise; however, a decrease might have been masked by the increased residual volume.

Changes in pulmonary parameters after intense exercise may reflect the occurrence of transient interstitial lung edema. Because the peak expiratory flow was significantly reduced at 30 minutes of recovery, it may be that exercise-induced bronchoconstriction is related to the cardiopulmonary response. The increase in pulmonary extravascular water volume might have been caused by distention of the lung capillaries that resulted from increased blood volume in the lung. Changes might also have been caused by impaired myocardial contractility, which was indicated by a split impedance dZ/dt waveform that occurred in all 6 subjects immediately after exercise and has not been described previously in healthy subjects.

▶ The competitive athlete who pursues competition to total exhaustion is almost inevitably stopped by the progressive development of near cardiac failure. Humans, fortunately, tend to collapse before the failure becomes irreversible, but there have been reports of greyhound dogs that have died after treadmill running to exhaustion.

There have been scattered reports suggesting that the impending cardiac failure leads to pulmonary congestion and edema formation. After very prolonged events there have been observations of decreased mechanical function of the lungs (vital capacity, forced expiratory volume), but this could reflect respiratory muscle fatigue rather than edema. Other reports of cough and expectoration, although suggestive, could also be caused by exercise-induced bronchospasm, or an increased inhalation of air pollutants.

Many of the reports that have denied the existence of edema have been based on relatively short periods of exercise, and an effect might seem more probable after a prolonged event such as a marathon run (1). Others have argued that most distance competitors pace their efforts better than those competing for shorter times. The data presented here relate to a 4-minute simulated rowing event and are thus analogous to other "maximal" tests in which pulmonary edema is not normally suggested.

One major problem is the lack of any good test for the development of edema. A decrease of diffusing capacity and an increase of residual volume, as proposed here, are the usual clinical methods. But both are also susceptible to exercise-induced bronchospasm. The third method that was used, transthoracic impedance, showed no change, although the authors argue that an increased fluid content may have been masked by an increase of residual volume. Plainly, resolution of this important question must await the availability of better diagnostic tools.—R.J. Shephard, M.D., Ph.D.

Reference

1. Miles DS, et al: *Respir Physiol* 52:349, 1983.

Reduced Exercise Capacity of Chronic Obstructive Pulmonary Disease Patients Exercising With Noseclip/Mouthpiece
Morrison DA, Collins M, Stovall JR, Friefeld G, Barbiere C, Carlson P, Carpenter B, Clegg L, DeLong J, Olsen MA, Pantoja P, Powell D, Wolf D (Denver VA Med Ctr; Univ of Colorado)
Am J Cardiol 64:1180–1184, Nov 15, 1989   3–7

The results of a number of studies have demonstrated that ventilatory abnormalities are the cause of exercise limitation in patients with chronic obstructive pulmonary disease (COPD). A major ventilatory abnormality in these patients is pathologically increased airway resistance. Approximately 50% of airway resistance appears to be in the nose and mouth, even in normal subjects. To examine the relationship between airway resistance and exercise capacity, 12 patients with stable COPD were studied.

The patients performed supine cycle ergometer exercise tests with and without noseclip and mouthpiece. During each of the tests, right-sided cardiac hemodynamic measurements, radionuclide ventriculography, and arterial and mixed venous gas sampling were performed. During the noseclip/mouthpiece exercise exhaled gases were collected and analyzed.

Rest and Exercise Comparison of Room Air vs. Noseclip

	Rest Without Noseclip	Rest With Noseclip	Rest Difference (p Value)	Exercise Without Noseclip	Exercise With Noseclip	Exercise Difference (p Value)
Duration	—	—	—	397 ± 270	300 ± 230	<0.01
VO_2	234 ± 32	244 ± 53	NS	780 ± 279	658 ± 200	<0.01
Cardiac output (liters/min)	4.4 ± 1.3	4.5 ± 1.1	NS	8.4 ± 2.7	7.3 ± 2.0	<0.05
RVEF	0.40 ± 0.09	0.40 ± 0.10	NS	0.39 ± 0.08	0.43 ± 0.08	<0.01
LVEF	0.56 ± 0.10	0.56 ± 0.12	NS	0.61 ± 0.12	0.60 ± 0.14	NS
Heart rate (beats/min)	0.73 ± 0.16	75 ± 16	<0.05	106 ± 14	106 ± 14	NS
Radial artery blood pressure (mm Hg)	95 ± 14	102 ± 14	NS	118 ± 16	118 ± 17	NS
PAP (mm Hg)	22 ± 4	22 ± 5	NS	40 ± 8	41 ± 10	NS
RAP (mm Hg)	5 ± 2	4 ± 2	NS	12 ± 5	12 ± 4	NS
paO_2 (mm Hg)	56 ± 7	57 ± 6	NS	50 ± 8	51 ± 6	NS
$paCO_2$ (mm Hg)	35 ± 5	36 ± 7	NS	36 ± 5	37 ± 7	NS
SvO_2 (%)	63 ± 5	64 ± 4	NS	40 ± 10	41 ± 10	NS
Ca-VO_2	5.4 ± 1.3	5.6 ± 1.4	NS	9.5 ± 3.0	9.3 ± 2.8	NS

Abbreviations: Ca-VO$_2$, arterial mixed venous content difference; LVEF, left ventricular ejection fraction; NS, not significant; paCO$_2$, arterial carbon dioxide tension; paO$_2$, arterial oxygen tension; PAP, mean pulmonary artery pressure; RAP, mean right pulmonary atrial pressure; RVEF, right ventricular ejection fraction; SvO$_2$, mixed venous oxygen saturation; VO$_2$, oxygen consumption (mL per minute) calculated from cardiac output and Ca-VO$_2$.
(Courtesy of Morrison DA, Collins M, Stovall JR, et al: Am J Cardiol 64:1180–1184, Nov 15, 1989.)

At rest, breathing with a noseclip resulted in a higher mean radial artery pressure. No other significant differences were noted at rest between breathing with and without a noseclip. Patients were able to exercise longer without the noseclip. The peak exercise oxygen consumption was significantly higher without the noseclip (780 mL/min) than with the noseclip (658 mL/min). A significant difference was also noted in the peak exercise cardiac output, which averaged 8.4 L/min without the noseclip and 7.3 L/min, with the device. The right ventricular ejection fraction during exercise was 0.39 without the noseclip and 0.43 with it. The left ventricular ejection fraction, exercise heart rate, and arterial and mixed venous blood gases did not differ significantly between the 2 exercise tests (table).

Exercise tolerance can be limited by a noseclip/mouthpiece in patients with advanced COPD. Decreased right-sided cardiac preload (venous return) might be the cause of this limitation.

▶ Respiratory and exercise physiologists have traditionally begun their observations by forcing a mouthpiece into a patient's mouth and applying an uncomfortable clip to the nose. Several previous authors have suggested that such an approach inevitably modifies respiration. At rest and in light effort, breathing normally occurs exclusively through the nose(1) so that the forcing of a large mouthpiece between the gums may actually lower airflow resistance. During more vigorous exercise the subject usually switches from nose to mouth breathing, because the nose is a much higher resistance pathway. The transition occurs at a ventilation of 30–40 L/min; unfortunately, the present authors did not state respiratory minute volumes, but given an exercise intensity of 2.5–3 METS in patients with COPD, they were probably at or beyond the switch-point to mouth breathing. Any effect from added respiratory impedance is thus attributable to the mouthpiece rather than to the noseclip as they suggest. Another major omission in this paper is a clear statement of the impedance offered by either the airways or the respiratory equipment. Given the nature of the disease, the respiratory equipment probably added between 10% and 20% to total airflow resistance, a figure compatible with the observed decrement of peak oxygen intake and peak cardiac output.—R.J. Shephard, M.D., Ph.D.

Reference

1. Niinimaa V, et al: *Respir Physiol* 43:69, 1981.

Hypoxic Ventilatory Response and Arterial Desaturation During Heavy Work

Hopkins SR, McKenzie DC (Univ of British Columbia, Vancouver)
J Appl Physiol 67:1119–1124, September 1989   3–8

Both a blunted ventilatory response to exercise and arterial desaturation with oxygen have been reported in athletes trained in endurance

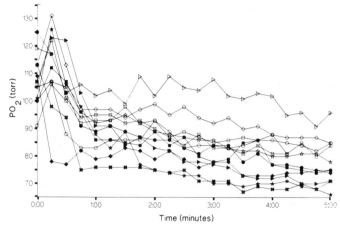

Fig 3–3.—Individual subject arterial PO_2 obtained during 5 minutes of running at a velocity corresponding to maximal O_2 uptake ($\dot{V}O_{2\ max}$). *Open squares* indicate subject 1; *open diamonds*, subject 2; *open triangles*, subject 3; *open circles*, subject 4; *open stars*, subject 5; *open crosses*, subject 6; *filled squares*, subject 7; *filled diamonds*, subject 8; *filled triangles*, subject 9; *filled circles*, subject 10; *filled stars*, subject 11; *filled crosses*, subject 12. (Courtesy of Hopkins SR, McKenzie DC: *J Appl Physiol* 67:1119–1124, September 1989.)

sports. To determine whether ventilatory response causes inadequate pulmonary ventilation, resulting in arterial desaturation, 12 healthy men trained in endurance or nonendurance sports were studied. Their mean age was 23.8 years and their mean maximal oxygen uptake was 63.0 mL $\cdot$ kg^{-1} $\cdot$ min^{-1}. Measurements were made during 5-minute treadmill runs at speeds corresponding to 100% of maximal oxygen uptake, except for ventilatory response to isocapnic hypoxia, which was measured separately.

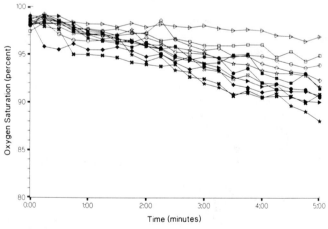

Fig 3–4.—Individual subject arterial O_2 saturation of hemoglobin obtained during 5 minutes of running at a velocity corresponding to maximal O_2 uptake. See Figure 3–3 for definition of symbols. (Courtesy of Hopkins SR, McKenzie DC: *J Appl Physiol* 67:1119–1124, September 1989.)

With exercise the arterial oxygen pressure declined to 78 mm Hg and arterial blood saturation with oxygen decreased to 92% (Figs 3–3 and 3–4). Calculated alveolar oxygen pressure was maintained. Carbon dioxide pressure was low at onset of exercise but then remained steady despite declining pH values. Peak ventilation was less than 95% of maximal ventilation determined by maximal oxygen uptake. The baseline hypoxic ventilatory response was normal in 6 athletes and diminished in 6. The hypoxic ventilatory response did not correlate significantly with arterial desaturation, maximal ventilation, ventilation to oxygen uptake ratio, or sport during exercise.

The genesis of exercise-induced hypoxemia appears to include the alveolar-arterial difference in partial pressure of oxygen and, to a lesser extent, alveolar hypoventilation. Endurance performance does not seem to be related to chemosensitivity. The hypoxemia is most likely caused by limitation of diffusion.

▶ For 50 years we have known that exercise can cause arterial hypoxemia. This phenomenon, paradoxically, is striking in elite athletes going all-out, whose hemoglobin saturation (can fall to the range of 93% to 87%. Why? This report suggests that the responsible mechanism is a limitation of diffusion of oxygen in the lung. In other words, when an elite athlete goes all-out and the cardiac output rises, e.g., to an astronomical 40 L/min, the red blood cells zip through the lung capillaries too fast to take up their full complement of oxygen. As Dempsey has asked, "Is the lung built for exercise?" (1). Does the real physiologic limit to human aerobic capacity lie not in the heart or in the muscles, but in the lung?—E.R. Eichner, M.D.

Reference

1. Dempsey JA: *Med Sci Sports Exerc* 18:143, 1986.

Influence of Plasma Catecholamines on the Lactate Threshold During Graded Exercise
Mazzeo RS, Marshall P (Univ of Colorado)
J Appl Physiol 67:1319–1322, October 1989   3–9

A number of mechanisms possibly responsible for the inflection in blood lactate found with increasing workloads have been suggested. During strenuous exercise, epinephrine, the catecholamines, and norepinephrine are involved in adjustment to disturbances in homeostasis. Studies have shown an association between plasma catecholamines and lactate production, but the dimensions of this relationship are unclear.

Six male competitive cyclists and 6 cross-country runners were tested after an overnight fast. They underwent graded exercise testing to exhaustion on both a treadmill and a bicycle ergometer. Oxygen consumption, carbon dioxide production, and ventilation each minute were measured. During the last minute of each workload, 5 mL of blood was sampled and analyzed for lactate and catecholamine concentrations.

Among the cyclists, maximal oxygen consumption did not differ significantly between treadmill running and cycling; however, both blood lactate and ventilatory thresholds were reached at a relatively earlier workload during treadmill running (Fig 3–5). For the runners these thresholds were reached earlier during the cycling test. The inflection in plasma epinephrine shifted in a similar manner and occurred simultaneously with that of the blood lactate threshold regardless of training status or testing protocol (Fig 3–6). There was also a high correlation between the shift in the ventilatory threshold and the blood lactate threshold, but the relationship was not as strong as that between plasma epinephrine and the blood lactate threshold.

There appears to be a causal relationship between the inflection in plasma epinephrine and the blood lactate threshold during graded exercise testing in competitive athletes. There seems to be a less pronounced

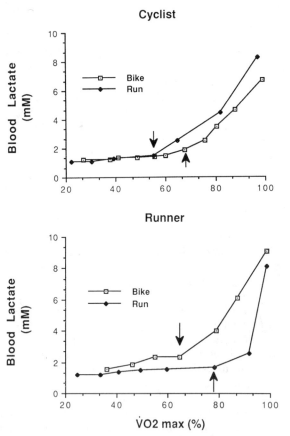

Fig 3–5.—Blood lactate concentrations during treadmill running and bicycle ergometry for both a cyclist and a runner as a function of $\dot{V}O_2$max. *Arrows* indicate lactate threshold. (Courtesy of Mazzeo RS, Marshall P: *J Appl Physiol* 67:1319–1322, October 1989.)

r = 0.974 ± 0.007

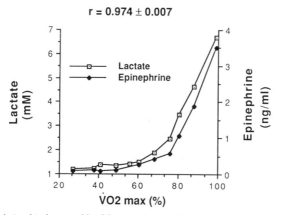

Fig 3–6.—Relationship between blood lactate concentration and plasma epinephrine content in a person during a graded exercise test. The correlation between these variables across all 24 exercise tests (both runners and cyclists) was .974 ± .007. (Courtesy of Mazzeo RS, Marshall P: *J Appl Physiol* 67:1319–1322, October 1989.)

relationship between the blood lactate threshold and the ventilatory threshold.

▶ Just as the fictitious anaerobic threshold was being put to sleep another threshold has reared its ugly head. The catecholamine threshold! Well, not really. These authors have made some interesting observations, relating catecholamines and blood lactate. Although each is present in blood, the site of origin of each is quite different—the adrenal medulla and glycogenolysis in muscle. Nevertheless, the very close temporal relationship between changes in epinephrine and lactate tempts one to invoke a causal relationship, as these authors do.—J.R. Sutton, M.D.

Acute Changes in Lipid, Lipoprotein, Apolipoprotein, and Low-Density Lipoprotein Particle Size After an Endurance Triathlon
Lamon-Fava S, McNamara JR, Farber HW, Hill NS, Schaefer EJ (Tufts Univ; Boston Univ; New England Med Ctr Hosp, Boston)
Metabolism 38:921–925, September 1989   3–10

Most studies of the effects of exercise on plasma lipid parameters have been done with regularly exercising subjects. The effects of acute prolonged exercise on plasma lipids, lipoproteins, apolipoproteins, and the size of low-density lipoprotein (LDL) particles, were evaluated in 6 women and 34 men who participated in an endurance triathlon. All were examined 6–12 hours before and just after the triathlon.

All 40 athletes lost weight, but mean posttriathlon body weight was significantly lower than mean pretriathlon value only in men. After the event plasma levels of triglyceride decreased by a mean of 67% in men and by 70% in women (table). Total plasma levels of cholesterol did not

Plasma Lipid, Lipoprotein, and Apolipoprotein Measurements
in Male *(M)* and Female *(F)* Athletes Before
and After Triathlon

	Gender	Before	After	P Value
Triglycerides	M	139 ± 83	46 ± 39	.0001
(mg/dL)	F	88 ± 33	26 ± 11	.001
Total cholesterol	M	205 ± 44	201 ± 45	NS
(mg/dL)	F	209 ± 38	189 ± 30	.005
HDL cholesterol	M	55 ± 13	65 ± 12	.0001
(mg/dL)	F	74 ± 12	78 ± 12	.01
LDL cholesterol	M	122 ± 40	127 ± 40	NS
(mg/dL)	F	118 ± 30	105 ± 25	.01
Apo A-I (mg/dL)	M	172 ± 34	186 ± 36	.005
	F	227 ± 33	230 ± 34	NS
Apo B (mg/dL)	M	69 ± 20	63 ± 21	.0005
	F	57 ± 13	47 ± 12	.0005
Apo A-I/Apo B	M	2.66 ± 0.76	3.21 ± 1.04	.0001
	F	4.13 ± 1.18	5.17 ± 1.49	.005
Apo A-I/HDL cho-	M	3.15 ± 0.38	2.87 ± 0.31	.0001
lesterol	F	3.08 ± 0.20	2.94 ± 0.18	.01
Apo B/VLDL+LDL	M	0.46 ± 0.06	0.46 ± 0.05	NS
cholesterol	F	0.43 ± 0.06	0.42 ± 0.05	NS

Values are means ± SD.
(Courtesy of Lamon-Fava S, McNamara JR, Farber HW, et al: *Metabolism* 38:921–925, September 1989.)

change in men but dropped by 9.7% in women. Plasma levels of high-density lipoprotein (HDL) rose by 18% in men and by 5% in women. Although the level of LDL-cholesterol did not change in men, it dropped significantly (11%) in women. In 6 athletes sampled randomly for up to 6 days after the event all values had returned to baseline levels by day 6.

Acute strenuous exercise is accompanied by marked reductions in serum levels of triglyceride and marked increases in levels of HDL-cholesterol. These changes are accompanied by alterations in the protein constituents of lipoproteins. The increase in HDL-cholesterol is paralleled by a rise in the plasma concentration of apolipoprotein A-I. The decrease in apolipoprotein B appears to be explained by the accelerated catabolism of very-low-density lipoprotein. The elevated catabolism of triglyceride in some persons with high baseline levels of triglyceride is associated with a rise in size of LDL particles.

▶ As has been described after a marathon (see the 1987 YEAR BOOK OF SPORTS MEDICINE, pp 81–83), this comprehensive study shows that a single, strenuous triathlon quickly improves the lipoprotein profile. The race caused a sharp decline in plasma triglyceride levels, a rise in plasma HDL-cholesterol, and, in women, a fall in LDL-cholesterol and total cholesterol. The responsible mechanisms seem to be related to enhanced lipolysis. Alas, by 6 days later all lipoprotein values were back to pre-race levels. We learn again: Use it or lose it. Regarding the rapid exercise-induced rise in HDL-cholesterol, recent research, using arteriovenous fluxes across the human forearm, suggests that exercising muscle itself acutely makes HDL-cholesterol (see Abstract 3–11).—E.R. Eichner, M.D.

Effects of Exercise and Fat Ingestion on High Density Lipoprotein Production by Peripheral Tissues

Ruys T, Sturgess I, Shaikh M, Watts GF, Nordestgaard BG, Lewis B (United Medical and Dental Schools of Guy's and St Thomas' Hosps, London)
Lancet 2:1119–1122, Nov 11, 1989   3–11

High-density lipoprotein (HDL)-cholesterol is thought to have a protective role against atherosclerosis, although the mechanism of this effect is not clear, nor are the roles of the subclasses of HDL. The peripheral production of HDL-cholesterol and of the subclasses HDL_2 and HDL_3 was evaluated by measurement of the arteriovenous fluxes across the human forearm in 9 healthy men with normal levels of cholesterol and triglycerides. Eight men were examined twice—once after an overnight fast and once after a 75-g fat load; the other man was studied only after fat loading. Blood samples were taken at 0 time and after 20 minutes of isometric exercise in the left forearm. Two patients with familial lipoprotein lipase deficiency also were studied, but only after fasting.

Exercise after fasting did not significantly affect the production or removal of any of the lipids and lipoproteins studied. After fat loading, the arteriovenous flux for total HDL, HDL_2, and HDL_3 was increased by exercise; only the positive flux for HDL_3, however, reached significance. Exercise produced an increase in forearm blood flow in the 2 patients with lipoprotein lipase deficiency, but a positive net flux of HDL_3- or HDL_2-cholesterol was not shown in either one.

The net fluxes of HDL_2- and HDL_3-cholesterol become positive during exercise. A high-fat meal increased the effects of exercise, especially the production of HDL_3. These findings, and the lack of an exercise effect on patients with lipoprotein lipase deficiency, suggest that muscle blood flow is an important determinant of peripheral HDL-cholesterol formation, but that lipoprotein lipase plays a role in mediating the normal production of HDL in exercising muscle.

▶ One of the most powerful tools in clinical physiology to establish the mechanism whereby a particular process occurs is by stimulation or inhibition and the observation of a specific outcome. So it is with the present study of the effect of exercise on cholesterol metabolism. The dual stimuli of exercise and fat loading were necessary to reveal that cholesterol flux-arteriovenous differences for HDL-, HDL_2-, and HDL_3-cholesterol were increased by exercise.

This is important, as HDL is key in initiating the reverse transport of cholesterol from peripheral tissues to the liver for metabolism and biliary excretion.— J.R. Sutton, M.D.

Hyperlipemic Response of Young Trained and Untrained Men After a High Fat Meal

Merrill JR, Holly RG, Anderson RL, Rifai N, King ME, DeMeersman R (Med College of Virginia, Richmond; Univ of California, Davis; Children's Hosp, Washington, DC; Medical Products, Wilmington, Del; Columbia Univ)

Arteriosclerosis 9:217–223, March–April 1989   3–12

Most studies of the etiology of atherosclerotic vascular disease, a major cause of death and disability in Western societies, have linked increased postabsorptive blood cholesterol and low-density lipoproteins with an increased risk for development of the disease. Little attention has been given to fat tolerance—the plasma triglyceride (TG) response to a fatty meal. Chronic endurance exercise may improve fat tolerance.

To test the hypothesis that endurance exercise training is associated with a reduced lipemia after the ingestion of a high-fat meal, 16 men aged 22–34 years were studied. Nine were trained and 7 were untrained (Fig 3–7). The trained group ran more than 48 km or biked more than 160 km weekly. The untrained group had been sedentary for at least the 3 months preceding study entry. Daily energy intake was 35% greater and daily energy expenditure during exercise was 704% greater in the trained than in the untrained men. Maximal oxygen intake ($\dot{V}O_{2max}$) was 31% higher and percent body fat 36% lower in the trained men. Dietary composition and body height and weight were comparable in the 2 groups.

A fasting blood sample was obtained, and the men ate a high-fat meal. Blood samples were obtained again every hour for 8 hours. Fasting lipids were similar in both groups. The postprandial peak triglyceride (TG_{max}) concentration was 42% higher, percent TG increase was 54% higher, and total lipemic response was 75% higher in the untrained men than in the trained men. The same 3-variable model—training status, fasting TG content, and $\dot{V}O_{2max}$—described the variation in TG_{max}, percent TG increase, and total lipemic response. This analysis also showed that, after

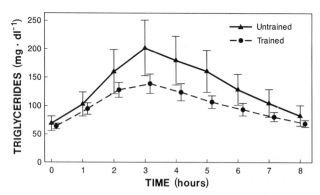

Fig 3–7.—Lipemic response to a high fat meal in trained and untrained persons. Values are the mean ± 1 SD. (Courtesy of Merrill JR, Holly RG, Anderson RL, et al: *Arteriosclerosis* 9:217–223, March–April 1989.)

adjusting for fasting TG and $\dot{V}O_{2max}$, the untrained men had significantly higher postprandial lipemia, whether expressed as TG_{max}, percent TG increase, or total lipemic response.

Exercise, specifically habitual endurance-type exercise, appears to attenuate the postprandial lipemia that follows a high-fat meal. The exact mechanism for this is not known. Exercise-induced adaptations seem to be mediated by changes in enzymes involved in cholesterol and TG synthesis, transport, and catabolism.

▶ Detailed studies of high-density lipoprotein-cholesterol subfractions and the associated apo-proteins have diverted attention away from triglycerides in recent years, although it was early recognized that a high fasting TG level was an independent risk factor for atherosclerosis (1). Nevertheless, there have been previous suggestions that regular exercise improves fat tolerance, at least in older individuals (2, 3). Such studies have been criticized for lack of control of other variables affecting lipid metabolism, such as sex, alcohol intake, cigarette smoking, medications, overall energy intake, and obesity.

The present study extended these observations by using younger subjects and attempting to control for extraneous variables by matching subjects and using multiple regression techniques. However, the comparison between trained and untrained subjects remains somewhat flawed, because the "untrained" group was jogging about 10–11 km per week and had an average maximal oxygen intake of 51.6 mL/kg · min. Nevertheless, the data confirm the observations of Altekruse and Wilmore (2), showing a clear difference of peak postprandial TG levels between the 2 groups. Presumably, the effects of training would have been more dramatic if the authors had succeeded in recruiting a truly sedentary control group.—R.J. Shephard, M.D., Ph.D.

References

1. Cohn PF, et al: *Ann Intern Med* 84:241, 1976.
2. Altekruse EB, Wilmore JH: *J Occup Med* 15:110, 1973.
3. Patch JR, et al: *Proc Natl Acad Sci USA* 80:1449, 1983.

Effects of Exercise-Induced Weight Loss on Low Density Lipoprotein Subfractions in Healthy Men
Williams PT, Krauss RM, Vranizan KM, Albers JJ, Terry RB, Wood PDS (Stanford Univ; Univ of California, Berkeley; Univ of Washington)
Arteriosclerosis 9:623–632, September–October 1989   3–13

Running increases concentrations of plasma high-density lipoprotein (HDL), but the effects of running on low-density lipoprotein (LDL) has yet to be established. One-year changes in LDL and very-low-density lipoprotein (VLDL) subfraction concentrations were compared between runners and sedentary controls.

Eighty-one sedentary men aged 30–55 years were randomly assigned to either a supervised running group—48 men—or to a sedentary control group—33 men. After 6 weeks the exercise group was asked to run

45 minutes daily for 5 days each week. Laboratory measurements were taken at baseline and at 3, 6, 9, and 12 months. Waist, hip, and thigh girths; estimated body composition; and calculated caloric intakes were also determined. Maximal oxygen uptake was measured by maximal treadmill testing.

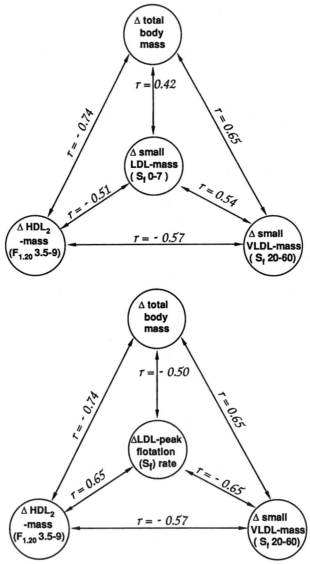

Fig 3–8.—Interrelationships between 1-year changes in total weight and 1-year changes in the serum mass concentrations of HDL_2, small VLDL particles of S_f 20 to 60, small LDL particles of S_f 0 to 7, and LDL peak flotation rate in 42 exercisers with complete data (includes both dieting and nondieting exercisers). All correlations are significant at $P < .01$ or less. (Courtesy of Williams PT, Krauss RM, Vranizan RM, et al: *Arteriosclerosis* 9:623–632, September–October 1989.)

The distances that exercisers ran varied considerably. Mean changes in any LDL and VLDL measures did not differ significantly among runners and controls; however, within the exercise group the distance run correlated negatively with changes in mass concentrations of small LDL. Weight loss and reduced upper-body weight correlated positively with changes in small LDL, intermediate-density lipoprotein, and VLDL mass, and negatively with change in the LDL peak-flotation rate (Fig 3–8).

Weight loss may primarily affect LDL mass distributions through metabolic processes related to HDL or small VLDL. The decrease in small LDL concentrations, coupled with the increase in the LDL peak-flotation rate, suggests that exercise-induced weight loss might effectively reduce the risk of coronary heart disease in persons with a high-risk lipoprotein profile.

▶ In part through the work of Peter Wood and his associates (1), it is now well recognized that it is advantageous to develop increased HDL-cholesterol concentrations through running, jogging, or walking a minimum of 18–20 km per week. However, less is known about the LDL subfractions; high concentrations of small, dense LDL particles seem to be associated with premature coronary disease (2) and with familial combined hyperlipidemia (3). Decreases in this component of LDL seem to be related mainly to loss of the fat component of body mass; although the present study found some significant correlations between the distance run and small LDL levels among the exercisers, differences between the exercisers and the nonexercisers were not statistically significant for either HDL or small LDL. This reinforces the earlier conclusion of Wood et al., i.e., if reliance is placed on exercise alone, a considerable weekly jogging distance is needed to assure benefit.—R.J. Shephard, M.D., Ph.D.

References

1. Wood PD, et al: Physical activity and high density lipoproteins, in Miller NE, Miller GJ (eds): *Clinical and Metabolic Aspects of High Density Lipoproteins.* Amsterdam, Elsevier Science Publishers, 1984, pp 133–165.
2. Crouse JR, et al: *J Lipid Res* 26:566, 1985.
3. Krauss RM, et al: *Clin Res* 31:503a, 1983.

Ventromedial Hypothalamic Regulation of Hormonal and Metabolic Responses to Exercise
Vissing J, Wallace JL, Scheurink AJW, Galbo H, Steffens AB (Univ of Copenhagen; State Univ of Groningen, Haren, The Netherlands)
Am J Physiol 256:R1019–R1026, May 1989   3–14

Traditionally, the exercise-related mobilization of extramuscular fuel stores has been thought to be regulated by bloodborne metabolic feedback mechanisms, chiefly the plasma glucose. More recently, studies have suggested a neural feed-forward regulation of substrate mobilization during exercise. The hormonal and metabolic responses to treadmill running were examined in brain-cannulated conscious rats during bilateral anesthesia of the ventromedial hypothalamus (VMH).

Anesthesia of the VMH increased plasma lactate, glycerol, catecholamine, and corticosterone levels in animals at rest. Hepatic and muscular glycogenolysis also increased. During treadmill exercise, glucose turnover, glycogenolysis, and plasma levels of glucose, lactate, catecholamines, and corticosterone all increased in both VMH-anesthetized and control animals. Insulin levels declined. Initial hepatic glucose production and subsequent plasma glucose levels were lower in the study animals, as was overall hepatic glycogenolysis.

Apparently, the VMH plays a role in the regulation of glucose metabolism during exercise. Sympathoadrenal activity is stimulated early in the course of exercise. Probably, activity in areas of the VMH that facilitate sympathetic activity is increased, whereas that in areas inhibiting sympathetic activity is lowered.

▶ The hormonal and neural responses to exercise are complex and the role of central factors in regulating these responses and the subsequent metabolic changes are poorly understood. This study explores the role that the VMH plays in metabolism during exercise. In an elegant series of studies on rats using stereotaxic procedures, the authors examined glucose metabolism during exercise. The principal conclusions derive from a role of the VMH in mediating the catecholamine response to exercise, which in turn affects glucose metabolism.—J.R. Sutton, M.D.

Hypothalamic-Pituitary-Adrenal Responses to Short-Duration High-Intensity Cycle Exercise

Kraemer WJ, Patton JF, Knuttgen HG, Marchitelli LJ, Cruthirds C, Damokosh A, Harman E, Frykman P, Dziados JE (US Army Research Inst of Environmental Medicine, Natick, Mass; Boston Univ)
J Appl Physiol 66:161–166, January 1989   3–15

Endurance exercise and short-term high-intensity exercise significantly increase β-endorphin (β-EP), adrenocorticotropin (ACTH), and cortisol plasma concentrations. The hormonal responses to 4 exercise intensities of high-power output were examined. The possible relationships between skeletal muscle fiber morphology and peripheral blood hormone levels after very high-intensity exercise also were assessed.

Ten normally active, healthy men (mean age, 24 years) performed maximal exercises at 36%, 55%, 73%, and 100% of maximal leg power on a computerized cycle ergometer. All exercise intensities were greater than those eliciting peak oxygen uptake for the individual subjects. Blood samples were collected at rest, immediately after exercise, and at 5 minutes and 15 minutes post exercise. One week before testing, muscle biopsy samples were obtained from the superficial portion of the vastus lateralis muscle of the dominant leg. The 4 exercise intensities were performed in random order. Plasma β-EP, ACTH, and cortisol levels were measured by radioimmunoassay techniques.

Plasma β-EP and ACTH levels were significantly increased immediately after exercise and at 5 minutes and 15 minutes post exercise at 36% maximal leg power. Plasma cortisol levels were increased at 15 minutes post exercise at 36% maximal leg power. Significant increases in blood lactate levels were observed after all 4 exercise intensities. Plasma β-EP levels at 36% maximal leg power correlated significantly with capillary density. Cortisol levels at 36% maximal leg power were significantly related to percentage of type II muscle fibers. Other significant relationships were not seen.

The plasma responses of β-EP, ACTH, and cortisol do not increase as the intensity of exercise is systematically increased at power productions in excess of maximal aerobic power. At high exercise intensities, blood lactate levels do not appear to be related to the plasma concentrations of β-EP, ACTH, or cortisol.

▶ This is an interesting study because, unlike most previous attempts to examine exercise-hormonal relationships, it uses very-short-term exercise—4 different work levels lasting from 0.1 to 3.15 minutes at intensities of 318% to 115% of $\dot{V}O_{2max}$. These were the maximum times possible at the exercise intensities used. For β-EP, ACTH, and cortisol only the lowest exercise intensity (which lasted the longest time) produced any elevation in the plasma concentration. The paper does not pretend to examine the mechanisms of hormonal secretion and is included here simply for the unique nature of its observations and the findings that appear unusual at first glance, i.e., that the lowest, not the highest, exercise intensities elicited the greatest endocrine response.—J.R. Sutton, M.D.

The Effects of Acute Exercise on Pulsatile LH Release in High-Mileage Runners
McColl EM, Wheeler GD, Gomes P, Bhambhani Y, Cumming DC (Univ of Alberta, Edmonton)
Clin Endocrinol 31:617–621, November 1989   3–16

The results of previous studies have shown a relationship between intense physical exercise and reproductive dysfunction in men as well as in women. How endurance training causes a decrease in sex steroid levels was investigated. Pulsatile luteinizing hormone (LH) release was assessed in 6 male runners to determine whether acute exercise influences the neuroendocrine regulation of the hypothalamic-pituitary-gonadal (HPG) axis. The runners' training included at least 80 km per week. Six age-matched, sedentary men served as controls.

Blood samples were obtained from the runners during 2 sampling sessions. Initially, sampling was performed every 15 minutes for 6 hours after a 24-hour period without significant exercise. Samples were then obtained after 60 minutes of running at a speed equivalent to 5% below the anaerobic threshold.

Controls had significantly higher levels of serum testosterone, a significantly higher LH pulse amplitude, and a significantly greater area under

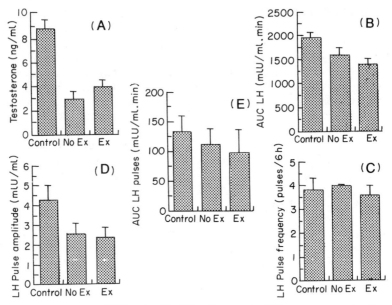

Fig 3–9.—**A,** mean (± SEM) resting *(No Ex)* and preexercise *(Ex)* testosterone levels; **B,** mean (± SEM) resting *(No Ex)* and postexercise *(Ex)* areas under the LH curve; **C,** LH pulse frequency; **D,** LH pulse amplitude; and **E,** area under the LH pulses in 6 trained male runners. Mean resting values in controls are also shown for each of the variables. Conversion factor: testosterone ng/mL × 3.46 = nmol/L. (Courtesy of McColl EM, Wheeler GD, Gomes P, et al: *Clin Endocrinol* 31:617–621, November 1989.)

the LH curve (Fig 3–9). Basal serum testosterone levels in the endurance runners were at the lower edge of normal. Preexercise serum testosterone levels were significantly higher than basal levels. Some basal variables of pulsatile LH release in the runners differed significantly from those in controls, suggesting that intense physical exercise can influence pulsatile LH release.

Men appear to have a higher threshold than women for exercise-induced hypothalamic-pituitary suppression. Although female runners have reductions in both LH pulse amplitude and frequency, exercise does not inhibit LH pulsatile release in males.

▶ The phenomenon of exercise-associated amenorrhea has received widespread publicity and has been established as a hypothalamic syndrome with a lack of pulsatility of LH (1). In the female, cessation of menses is fairly obvious. Not so for a male counterpart—but does it even exist?

Acute bouts of exercise result in a significant elevation of serum testosterone in normal subjects (1), but in the chronically active, endurance athletes (80 km/wk) the serum testosterone level appears depressed. Furthermore, as the present study shows, there is impairment of LH pulsatility in some of these runners. An even more subtle hypothalamic pituitary defect was demonstrated by MacConnie et al. in moderately active endurance athletes who had normal resting testosterone concentrations but diminished LH responsiveness to increasing doses of gonadotrophin releasing hormone (2). The apparent discrepancies between the MacConnie studies and those of the present paper may simply be the result of the differences in the training intensity of the subjects. The training regimen of the MacConnie subjects was less severe. Perhaps, then, the hypothalamic-pituitary-testicular dysfunction observed in the latter group is an intermediate stage in the development of these abnormalities.— J.R. Sutton, M.D.

References

1. Sutton JR, et al: *Br Med J* 1:520, 1973.
2. MacConnie SE, et al: *N Engl J Med* 315:411, 1986.

Effects of Propranolol and Pindolol on Plasma ANP Levels in Humans at Rest and During Exercise
Bouissou P, Galen F-X, Richalet JP, Lartigue M, Devaux F, Dubray C, Atlan G (Institut National de la Santé et de la Recherche Médicale, Créteil; Unité de Formation et de Recherche Pharmacie, Limoges, France)
Am J Physiol 26:R259–R264, August 1989   3–17

The regulation of atrial natriuretic peptide (ANP) in humans is not clear. Significant elevations in peripheral plasma ANP concentrations have been seen during intense physical exercise but not after mild physical exertion. Whether β adrenoceptors are directly involved in the regulation of tonic and exercise-induced secretion of ANP was investigated in 9 healthy men who underwent 3 experimental conditions.

Three days before each study session the men were randomized to receive either propranolol, pindolol, or placebo in a double-blind crossover fashion. Maximal oxygen consumption ($\dot{V}O_{2max}$) was determined by pretest on a bicycle ergometer, and baseline measurements of heart rate and blood pressure were taken in both the supine and upright positions. Blood samples were drawn at both times. The men then exercised to exhaustion on the bicycle ergometer at 45%, 65%, 80%, and 100% $\dot{V}O_{2max}$. Ventilatory and gas-exchange data were obtained during exercise, and the heart rate was monitored. Blood pressure was measured twice at each stage, and blood samples were drawn in the last minute of each workload.

The $\dot{V}O_{2max}$ during β blockade was not significantly different from the placebo value. Pindolol treatment did not affect resting heart rates; however, resting heart rates were decreased with propranolol. At all exercise intensities, both β blockers caused a reduction in heart rate. Mean blood pressure was unaffected by β blockade at rest but was reduced during exercise. The increase in the plasma ANP level corresponded to exercise intensities with placebo treatment, but with β blockade there was a marked elevation in the plasma ANP concentration at all levels of activity (Fig 3–10). Although the men had different hemodynamic responses to pindolol and propranolol, both β blockers produced similar increases in the basal level of plasma ANP.

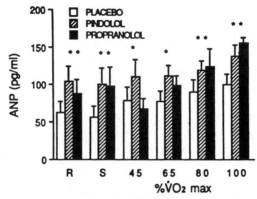

Fig 3–10.—Plasma ANP levels in 9 subjects treated with placebo and β blockers at rest in recumbent *(R)* and upright sitting *(S)* positions and during graded exercise. *P < .05 propranolol or pindolol vs. placebo. (Courtesy of Bouissou P, Galen F-X, Richalet JP, et al: *Am J Physiol* 26:R259–R264, August 1989.)

Apparently, β-adrenoceptor mechanisms are not directly responsible for tonic and exercise-induced ANP secretion in humans. During exercise with β blockade, higher plasma ANP values may result from an increase in preload secondary to altered inotropic function.

Plasma Atriopeptin During Exercise in Dogs Under β-Blockade

Péronnet F, Abrafi Adjoa S, Béliveau L, Bichet D, Nadeau R, Brisson G (Univ of Montréal; Hôp du Sacré-Coeur, Montréal)
Am J Physiol 256:R1098–R1102, May 1989   3–18

The release of atriopeptin (atrial natriuretic peptide, ANP) appears to be related to the atrial stretch. Plasma ANP concentrations were described at rest and after moderate treadmill exercise in dogs. Measurements were repeated after β-adrenergic blockade with propranolol, known to impair central hemodynamic responses in dogs during exercise.

Exercise without administration of propranolol was associated with a significant increase in heart rate and systolic blood pressure, but no change was noted in diastolic blood pressure. Propranolol significantly reduced systolic blood pressure in response to exercise and heart rate, at rest as well we during exercise. Blood pressure at rest and diastolic pressure during exercise were not significantly modified, however, with propranolol. The serum potassium concentration rose significantly in response to exercise and was even higher with propranolol. Exercise without β blockade resulted in a small but significant increase in the plasma ANP concentration (Fig 3–11).

The hypothesis that ANP release during exercise is under the control of atrial stretch is supported. Reduction of the response of plasma renin activity and the aldosterone concentration during exercise with β blockade may result in part from the higher plasma ANP concentration. The low

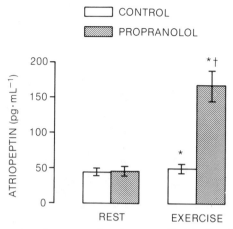

CONTROL

PROPRANOLOL

Fig 3–11.—Plasma atriopeptin concentrations (means ± SE; *significantly different from rest; †significantly different from corresponding control; $P < .05$). (Courtesy of Péronnet F, Abrafi Adjoa S, Béliveau L, et al: *Am J Physiol* 256:R1098–R1102, May 1989.)

concentrations of vasopressin with propranolol administration may reflect a dissociation between activity of the renin-angiotensin system and vasopressin release.

Effect of β-Adrenoceptor Blockade on Renin-Aldosterone and α-ANF During Exercise at Altitude

Bouissou P, Richalet J-P, Galen FX, Lartigue M, Larmignat P, Devaux F, Dubray C, Keromes A (Faculté de Médecine Créteil, INSERM, Paris; UFR Pharmacie, Limoges)
J Appl Physiol 67:141–146, July 1989   3–19

Plasma renin and aldosterone responses are altered during exercise at high altitude. Whether the β adrenoceptors are involved in the renin-aldosterone response to exercise at high elevations was investigated by comparing the effects of β blockade on exercisers at high and low altitudes. The interactions among plasma renin activity, plasma aldosterone concentration, and α-atrial natriuretic factor (α-ANF) also were explored.

At sea level 6 healthy men and 6 healthy women performed maximal standardized exercise on a bicycle ergometer with and without treatment with the β blocker, pindolol. The same protocol was followed for 5 days at an altitude of 4,350 m.

At sea level pindolol caused a reduction in plasma renin activity and an increase in the plasma α-ANF level, but there was no change in the plasma aldosterone concentration. During exercise at high altitude without β blockade, plasma renin activity and the plasma aldosterone level were significantly lower than at sea level. However, α-ANF was unaffected by hypoxia (Fig 3–12). After β blockade at high altitude, exercise-

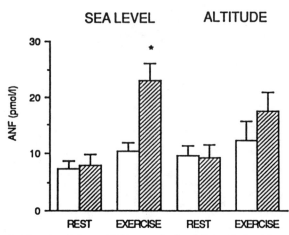

SEA LEVEL   ALTITUDE

Fig 3–12.—Atrial natriuretic factor (ANF) at sea level and high altitude with no treatment *(open bars)* and with pindolol *(hatched bars)*. *$P < .05$, pindolol vs. control. (Courtesy of Bouissou P, Richalet J-P, Galen FX, et al: *J Appl Physiol* 67:141–146, July 1989.)

induced elevation in plasma renin activity disappeared, but there was no additional decline in the plasma aldosterone concentration. Subjects tended to have lower plasma norepinephrine and epinephrine concentrations during maximal exercise at altitude, but the differences were not statistically significant.

Hypoxia apparently has a suppressive effect on the renin-aldosterone system. However, β blockade does not appear to be responsible for the inhibition of renin secretion at high altitude.

▶ These 3 papers (Abstracts 3–17, 3–18, and 3–19) explore the role of the adrenoceptor in mediating the release of ANF on exercise. Two studies (Abstracts 3–17 and 3–18) in humans and dogs at sea level suggest that although β blockade increases the tonic and exercise responses of ANF, this can be adequately explained by changes in atrial stretch. Abstract 3–19 examines renin, aldosterone, and ANF during exercise at altitude in humans and, although a significant increase in ANF was observed at sea level, the magnitude of the response tended to be less at altitude and not dependent on the β receptor. As with sea level, the observations are explicable on the basis of the Frank-Starling mechanism with atrial stretch as the mediator, which was invoked from differences in stroke volume.—J.R. Sutton, M.D.

Effects of Insulin and Exercise on Muscle Lipoprotein Lipase Activity in Man and Its Relation to Insulin Action
Kiens B, Lithell H, Mikines KJ, Richter EA (Univ of Copenhagen, Royal Veterinary and Agricultural Univ, Copenhagen; Uppsala Univ, Sweden)
J Clin Invest 84:1124–1129, October 1989   3–20

Muscle lipoprotein lipase (LPL) activity may be sensitive to variations in plasma insulin concentrations. The effects of exercise and physiologic increase in plasma insulin concentration on muscle LPL activity, leg exchange of glucose, and serum lipoprotein levels were studied in 8 physically fit young men. Seven were assigned to a clamp-study group to receive intravenous insulin and glucose and 6 were assigned to a control group to receive saline infusion. Five men participated in both groups. Individuals performed 60 minutes of repeated dynamic knee extensions with 1 leg at 75% of maximum work capacity. Blood flow was measured and blood was sampled from 1 femoral artery, both femoral veins, and both thighs. Muscle biopsy specimens were also obtained from each thigh.

The muscle-glycogen concentration increased significantly in the exercised thigh after insulin infusion. Glucose uptake in the nonexercised thigh increased after insulin infusion. Both basal muscle LPL activity and decrease in muscle LPL activity correlated significantly with the increase in thigh glucose uptake. In the exercised thigh there was no significant correlation between the decrease in muscle LPL activity and the increase in glucose uptake (Fig 3–13). The triacylglycerol content of serum lipoproteins decreased during insulin infusion.

In the control group, muscle LPL activity was similar in the nonexercised and exercised thighs immediately after exercise. After 4 hours of recovery, muscle LPL activity was significantly higher in the exercised muscle. After 8 hours of recovery the LPL activity had decreased significantly

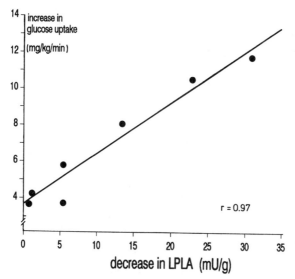

Fig 3–13.—Relationship between increase in glucose uptake (mg · kg^{-1} · minute^{-1}) and decrease in muscle LPL activity (mU · g^{-1}) after insulin infusion at the second clamp step (44 mU · L^{-1}; r = .97, P < .05). (Courtesy of Kiens B, Lithell H, Mikines KJ, et al: *J Clin Invest* 84:1124–1129, October 1989.)

in the exercised thigh but remained unchanged in the nonexercised thigh. The muscle glycogen content decreased during the exercise period and did not increase during recovery.

Physiologic concentrations of insulin decreased muscle LPL activity in proportion to the effect of insulin on muscle glucose uptake. In contrast, muscle contractions cause a local, delayed, and transient increase in muscle LPL activity. Basal muscle LPL activity is an indicator of muscle insulin sensitivity.

▶ This elegant invasive study contrasts the different physiologic concentrations of insulin on muscle LPL activity and compares this with the effect of muscle contractions, using a combination of femoral arterial and venous catheterization, muscle biopsies of the vastus lateralis, and a 2-step sequential euglycemic glucose-insulin clamp procedure.—J.R. Sutton, M.D.

Physical Exercise: Evidence for Differential Consequences of Tryptophan on 5-HT Synthesis and Metabolism in Central Serotonergic Cell Bodies and Terminals
Chaouloff F, Laude D, Elghozi JL (Centre Hospitalier Universitaire Necker-EM, Paris)
J Neural Transm [GenSect] 78:121–130, 1989   3–21

Brain serotonin or 5-hydroxytryptamine (5-HT) synthesis is dependent on the concentration of the 5-HT precursor tryptophan (TRP) in the brain. Exercise may affect central transmitter synthesis. The effects of physical exercise on 5-HT synthesis and metabolism in the midbrain, and on the striatum and hippocampus, were assessed in exercising rats.

Male Wistar rats trained to run on a horizontal treadmill were randomly divided into 2 groups. Control rats rested for 90 minutes and study rats exercised for 90 minutes on a treadmill after which they were all killed. Resting and exercising rats were subdivided into 3 subgroups. At 1 hour after the start of exercise, a subgroup of resting and running rats was injected with the 5-HT synthesis inhibitor NSD 1015. Thirty minutes after the start of exercise, another subgroup of resting and running rats was injected with TRP. A third subgroup was injected with saline 30 minutes after the start of exercise. Tryptophan 5-HT, 5-hydroxytryptophan, and 5-hydroxyindolacetic acid levels in the midbrains, striata, and hippocampi were analyzed by liquid chromatography with on-line amperometric and ultraviolet detections.

Running triggered a 30% increase in TRP concentrations in the 3 brain regions examined. After 5-HT synthesis inhibition by NSD 1015 injection, running promoted 5-hydroxytryptophan accumulation in the midbrain, did not affect these 5 levels in the striatum, and decreased them in the hippocampus, when compared with values measured in the resting rats (Fig 3–14). Therefore, the increased TRP concentration after exer-

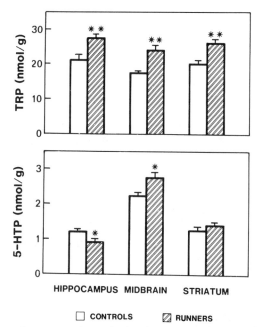

Fig 3–14.—Tryptophan (TRP) and 5-HT levels in brain regions of resting and exercising rats pretreated for 30 minutes with NSD 1015 (100 mg/kg). Exercise duration was 90 minutes. Data are the means ± SEM of 6 animals/group. Differences between resting and running rats are indicated as $*P < .05$; $**P < .01$. (Courtesy of Chaouloff F, Laude D, Elghozi JL: *J Neural Transm (GenSect)* 78:121–130, 1989.)

cise was not associated with an increased 5-hydroxytryptophan accumulation in the striatum and hippocampus. On the other hand, the TRP loading experiments showed that running differentially affected TRP utilization in the 5-HT synthesis pathway.

Under certain pharmacologic conditions, exercise alters the relationship between TRP availability and its utilization in the 5-HT synthesis pathway of serotonergic nerve terminals but not in the cell bodies.

▶ Ever since the elegant brain catecholamine studies during exercise by Gordon et al. in 1966 (1) we have been aware of the importance of exercise in stimulating central neurotransmitters. This was extended to dopamine by Bliss and Ailion (2) in 1971 and by the present authors to serotonin metabolism in 1985 (3). In the present study the authors examined the relationships between tryptophan availability (the precursor of 5-HT, or serotonin) and 5-HT synthesis in the serotonergic cell bodies in the midbrain, which contains various raphe nuclei and nerve endings, e.g., the hippocampus and the striatum. Although elegant and very interesting, none of these studies addressed the question of what effect perturbation of the central neurotransmitters has on exercise performance, a topic addressed in a most novel manner by Heyes and colleagues (4), who also demonstrated an important role for dopamine in the actual performance of exercise and the time to exhaustion.—J.R. Sutton, M.D.

References

1. Gordon R, et al: *Pharmacol Exp Ther* 153:440, 1966.
2. Bliss EL, Ailion J: *Life Sci* 10:1161, 1971.
3. Chaouloff F, et al: *Br J Pharmacol* 86:33, 1985.
4. Heyes MP, et al: *Life Sci* 36:671, 1988.

Increase in Plasma Melatonin, β-Endorphin, and Cortisol After a 28.5-Mile Mountain Race: Relationship to Performance and Lack of Effect of Naltrexone

Strassman RJ, Appenzeller O, Lewy AJ, Qualls CR, Peake GT (Univ of New Mexico; Oregon Health Sciences Univ, Portland)

J Clin Endocrinol Metab 69:540–545, September 1989   3–22

Intense exertion increases the plasma melatonin, β-endorphin, and cortisol concentrations. There may also be an association between melatonin and endogenous opioids. Exercise may stimulate endogenous opioid release and thereby inhibit reproductive function by augmenting melatonin secretion and/or by directly inhibiting the gonadal axis.

Plasma melatonin, cortisol, and β-endorphins were measured in 12 men and 39 women before and after a 46-km mountain race. The women were aged 25–55 years; the men were aged 24–63 years. The menstrual cycle status of women was not considered. Immediately before the race, 12 men and 1 woman received 50 mg of naltrexone orally.

Mean plasma levels of melatonin (Fig 3–15), cortisol, and β-endorphin were higher after the race than before it. Gas chromatography-mass spectrometry assay was used to confirm the melatonin results in 12 indi-

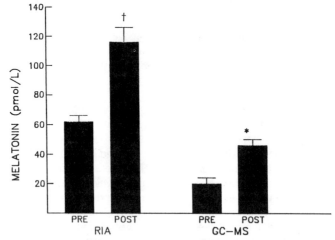

Fig 3–15.—Mean (±SE) plasma melatonin values before and after a 28.5-m high altitude mountain race, measured by radioimmunoassay in 43 subjects and gc-ms in 12 subjects. *$P < .02$; †$P < .001$ (vs. to prerace values). (Courtesy of Strassman RJ, Appenzeller O, Lewy AJ, et al: *J Clin Endocrinol Metab* 69:540–545, September 1989.)

viduals. Naltrexone did not affect the increase in any of the 3 hormones. Increased levels of plasma melatonin, cortisol, and β-endorphin were negatively correlated with finishing time; however, only cortisol and β-endorphin elevations correlated with each other. In trained athletes, prolonged exercise can increase the plasma melatonin concentration. However, this increase is not caused by concomitant opioid release.

▶ Exercise-induced melatonin secretion has been suggested as a factor in the disturbances of reproductive function seen in both sexes with repeated bouts of heavy exercise (1). Although others have argued that β-endorphins are implicated in this chain of events, Strassman and associates argue against this possibility. Their evidence is drawn from a 46-km mountain race; race times were negatively correlated with speeds, but melatonin and β-endorphin levels were not correlated with each other. Given the considerable difficulty in making the analyses, the variable times of sampling, and the scatter in the data, it remains conceivable that there was a relationship between the 2 data sets that the authors were unable to reveal. The lack of effect of naltrexone on melatonin levels supports the authors' hypothesis, although, again, it is conceivable that opioid blockade was incomplete with the doses of naltrexone that were used.— R.J. Shephard, M.D., Ph.D.

Reference

1. Bullen B, et al: *Can J Appl Sports Sci* 7:90, 1982.

Plasma Volume Responses Associated With a Sprint Triathlon in Novice Triathletes
McNaughton LR (Tasmanian State Inst of Technology, Launceston, Australia)
Int J Sports Med 10:161–164, June 1989   3–23

In Australia novice athletes often compete in short-course triathlons. These athletes seemed to be appropriate subjects for a study of the cardiovascular and plasma volume changes associated with swimming, cycling, and running over short distances. Ten male novice triathletes with an average age of 24.3 years completed a 1-km swim, a 30-km cycle ride, and a 10-km run on a cool and overcast day. Blood samples were obtained and weight was recorded before the triathlon and after each leg was completed. Changes in plasma volume were determined according to the formula of Dill and Costill.

Weight decreased significantly over the time-frame of the event, with the most significant change occurring during the running stage. During the swimming phase plasma volume decreased by 3.8%. There was a further decrease of 4.3% during the cycling stage and another 6.2% decrease during running, for a total decrease in plasma volume of 14.3% (Fig 3–16). The variations in reduced plasma volume are attributable to the differences in posture adopted for each of the exercise states.

Novice athletes in particular should be aware of the changes that take

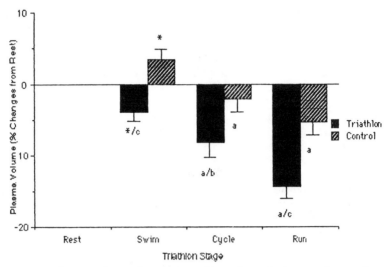

Fig 3–16.—Changes in plasma volume during triathlon and control. (Courtesy of McNaughton LR: *Int J Sports Med* 10:161–164, June 1989.)

place during events of this type. They should take care to be sufficiently hydrated during each event, especially when the weather is hot and humid.

Relation of Plasma Volume Change to Intensity of Weight Lifting

Collins MA, Cureton KJ, Hill DW, Ray CA (Univ of Georgia, Athens)
Med Sci Sports Exerc 21:178–185, April 1989   3–24

To determine the relationship between changes in plasma volume and exercise intensity, 15 men with a mean age of 22.3 years were studied. All had experience in weight lifting, but none was currently involved in a weight-lifting program. Blood samples were obtained before and during a 60-minute period after weight lifting at intensities of 40%, 50%, 60%, and 70% of a 1-repetition maximum (1-RM).

The 1-RM was determined by 2 trials on separate days in which the supine bench press, bent-over row, standing 2-arm curl, and parallel squat were used. For the test itself the men performed 3 circuits consisting of 10 repetitions of each of the 4 exercises performed over 30 seconds followed by 30 seconds of rest. Each session lasted for 11.5 minutes. Lifting at each intensity was performed on separate days in random fashion. The method of Dill and Costill was used to calculate changes in plasma volume.

Plasma volume was significantly reduced immediately after exercise at all 4 intensities (Fig 3–17). The changes were linearly related to the intensity of the weight lifting.

One factor that affects the degree of change in plasma volume is capil-

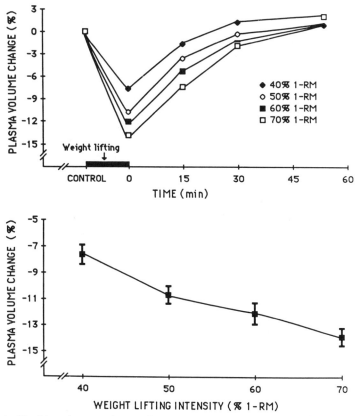

Fig 3–17.—Mean change in plasma volume immediately post exercise and during recovery after weight lifting at 4 intensities (A) and relationship between mean change in plasma volume immediately post exercise and weight-lifting intensity (B). For all intensity conditions the plasma volume decreased significantly immediately after exercise. In B, all means are significantly different from one another. (Courtesy of Collins MA, Cureton KJ, Hill DW, et al: *Med Sci Sports Exerc* 21:178–185, April 1989.)

lary fluid pressure. Increased arterial pressure induces filtration of plasma into interstitial space. During heavy-resistance exercise the mean arterial pressure would be expected to increase in proportion to exercise intensity. Shifts in plasma volume are also affected by osmotic gradients. Lactate accumulation during weight lifting appears to be greater than during dynamic low-resistance exercise at a given oxygen uptake.

Regardless of the level of intensity or degree of change, plasma volume was restored to baseline in approximately 30 minutes, a recovery time similar to that for blood lactate. Recovery reflects a decline in intravascular hydrostatic pressure, clearance of lactates and other metabolites from muscles and the interstitium, and the return of fluid to circulation through the lymphatics. In this study the contribution of sweat loss to reduced plasma was probably negligible because exercise bouts were brief and the laboratory was air conditioned.

Plasma decreases linearly in relation to intensity of weight lifting. The relationship is similar to that reported for dynamic low-resistance exercise.

▶ The 2 articles reviewed in Abstracts 3–23 and 3–24 present valuable information on plasma volume changes during diverse exercises and postures. Weight lifting decreases plasma volume fast and in proportion to intensity; lifting 70% of the 1-repetition maximum, for example, decreases plasma volume by 14%. After only 30 minutes of rest most of the lost plasma is already back in the circulation. The fast fall in plasma volume is caused by the steep rise in mean arterial blood pressure, which boosts the capillary hydrostatic pressure, and the generation of lactic acid and other small metabolites in the muscles, which boost the osmotic pull. Result: "Bulking up." The fast return occurs because, in this experiment, little fluid was lost as sweat: When the arterial pressure falls to normal and the waste metabolites are cleared, the plasma volume returns quickly to normal.

The triathlon study (Abstract 3–23) reminds us that plasma volume changes associated with exercise are influenced by the posture of the exerciser. During the race the plasma volume fell by 14.3%: 3.8% during the swim, 4.3% during the cycle portion and 6.2% during the run. But during the "mock race," when the athletes spent equivalent time resting in the "race postures," the plasma volume also changed: It actually rose by 3.6% during immersion, but then fell by 5.6% while the subject was sitting and 3.2%, while the subject was standing, for a total fall of 5.2% from baseline. In other words, more than one third of the fall in plasma volume during the race stems not from the exercise but from the postures assumed while exercising.—E.R.Eichner, M.D.

Influence of Polyunsaturated Fatty Acid Diet on the Hemorrheological Response to Physical Exercise in Hypoxia
Guezennec CY, Nadaud JF, Satabin P, Leger F, Lafargue P (Centre d'Etudes et de Recerces de Médecine Aérospatiale, Paris; Institut National de Recherche Agronomique, Paris)
Int J Sports Med 10:286–291, August 1989   3–25

Hemorrheologic parameters are altered by physical exercise and exposure to high-alitutde hypoxia. Changes result in a decrease in red blood cell deformability (RCD). However, RCD can be increased by a daily dietary supplement of fish oil. The influence of fish oil supplementation on RCD after exercise was evaluated in 14 men who were randomized to consume either a standard diet rich in lipids or a diet supplemented with 6 g of MaxEPA fish oil for 6 weeks. Before and immediately after the 6 weeks of experimental diet, both groups underwent 1 hour of cycling at 70% of maximal capacity both at sea level and at a simulated altitude of 3,000 m in a hypobaric chamber. Blood samples were drawn before and after exercise for evaluation of RCD, plasma viscosity, and erythrocyte phospholipid composition.

In the control group, RCD was unchanged after exercise at sea level;

Plasma Viscosity (CP) Changes Under Effect of Normoxic and
Hypoxic Exercise After MaxEPA Diet and Control Diet

	Normoxy		Hypoxy	
	Rest	Post-exercise	Rest	Post-exercise
Control	1.08	1.17	0.89	0.88
	± 0.15	± 0.25	± 0.21	± 0.19
MaxEPA	0.85	1.12	0.82	0.84
	± 0.12	± 0.16	± 0.09	± 0.17

(Courtesy of Guezennec CY, Nadaud JF, Satabin P, et al: *Int J Sports Med* 10:286–291, August 1989.)

however, it was decreased by an average of 53% after the same exercise under hypoxic conditions. In study subjects, the 6-week diet of fish oil abolished the decrease in RCD induced by hypoxic exercise. Total polyunsaturation of the erythrocyte membrane was enhanced by the MaxEPA diet as well. Plasma viscosity was unchanged regardless of diet or physical exercise conditions (table).

Physical exercise at an altitude of 3,000 m decreases RCD, but the same workload at sea level does not. However, the consequences of hypoxic exercise on erythrocytes can be prevented by adding a fish oil supplement to the diet for 6 weeks.

▶ The exercise-induced reduction of RCD is typically associated with very prolonged exercise, i.e., a marathon, or a 100-km run (1) but it could also occur over shorter distances if exercise was combined with hypoxia, as in mountain climbing. Potential adverse consequences include a reduction of capillary blood flow, increased pulmonary vascular resistance, and peripheral red blood cell hemolysis (2); the presence of red blood cells with altered mechanical properties also enhances platelet adhesion to the vessel wall (3). The mechanism of dietary protection seems to be the entry of the fish oil into the red blood cell membrane, which makes it more flexible. The impact on such problems as exercise-induced myocardial infarction would seem to warrant further study.—R.J. Shephard, M.D., Ph.D.

References

1. Galea G, Davidson R: *Int J Sports Med* 6:136, 1985.
2. Simchon S, et al: *Am J Physiol* 253:4898, 1987.
3. Aarts PP, et al: *Blood* 62:214, 1983.

Iron Deficiency in Athletes: Insights From High School Swimmers
Rowland TW, Kelleher JF (Baystate Med Ctr, Springfield, Mass)
Am J Dis Child 143:197–200, February 1989   3–26

Although nonanemic iron deficiency often occurs in high school distance runners, data on the incidence in other athletes is sparse. The hematologic and iron status of 15 male and 15 female high school swimmers was assessed at the beginning and end of a competitive season.

Red blood cell distribution width, mean corpuscular volume, and free erythrocyte protoporphyrin values were normal in all of the swimmers. The initial serum ferritin level in 46.7% of the girls was less than 12 µg/L but was normal in all of the boys. Serum haptoglobin values were normal. The amount of menstrual flow and initial ferritin levels were inversely related. In the girls the average daily available iron intake was 43.3% of the Recommended Daily Allowance; it was higher but still deficient among boys. The iron status and hematologic values did not change during the swimming season.

Female high school competitive swimmers have hypoferritinemia that apparently is the result of menstrual blood flow and low dietary iron intake. Athletes do not appear to have major hemolysis from muscle compression in the course of physical activity.

Causes of Iron Deficiency in Adolescent Athletes

Nickerson HJ, Holubets MC, Weiler BR, Haas RG, Schwartz S, Ellefson ME (Marshfield Clinic and Marshfield Med Research Found, Marshfield, Wisc; Minneapolis Med Research Found, Inc)
J Pediatr 114:657–663, April 1989   3–27

Previous studies have documented nonanemic iron deficiency in 20% to 40% of adolescent female cross-country runners. Iron-deficient anemia decreases athletic performance, but there is controversy over the role of nonanemic iron deficiency in athletic performance. An attempt was made to identify the causes of iron deficiency in cross-country runners. Iron deficiency was defined as a serum ferritin level of 12 ng/mL or lower, concomitant with a transferrin saturation of 16% or less.

The series included 41 female and 25 male cross-country runners aged 15–18 years. Females with iron-deficiency anemia were excluded. Fourteen females and 9 males were randomly assigned to an oral iron supplement plus an iron-rich diet; 13 females and 8 males were given a placebo plus an iron-rich diet; and 14 females and 8 males received neither. Runners averaged 20–30 miles per week during the running season, but during preseason training females averaged 14 miles per week and males averaged 18 miles per week. Urine and plasma were collected before and immediately after competitive runs of 2 miles.

In the first test of the season, 8 females in the iron-supplemented group, 2 in the diet-only group, and 2 in the control group had low initial serum ferritin levels, whereas only 3 males had initial low iron stores. By the second or third test during the running season, 34% of the females had become iron deficient, compared with only 8% of the males. The 14 females who became iron deficient had significantly lower initial serum ferritin levels than the 27 females who remained iron sufficient. Serum

Fecal Blood Loss in 20 Female Runners With at Least 1
Stool >4 mg of Hemoglobin per Gram of Stool by
Heme-Compound Testing*

Runners	Total	Yes	No
Iron deficient during season	9	7	2
Not iron deficient during season	11	2	9
TOTAL	20	9	11

*Fisher exact test: $P = .02$.
(Courtesy of Nickerson HJ, Holubets MC, Weiler BR, et al: *J Pediatr*
114:657–663, April 1989.)

ferritin levels also decreased significantly during training in the 18 iron-sufficient females assigned to diet alone or to no treatment.

Of 90 stool specimens collected from 20 females, 14 specimens from 9 females were abnormal, containing more than 4 mg of hemoglobin per g of stools (table). Seven of these 9 were iron deficient. Sixty of the 61 stool specimens from 13 male runners were normal. All females initially had a low dietary iron intake, and dietary instruction did not significantly improve this. Daily supplementation with 60 mg of elemental iron did not prevent iron deficiency in 35% of the females, but a daily dose of 180 mg was adequate.

Initially decreased iron stores and gastrointestinal bleeding are responsible for the high incidence of iron deficiency seen in young female cross-country runners.

The Frequency of Anemia and Iron Deficiency in the Runner
Balaban EP, Cox JV, Snell P, Vaughan RH, Frenkel EP (Univ of Texas, Dallas)
Med Sci Sports Exerc 21:643–648, December 1989   3–28

The presence of anemia in endurance athletes remains controversial. The frequency of anemia and iron deficiency was investigated in 35 highly competitive men and 37 women runners. The mean age of the male runners was 36 years; 57% were principally long-distance runners, 27% were middle-distance runners, and 16% were sprinters. The mean age of the female runners was 29 years; 67% were long-distance runners, 25% were middle-distance runners, and 9% were sprinters. Hematologic parameters were compared in the athletes and in 27 male and 21 female nonrunners. The impact of iron supplementation was also assessed.

The mean hemoglobin concentrations in male runners was 14.6 g/dL^{-1} and in nonrunners, 15.3 g/dL^{-1} (Fig 3–18). In women the mean hemoglobin value was 13.5 g/dL^{-1} in runners and 12.8 g/dL^{-1} in nonrunners (Fig 3–19). Anemia was present in 2 male runners, 2 female runners, and 1 female nonrunner. One male runner was taking iron supplementation

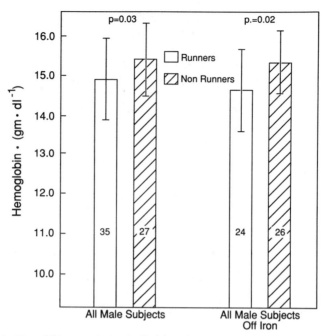

Fig 3–18—Hemoglobin concentrations in all of the male runners compared with all of the male controls (nonrunners), and all of the male runners not taking iron compared with all of the male controls taking iron. (Courtesy of Balaban EP, Cox JV, Snell P, et al: *Med Sci Sports Exerc* 21:643–648, December 1989.)

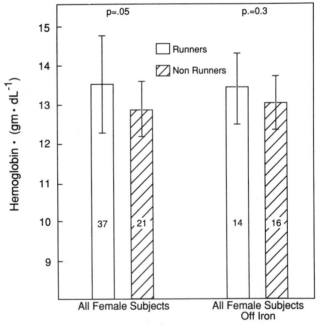

Fig 3–19.—Hemoglobin concentrations of all of the female runners compared with all of the female controls (nonrunners), and all of the female runners not taking iron compared with all of the female controls taking iron. (Courtesy of Balaban EP, Cox JV, Snell P, et al: *Med Sci Sports Exerc* 21:643–648, December 1989.)

because of a duodenal ulcer; this runner was not iron deficient. The other male runner was iron deficient, but iron supplementation corrected the problem. Iron depletion was present in 9 female runners and 7 female nonrunners; 2 runners were taking iron supplements. Iron depletion was present in 3 male runners and 2 male nonrunners; none was taking iron supplements. There were no significant iron storage parameter differences when either male or female runners not taking iron were compared with controls not taking iron.

Hemoglobin concentrations are thought to be lower in endurance athletes than in nonathletes. In this study, measured hemoglobin concentrations were unpredictably lower in male runners than in controls and unpredictably higher in female runners than in controls. There were no significant differences in iron storage parameters between runners taking supplemental iron, runners not taking supplemental iron, and controls taking or not taking iron. Iron absorption and loss were virtually the same in runners and nonrunners.

Anemia is not a statistically common condition in runners, nor is iron depletion more common in runners than in nonrunners. In runners, evidence of anemia or iron depletion should be regarded as an independent clinical incident and not as a consequence of the activity.

▶ The 3 articles reviewed in Abstracts 3–26, 3–27, and 3–28 yield needed insight into iron and anemia in athletes. In Abstract 3–26 it is seen that almost half of female high-school swimmers have low iron stores, i.e., a serum ferritin level of less than 12 ng/mL, but that 10 weeks of swim training does not change either iron or hematologic status. Missing is a nonathletic control group, which probably would have shown the same prevalence of low iron stores.

Abstract 3–27 illustrates key problems in interpreting iron status in female athletes. The study claims that 14 of 41 adolescent runners (34%) became "iron deficient" during the season. One problem is the unduly stringent definition of iron deficiency. In fact, 12 of the 14 girls had iron deficiency (ferritin level of 12 ng/mL or lower) at the outset, and any further fall in serum iron values was likely the result of hemodilution from the training-induced rise in plasma volume. Another problem is the putative link between gastrointestinal bleeding and iron deficiency. Not only was there no evidence of gastrointestinal blood loss after races, but almost all (60 of 61) of the specimens obtained from boys were negative for blood. In contrast, almost half of the girls tested (9 of 20) had blood in stool specimens. Such testing is merely a novel way to detect those females with heavy menses. The iron deficiency here is not from gastrointestinal bleeding but from insufficient dietary iron to replace menstrual loss.

The third article begins to clear the air. Male runners had significantly lower hemoglobin values than nonrunners. Why? Hemodilution from the running. In contrast, female runners had higher hemoglobin values than nonrunners. Why? Because female runners, as a group, were more than twice as likely to be taking iron pills and so were less likely to have even mild iron-deficiency anemia.

The authors rightly conclude that the iron status of runners is similar to that in the general population.

That "nonanemic iron deficiency" curbs athletic performance is a myth that dies hard. Two recent studies will help to kill it. In one, iron-deficiency anemia was induced in men by venesection. When the anemia, but not the iron deficiency, was obviated by transfusion, exercise capacity was the same as at baseline (1). In the other study, women with low ferritin levels but no anemia were randomly given placebo or iron therapy for 8 weeks. Iron therapy boosted ferritin levels but not hemoglobin levels or exercise capacity (2).—E.R. Eichner, M.D.

References

1. Celsing F, et al: *Med Sci Sports Exerc* 18:156, 1986.
2. Newhouse IJ, et al: *Med Sci Sports Exerc* 21:263, 1989.

Red Blood Cell Morphology After a 100-km Run
Reinhart WH, Bärtsch P, Straub PW (Univ of Bern, Switzerland)
Clin Lab Haematol 11:105–110, 1989   3–29

Red blood cell (RBC) values were investigated in 19 trained male athletes aged 36–63 years just after a 100-km run. In 9 runners RBC shape was studied in a wet preparation of fixed RBCs.

The hemoglobin value, RBC count, hematocrit level, and RBC indices were similar on race day and 4–6 days later. However, just after the race the percentage of stomatocytes in whole blood was increased significantly. The frequency of stomatocytes was especially high after the race in 3 runners whose values for RBCs, hemoglobin, and RBC indices were normal; the RBC shape later returned to normal. Stomatocytic shape transformation did not occur in RBCs from a universal donor when they were incubated in runners' plasma.

Long-distance running leads to stomatocytosis. This transformation is not caused by a factor in plasma but by a change in the RBC membrane. Stomatocytic transformation in the RBCs of runners has been reported elsewhere. The mechanism is not known, but it may be related to the presence of an echinocytic agent early in exercise that increases the sensitivity of RBCs to stomatocytic transformation. The transformation may contribute to the decreased RBC deformability and removal of older RBCs from circulation described after a 100-km run.

▶ The normal shape of the RBC, a diskocyte, embodies a dynamic equilibrium between 2 potential opposing shape changes, i.e., the echinocytic (spiny) vs. the stomatocytic (cupped) change. In vitro at least, normal diskocytes exposed to diverse amphipathic drugs or to alterations in pH or the plasma milieu can easily change shape in either direction. Depending in part on how they are formed, both echinocytes and stomatocytes tend to be less deformable than normal. The authors here report stomatocytes after a 100-km run, as one of them did earlier after a marathon (1).

Intriguingly, such "postmarathon stomatocytes" are apparently seen only in wet preparations of glutaraldehyde-fixed cells; they are rarely seen in standard blood smears (1). In contrast, we and other (2) have seen echinocytes (or at least "burr" cells) in standard blood smears after marathons. These "postmarathon echinocytes" may result in part from increases in the plasma levels of free fatty acids; such increases have been reported to cause echinocytes in patients undergoing coronary bypass surgery (3). One wonders here if the glutaraldehyde preparation itself either masks echinocytes, as has been reported previously (4), or even converts echinocytes to stomatocytes. In this respect, one might note that, in the above article, after the race, not only were stomatocytes significantly increased in number, but echinocytes were significantly decreased.—E.R. Eichner, M.D.

References

1. Reinhart WH, Chien S: *Am J Hematol* 19:201, 1985.
2. Gales G, Davidson RJL: *Int J Sports Med* 6:136, 1985.
3. Kamada T, et al: *Lancet* 2:818, 1987.
4. Feo CJ, et al: *Br J Haematol* 40:519, 1978.

White Blood Cell Response to Uphill Walking and Downhill Jogging at Similar Metabolic Loads
Smith LL, McCammon M, Smith S, Chamness M, Israel RG, O'Brien KF (East Carolina Univ, Greenville, NC)
Eur J Appl Physiol 58:833–837, 1989   3–30

To determine whether leukocytosis would occur in response to eccentric exercise, concentric exercise, and/or possible increases in serum cortisol levels, 8 healthy, untrained men were assessed after downhill running (eccentric exercise) and an equivalent bout of uphill walking (concentric exercise). The men performed the 2 bouts of exercise at 46% $\dot{V}O_{2max}$ for 40 minutes. Oxygen uptake measured at minutes 6–10 of both bouts was 45.8% $\dot{V}O_{2max}$ for uphill walking and 47.2% $\dot{V}O_{2max}$ for downhill jogging. The mean heart rate was significantly higher during downhill jogging than uphill walking. The total white blood cell response to the 2 bouts differed significantly. Within 1–3.5 hours after downhill jogging the counts were increased, compared with uphill walking (Fig 3–20). Within 1–2 hours after downhill jogging the neutrophil count was significantly higher than after uphill walking. Minimal muscle soreness was reported after uphill walking, but significant delayed-onset muscle soreness was reported after downhill jogging.

Eccentric exercise produced significant neutrophilia compared with concentric exercise in this study. Neutrophils were significantly higher than baseline values within 1–2 hours after eccentric exercise. At the

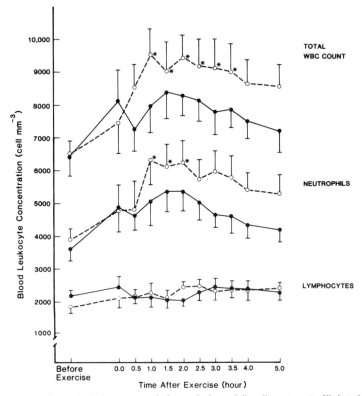

Fig 3–20.—Changes in leukocyte count before and after uphill walking (n = 8; *filled circles*) and downhill jogging (n = 8; *open circles*). Values represent means and SEM (*asterisk* indicates P < .05 compared with before exercise). (Courtesy of Smith LL, McCammon M, Smith S, et al: *Eur J Appl Physiol* 58:833–837, 1989.)

mild workloads studied, cortisol did not seem to be responsible for the increased neutrophils.

▶ The sustained neutrophilia and greater muscle soreness after downhill jogging here probably reflect ultrastructural muscle damage with attendant inflammation and acute-phase response. The acute-phase response releases a host of lymphokines, including interleukin-1, interleukin-2, and tumor necrosis factor (1). It is known that the eccentric action of downhill running damages muscles more than level or uphill running, and that 2 weeks of specific downhill training mitigates this damage (2,3). Downhill running also causes more intravascular hemolysis than uphill running (see the 1989 YEAR BOOK OF SPORTS MEDICINE, pp 288–289).—E.R. Eichner, M.D.

References

1. Dufaux B, Order U: *Int J Sports Med* 19:1, 1989.
2. Schwane JA, et al: *Med Sci Sports Exerc* 19:584, 1987.
3. Triffletti P, et al: *Med Sci Sports Exerc* 20:242, 1988.

Complement Activation After Prolonged Exercise

Dufaux B, Order U (Deutsche Sporthochschule Köln, Cologne, West Germany)
Clin Chim Acta 179:45–49, Jan 13, 1989   3–31

The inflammatory reaction associated with physical exertion results in elevated levels of several serum glycoproteins after intense and prolonged exercise. The concentrations of the complement cleavage products C3a, C4a, and C5a in serum after prolonged exercise were measured in 8 healthy young new aged 20–28 years.

All were moderately trained physical education students who ran for 2.5 hours and covered between 25 and 33 km. Blood samples were collected before, during, and after the race.

Compared to baseline, the mean plasma volume was reduced by 8%, 5%, and 4%, respectively, immediately after and 1 and 3 hours after running. In all participants the plasma concentration of C3a was raised during and immediately after running (Fig 3–21). The plasma concentration of C4a was raised during and immediately after the race and also at 1 and 3 hours afterward. The concentration of C5a was undetectable in most blood samples, suggesting that C5a binds rapidly to receptors on leukocytes and is quickly removed from the circulation.

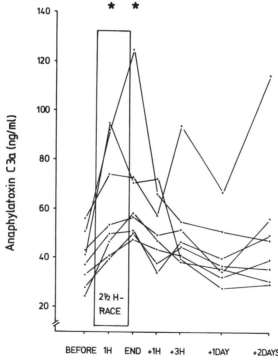

Fig 3–21.—Individual values of C3a in plasma before, during, and in first hours and days after 2.5-hour race in 8 runners. Concentrations during and after exercise were corrected for changes in plasma volume. Significant differences with preexercise values are indicated (*P = .01). (Courtesy of Dufaux B, Order U: *Clin Chim Acta* 179:45–49, Jan 13, 1989.)

Running for 2.5 hours increases the plasma concentrations of the complement cleavage products C3a and C4a, providing evidence of complement activation after prolonged exercise. Because C4a is generated, it is apparent that the classic pathway of the complement system is involved. Complement has the capacity to recruit humoral and cellular effector systems, and it modulates the extent and intensity of the immunologically induced inflammatory response. Activation of complement after exertion may be part of a mechanism to clear tissue debris released by mechanical or metabolic tissue alterations during exercise.

▶ This is the first demonstration that the complement system is activated by vigorous exercise, i.e., a 2.5-hour run. Exactly how it is activated remains unclear; presumably, it is triggered nonimmunologically by products from damaged muscle, by acute-phase reactants, or via the exercise-induced activation of fibrinolysis. Other research shows that serum complement (C3 and C4) levels, but not immunoglobin levels, are lower in marathoners than in age-matched, sedentary controls at rest, during graded maximal exercise, and during recovery (1).—E.R.Eichner, M.D.

Reference

1. Nieman DC, et al: *Int J Sports Med* 10:124, 1989.

Decreased Secretory Immunoglobulins Following Intense Endurance Exercise
Mackinnon LT, Chick TW, Van As A, Tomasi TB (Univ of New Mexico; VA Med Ctr, Albuquerque)
Sports Training Med Rehabil 1:209–218, 1989   3–32

Because of the high frequency of recurrent respiratory infections in competitive athletes after rigorous training, the effects of severe exercise on the mucosal immune response were studied. Results of a previous study showed decreased salivary IgA levels after a 50-km ski competition. To clarify the specific role of exercise rather than environmental conditions, 8 competitive bicyclists were studied under controlled ambient temperatures in a noncompetitive setting. Parotid saliva was collected so that the levels of secretory antibodies involved in resistance to respiratory illness could be assessed.

Salivary IgA and IgM levels decreased significantly immediately after exercise and remained significantly depressed at 1 hour later, returning to preexercise levels within 23 hours (Fig 3–22). Immunoglobulin levels in serum were unaffected by exercise.

Strenuous exercise apparently suppresses mucosal immunity. The mechanisms for such suppression are not clear. Chronic emotional stress can depress salivary levels of IgA. Results of previous studies have shown that upper respiratory symptoms after marathons were more common in the more rigorously trained athletes. Whether it is the intensity of exer-

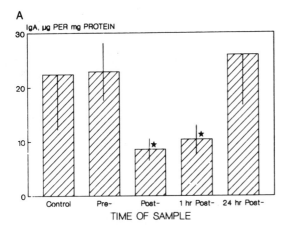

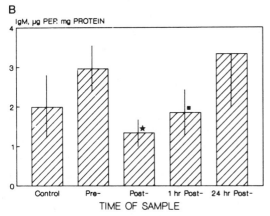

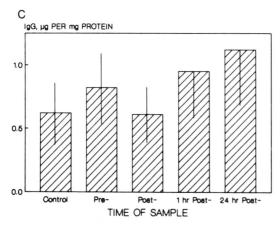

Fig 3–22.—Time course of parotid saliva Ig suppression and recovery after exercise. Values are mean microgram of each Ig per milligram of protein ± SEM *(bars)*. **A,** IgA; N = 5 controls, 8 cyclists; **B,** IgM; N = 5 controls, 5 cyclists; **C,** IgG; N = 3 controls, 3 cyclists. For IgG, only 3 of 5 controls and 3 of 8 cyclists had detectable levels of IgG. *Star* indicates $P < .01$; *square* indicates $P < .025$ vs. preexercise values; *t*-test for repeated measures, Bonferroni's method. (Courtesy of Mackinnon LT, Chick TW, Van As A, et al: *Sports Training Med Rehabil* 1:209–218, 1989).

cise, the level of training, or the duration of exercise that reduces secretory immunoglobulin levels remains to be determined.

The Effect of Exercise on Natural Killer Cell Activity in Young and Old Subjects

Fiatarone MA, Morley JE, Bloom ET, Benton D, Solomon GF, Makinodan T (VA Med Ctr, Sepulveda, Calif; VA Med Ctr, West Los Angeles; Univ of California, Los Angeles)
J Gerontol 44:M37–M45, March 1989   3–33

It is well known that in humans, immune function decreases with age. However, it is not clear how much of this age-related change is inevitable and irrevocable. Exercise in humans increases the antibody response to antigenic challenge. Human aging is usually accompanied by both a reduction in physical activity and impaired responsiveness of the immune system. Healthy young and elderly volunteers were studied to assess the effect of maximal physical exercise on antigenic and functional characteristics of peripheral blood lymphocytes possessing natural killer activity.

Eight women aged 21–39 years (mean, 30 years) and 9 women aged 65–79 years (mean, 71 years) who were moderately active and not significantly obese or malnourished underwent exercise testing with cardiac monitoring on a bicycle ergometer. Blood samples were drawn just before exercise, at peak exercise, and after a 15-minute recovery period. All blood samples were analyzed for the natural killer cell response to in vitro stimulation with recombinant interleukin-2.

At baseline there was no significant difference between young and elderly subjects with regard to the number and function of natural killer cells. Exercise significantly enhanced natural-killer cell activity immediately after exercise in the elderly women as well as in the young women. The effect was short lived, and all parameters had returned to baseline by the end of the 15-minute recovery period. Thus in healthy elderly persons, natural killer cell activity increases in response to acute exercise at least as effectively as in young persons.

▶ The articles reviewed in Abstracts 3–32 and 3–33 expand our information on exercise, immunity, and infections (see the 1989 YEAR BOOK OF SPORTS MEDICINE, pp 275–281). New evidence suggests that natural killer (NK) cells are the first line of defense against certain viruses, e.g., certain herpesviruses (1). If NK cells are "Minutemen" against bloodborne viruses, mucosal immunoglobulins (especially IgA) are "Minutemen" against microorganisms in the nose and throat. The above-described articles, which corroborate and extend earlier research, show that intense exercise decreases salivary IgA (and IgM) and increases the number and activity of NK cells in the blood. The problem is that, regarding immune defense, these results seem to be "opposite." See the Amsterdam Growth and Health Study for different results on IgA: Exercise decreased salivary IgA in women but increased it in men (2).

How important are such "exercise-induced immune changes"? Although running a marathon, for example, evokes changes in lymphocyte numbers and function, most of these changes return to normal within a day (3). A typical pattern for NK cells is to increase in number and activity during the first hour of a marathon, fall to subnormal values an hour or so after the marathon ends, and return to normal within 21 hours (4). Then, too, it is still unclear whether athletes contract fewer or more infections. A questionnaire survey of college athletes (wrestlers, swimmers, gymnasts), for example, found no increase in upper respiratory infections during the competitive season (5). Also, in our new world of "psychoneuroimmunology," almost any stress—physical or mental—can perturb "immunity." In dental students salivary IgA levels wax and wane with school stress. In medical students NK activity falls as exams approach. In college students NK activity correlates with how stress is handled: "Good" copers have higher NK activity than "poor" copers. Also, epidemiologic research in the general population ties the frequency of upper respiratory infections to life stress (6). So, exercise causes intriguing changes in immune factors, but we still do not know whether these modest, mixed, and transient changes are biologically important. It may depend on whether the exercise in question is a tonic or a stress.—E.R.Eichner, M.D.

References

1. Ritz J: *N Engl J Med* 320:1748, 1989.
2. Schouten WJ, et al: *Int J Sports Med* 9:289, 1988.
3. Nieman DC, et al: *Int J Sports Med* 10:317, 1989.
4. Berk LS, et al: *Med Sci Sports Exerc* 22:207, 1990.
5. Strauss RH, et al: *Am J Sports Med* 16:653, 1988.
6. Graham NMH, et al: *Am J Epidemiol* 124:389, 1986.

Physical Exercise Increases Natural Cellular-Mediated Tumor Cytotoxicity in Elderly Women

Crist DM, Mackinnon LT, Thompson RF, Atterbom HA, Egan PA (Univ of New Mexico)
Gerontology 35:66–71, March–June 1989   3–34

Aging has been linked to impairments in immune function, including changes in natural cellular-mediated cytotoxicity. The influence of acute treadmill exercise testing on natural killer (NK) cell tumor cytotoxicity in vitro was studied in 14 elderly women who were randomly assigned to either an exercise training group or a nonexercising control group. Exercisers performed aerobic exercise to 50% of maximum for 20 minutes 3 times per week for 16 weeks. The tumor cytotoxic activity of NK cells in vitro was measured in fresh peripheral blood lymphocytes obtained from venous blood samples taken immediately before and within 20 minutes after treadmill exercise.

There were no identifiable differences between exercisers and controls at baseline. The mean basal level of NK activity before treadmill exercise was greater in exercisers than in controls after the experimental period. After acute treadmill exercise in both groups, a significant increase in NK activity occurred. The acute increase in tumor cytotoxicity was significantly greater in the exercise group than in controls, however.

Natural cellular-mediated tumor cytotoxicity is increased in response to acute exercise and long-term exercise training in elderly women. Further studies are warranted to confirm results and to assess the relationship of augmented NK activity to health maintenance in the elderly.

▶ Both humans and experimental animals become increasingly vulnerable to tumors as they grow older. In humans, part of the problem is a cumulative exposure to such agents as cigarette smoke and industrial by-products. However, a second important factor is the age-related deterioration of immune function. As aging proceeds, the body becomes less able to recognize abnormal cells, resulting in increased vulnerability to viruses, tumors, and immune diseases. The immune system is quite complex, and there is disagreement as to the impact of aging on one important component of tumor cell destruction, i.e., natural killer cell activity; some observers find a decrease (1,2), whereas others observe no loss of killer cell activity with aging (3). Possibly, differences in habitual activity contribute to these discrepant findings. In the present study, the prescribed exercise, to 50% of heart rate reserve, was quite moderate and often performed from a chair; there were thus no other functional gains, and it is remarkable that such light activity nevertheless improved immune function. Others also have found that a little exercise suffices to improve immune responses (4, 5). Finally, it is worth stressing a point not made in this paper: An excess of activity can have a negative impact on immune function and has indeed been suggested as an indicator of overtraining.—R.J. Shephard, M.D., Ph.D.

References

1. Rabinowich H, et al: *Mech Ageing Dev* 32:213, 1985.
2. Mysliwska J, et al: *Mech Ageing Dev* 31:1, 1985.
3. Murasko DM, et al: *Am J Med* 81:612, 1986.
4. Targan S, et al: *Clin Exp Immunol* 45:352, 1981.
5. Edwards AJ, et al: *Clin Exp Immunol* 58:420, 1984.

Intravascular Hemolysis in Aerobic Dancing: The Role of Floor Surface and Type of Routine
Schwellnus MP, Penfold GK, Cilliers JF, Kuyl JM, van den Heever DP (Biokinetic Ctr, Pretoria, South Africa; Univ of Witwatersrand, Johannesburg)
Phys Sportsmed 17:55–67, August 1989   3–35

Intravascular hemolysis has been described as an etiologic factor in the anemia that occurs in endurance athletes. The excessive force applied to capillaries during footstrike appears to be one mechanism responsible for hemolysis. To determine whether intravascular hemolysis occurs during aerobic dancing and whether the type of aerobics, floor surface, and du-

TABLE 1.—Serum Concentrations of Haptoglobin in
65 Female Aerobic Dancers

	No.	At Rest	After Dancing 60 min
LISS	18	1.34 ± 0.19	1.24 ± 0.16
LIHS	15	1.57 ± 0.16	1.12 ± 0.12*
HISS	17	1.34 ± 0.12	0.76 ± 0.08*
HIHS	15	1.23 ± 0.16	0.76 ± 0.18*

In g/L; mean †SE.
*$P < .005$.
(Courtesy of Schwellnus MP, Penfold GK, Cilliers JF, et al: *Phys Sportsmed* 17:55–67, August 1989.)

ration of dancing also plays a role in its development, 65, healthy women aged 18–50 years were assigned to 1 of 4 groups according to the type of routine performed and the hardness of the floor surface. All 65 women participated in an hour-long dance session. A subgroup participated in 5 successive 1-hour sessions, with 1 hour of rest between sessions. Blood and urine were tested before and after exercise.

A highly significant decrease in the level of haptoglobin was noted after 1 hour of exercise in the low-impact, hard surface (LIHS) group; the high-impact, soft surface (HISS) group; and the high-impact, hard surface (HIHS) group, but not in the low-impact, soft surface (LISS) group (Table 1). There was a significant drop in the serum level of haptoglobin after the first hour and another significant drop after 5 hours of dancing (Table 2). After 1 hour of dancing the plasma level of hemoglobin remained similar in all groups, and there was no significant change after 5 hours of dancing. No evidence of hemoglobinuria could be found in any of the women after 5 hours of dancing. Results of all tests for methemalbuminemia were negative before and after dancing of any duration.

Aerobic dancing, especially high-impact dancing on hard floors, can

TABLE 2.—Serum Haptoglobin and Plasma Hemoglobin Values in 41
Female-Aerobic Dancers

	At Rest	After Dancing 60 Min	After Dancing 5 Hours
Serum haptoglobin (g/L, no. = 21)	1.33 ± 0.73	1.17 ± 0.58*	0.98 ± 49†
Plasma hemoglobin (μg/L, no. = 20)	0.48 ± 1.43	0.50 ± 0.87	0.38 ± 1.12

Mean ± SE.
*Differed significantly from resting value.
†Differed significantly from 60-minute value.
(Courtesy of Schwellnus MP, Penfold GK, Cilliers JF, et al: *Phys Sportsmed* 17:55–67, August 1989.)

cause minor intravascular hemolysis. However, it is not likely to contribute to iron loss, even if the dancing is done several times a day.

▶ We can now add aerobic dancing to sports that can cause intravascular hemolysis. Such hemolysis has long been considered to result from impact, either the "footstrike" (e.g., in running) or the "handstrike" (e.g., in karate). It is probably better thought of as "exertional hemolysis," however, because it has now been described in distance swimmers and in rowers. Presumably, turbulent blood flow in exercising muscle somehow bursts a few red blood cells in the bloodstream. Generally, such hemolysis is mild; as such, it rarely exhausts the serum haptoglobin and thus rarely causes urinary iron loss. It can easily be offset by mild reticulocytosis and thus is no threat to recreational athletes. In world-class marathoners, however, it may cap the adaptive rise in red blood cell mass that helps to make winners.—E.R. Eichner, M.D.

Gastrointestinal Bleeding in Athletes
Eichner ER (Univ of Oklahoma)
Phys Sportsmed 17:128–140, May 1989   3–36

In the past decade, gastrointestinal (GI) bleeding in distance runners has been the focus of increasing attention. A large survey of marathoners found that about 2% of respondents had bloody stools occasionally or frequently after running. Six studies of occult bleeding in runners found positivity rates ranging from 0% to 11% before races and from 13% to 30% after races, indicating that running-related minor bleeding is fairly common.

In another study of 6 male and 5 female runners, 55% had stools positive for occult blood more than once during the season. Bleeding episodes in this group were always minor and brief and did not cause either iron depletion or anemia. Episodes were significantly more frequent after greater exertion.

It is not yet known whether GI bleeding is a general threat to distance runners. However, running-related iron-deficiency anemia has been reported, principally in female runners. The preponderance of women in these reports may be the result of selection bias, however. Men tend to have greater iron stores, so it takes less bleeding in women to cause iron-deficiency anemia.

The site of GI bleeding varies, but it often seems to be the stomach. It is unclear how running causes or exacerbates peptic ulcer disease or gastritis. The cecum is increasingly reported as the site of bleeding. One report postulates that running causes hemorrhagic ischemic colitis to develop as a result of reduced blood flow to the proximal colon, citing studies showing that strenuous exercise can reduce visceral blood flow by as much as 80% in healthy persons. Rectal bleeding is rare, but all-out running has been reported to induce bleeding from underlying ulcerative proctitis. Sometimes, no bleeding site is found despite thorough investigation.

All-out exercise may impair hemostasis. Although the effect of exercise on platelet function and coagulation is debatable, there is no doubt that exercise enhances fibrinolysis. Because the risk of bleeding seems to correlate with the intensity of exercise, gradual conditioning may help to prevent GI bleeding during athletics. Athletes with symptoms of upper GI problems such as gastritis or ulcer may be treated with antacids or H_2 blockers to enable them to train hard and compete. Athletes should avoid nonsteroidal anti-inflammatory drugs for 24 hours and aspirin for 2 or 3 days before a race. Iron therapy may have a preventive role in female runners. In general, GI bleeding should be attributed to sports participation only after treatable lesions have been excluded.

▶ Bloody diarrhea cost Mark Allen victory in the 1987 Hawaii Ironman Triathlon. For most athletes, however, and even for most distance runners, GI bleeding is either not a problem or is only a minor, brief, and infrequent occurrence. Although the story is still evolving, exercise-related GI bleeding seems not to be a common cause of iron-deficiency anemia in athletes. See also the 1988 YEAR BOOK OF SPORTS MEDICINE, pp 130–133.—E.R. Eichner, M.D.

Exercise During Pregnancy: Current State of the Art
Shangold MM (Hahnemann Univ, Philadelphia)
Can Fam Physician 35:1675–1680, August 1989   3–37

A physically fit body is better able to meet the demands of pregnancy, and many women today are physically fit when they become pregnant. However, pregnant women need guidance about the level of exercise they can safely perform to maintain fitness without endangering the fetus.

One concern about exercise during pregnancy is blood distribution. Fetal bradycardia is much more likely to follow exercise that exceeds 67% of the maximum oxygen uptake. This workload corresponds to a maternal heart rate of more than 150 bpm. Although no cases have been documented, maternal hyperthermia during exercise or hot tub/sauna use might also endanger the fetus. Animal studies have shown that fetal temperature exceeds maternal temperature after maternal exercise, and fetal temperature can remain higher for longer than 60 minutes.

Pregnant women who exercise must ingest enough calories, vitamins, and minerals for themselves, their fetuses, and their exercise. Both pregnancy and exercise require more carbohydrates, for example. Fluid requirements are higher for exercise but not for pregnancy. Extra iron and calcium are also required by pregnant women who exercise.

Several recommendations can be made based on what is known about exercise during pregnancy. First, women should undertake fitness training before they become pregnant. Women who are used to aerobic exercise can probably continue their usual regimen at a comfortable pace during pregnancy as long as there are no complications. Pace should be judged by perceived exertion rather than heart rate. Women who were inactive before pregnancy should not undertake aerobic activities other than brisk walking. To avoid possible risks of hyperthermia, exercise should be limited to 30 minutes per session. Pregnant exercisers should check their temperatures rectally after routine exercise in early pregnancy. If the temperature does not exceed 38.3° C (101° F) that level of exercise can be safely continued. The use of hot tubs and saunas should be avoided during pregnancy. Both sedentary and active women can benefit from weight training and stretching exercises during pregnancy. Strengthening muscles can alleviate back pain and other muscular aches associated with pregnancy.

Pregnant women can benefit from exercise. However, they should avoid high-intensity or prolonged exercise, dehydration, hyperthermia, and regimens with a potential for abdominal trauma.

▶ This article contains some very useful practical advice regarding exercise for the pregnant patient. It quite correctly points out that because of the additional circulatory loop to the placenta, the heart rate no longer provides a reliable guide to the intensity of effort during pregnancy; rather, the rating of perceived exertion should be substituted. The risk of hyperthermia developing during an exercise session depends greatly on the amount of radiant sunlight, and it might be possible to increase core temperature to more than 38.3° C on a sunny day, even if exercise is held to only 30 minutes; the pregnant patient should thus be watchful if the ambient temperature exceeds 26° C, especially if the day is humid.—R.J. Shephard, M.D., Ph.D.

The Effects of Maternal Exercise on Early Pregnancy Outcome
Clapp JF III (Univ of Vermont)
Am J Obstet Gynecol 161:1453–1457, December 1989   3–38

The etiologic factors involved in spontaneous abortion are not well understood. It is estimated that approximately one third of all spontaneous abortions are associated with a chromosomal anomaly. Specific environmental factors (e.g., subchorionic hemorrhage and defective luteal function) account for fetal loss in some patients. Anomalous environmental circumstances may be responsible for loss in others. The hypothesis that vigorous aerobic exercise during the periconceptional period and early pregnancy increases the incidence of abnormal early pregnancy outcome was tested prospectively in 119 white women aged 25–38 years. All were in excellent general health and had physically active life-styles.

All 119 women were followed for several cycles before conception and then for 6 additional cycles, or throughout the subsequent pregnancy. Exercise performance was monitored prospectively in 49 recreational runners and 41 aerobic dancers who had exercised for at least 2 years at least 3 times a week for a minimum of 20 minutes at an intensity exceeding 50% of measured maximal oxygen intake. The control group consisted of 29 physically active, intermittently athletic women matched for age, weight, percent body fat, and multiple life-style factors. The controls had discontinued all forms of endurance exercise before attempting conception and did not resume exercising until after pregnancy. Pregnancy was diagnosed by an early test for β-subunit human chorionic gonadotropin; viability was confirmed by ultrasonography at 40 days' conceptional age.

Spontaneous abortions occurred in 17% of the runners, in 18% of the aerobic dancers, and in 25% of the controls; the overall incidence of spontaneous abortion was 19%. The remaining women all gave birth at term. One congenital abnormality was detected at term in each of the 3 groups.

These findings do not support the hypothesis that vigorous aerobic exercise during the periconceptional period and during early pregnancy increases the incidence of spontaneous fetal loss. Although this is reassuring, the data may not have general application, as all women selected for this study were physically active and in excellent general health.

▶ There have been fears that the cardiovascular, hormonal, and thermal perturbations induced by vigorous exercise might result in early fetal loss (1). Although the present observations were intended to answer this question, they do not do so entirely. The exercising women were involved in recreational running and aerobic dance. The runners were averaging a pace of 8 minutes per mile and were spending 1–6 hours per week at this pace, hardly enough to induce large cardiovascular, hormonal, or thermal changes, particularly as the women were young and healthy. Those involved in aerobic dance were in general involved in even less physical activity. Further studies of this sort are required including women who engage in more extensive bouts of activity and those who decide to begin exercising from an unfit state around the time of conception.—R.J. Shephard, M.D., Ph.D.

Reference

1. Clapp JF, et al: *Med Sci Sports Exerc* 19:124, 1987.

Slipped Upper Femoral Epiphysis in an Amenorrhoeic Athlete
Wolman RL, Harries MG, Fyfe I (Northwick Park Hosp, Harrow, Middlesex, England)
Br Med J 299:720–721, Sept 16, 1989   3–39

A slipped upper femoral epiphysis is a prepubertal disorder associated with various endocrine disorders. The condition is probably an important cause of osteoarthritis in later life. A 17-year-old girl with primary amenorrhea and a slipped upper femoral epiphysis was successfully treated with internal fixation.

Girl, 17 years, with primary amenorrhea, had a 9-month history of pain in the right thigh. She had been running 64 km a week as part of her training as a middle distance runner and had been training since age 10 years. Thigh pain had started gradually and was aggravated by exercise. There was no history of injury.

Treatment with physiotherapy had not relieved the symptoms. Clinical examination showed a physically immature girl with a 15.3% body-fat ratio. Pelvic radiographs revealed partial slipping of the right femoral epiphysis. Internal fixation was performed and the patient made a good postoperative recovery. She was advised to stop training to allow the epiphysis to close. Follow-up examination after a 2-month rest from training showed that her body fat had increased to 16.7%. Menarche had occurred, and a repeated pelvic radiograph confirmed that the epiphysis was closing.

It is unusual to see a slipped upper femoral epiphysis in girls older than 14 years. However, in this patient, the pubertal delay caused by intensive training started at a young age had retarded bone maturation. The resulting delayed closure of the femoral epiphysis had increased the period in which the slip could occur. Moreover, the intense physical activity may have increased the shearing forces placed on the hip and increased the risk still further.

▶ This case is instructive as it again brings home the importance of biologic rather than chronologic age when dealing with children and adolescents. A slipped upper femoral epiphysis is unusual in a 17-year-old girl, but she was prepubertal and when viewed from that perspective the findings were biologically plausible. An additional point of interest in this athlete with primary amenorrhea was the onset of menses after a 2-month rest from training.—J.R. Sutton, M.D.

Effect of Testosterone on Muscle Mass and Muscle Protein Synthesis
Griggs RC, Kingston W, Jozefowicz RF, Herr BE, Forbes G, Halliday D (Univ of Rochester; Clinical Research Ctr, Harrow, England)
J Appl Physiol 66:498–503, January 1989   3–40

Because the effect of androgens on muscle strength without muscle training has not been confirmed, the effect of a pharmacologic dose of testosterone on muscle mass, total-body potassium mass, muscle protein synthesis, whole-body protein synthesis, and muscle fiber size in the absence of any exercise training was investigated in 9 normal, healthy men aged 19–40 years. None of the men had participated in vigorous weight or exercise training during the month preceding the study. Each participant was given testosterone enanthate, 3 mg/kg intramuscularly weekly for 12 weeks. At the start of the study, stable isotopelabeled amino acids were infused to assess changes in muscle protein synthesis. A primed continuous infusion of labeled leucine was used to assess whole-body protein synthesis in 4 men. Urinary creatinine excretion was measured to assess changes in muscle mass. Whole-body scintillation counting was used to evaluate changes in total body potassium as a parameter of lean body mass. Muscle needle biopsy was performed to study morphological changes in muscle fiber.

Testosterone enanthate injections increased muscle protein synthesis as estimated by the incorporation of stable isotope into muscle in all 9 men. The mean increase in muscle protein synthesis was 27%. Whole-body protein synthesis did not change significantly. Testosterone enanthate increased muscle mass, as assessed by creatinine excretion, by a mean of 20%. The mean change in lean body mass, as reflected in changes in total body potassium, averaged 12%. However, testosterone administration did not increase muscle strength, as muscle needle biopsy specimens showed only a small and insignificant increase in muscle fiber diameter.

In men with normal gonadal function, the use of androgens without concomitant exercise training increases muscle protein synthesis, muscle mass, and lean body mass, but not muscle fiber size, suggesting that muscle strength is not increased.

▶ The use of stable isotope has proved to be an invaluable tool to examine various metabolic pathways, especially those associated with protein metabolism. Whenever there is an increase or decrease in muscle bulk, without such studies it is impossible to determine whether the observed changes result from altered protein synthesis, altered protein degradation, or a combination of both. Furthermore, not all tissues are equally affected by a pharmacologic intervention. Thus when infusion of stable isotopes is combined with multiple biopsies, as is possible using the needle biopsy techniques to sample muscle, a clearer picture of the dynamics emerges. This elegant study also attests to the value of interinstitution trans-Atlantic collaboration. The authors have clearly demonstrated that testosterone in normal males exerts its effect on muscle mass by enhancing protein synthesis in muscle with a tendency to increase muscle fiber size. Whole-body protein synthesis was not increased.

These authors previously demonstrated an increase in muscle protein synthesis in patients with myotonic dystrophy, in whom they found an increase in muscle RNA but not DNA. The authors also implied that the muscle was stronger after testosterone injections, but these data were not included in the paper!—J.R. Sutton, M.D.

4 Exercise Testing, Prescription, and Training

Influence of Age and Stature on Exercise Capacity During Incremental Cycle Ergometry in Men and Women
Jones NL, Summers E, Killian KJ (McMaster Univ, Hamilton, Ont)
Am Rev Respir Dis 140:1373–1380, 1989   4–1

Exercise testing is widely used to measure the severity of respiratory, neuromuscular, and cardiovascular disability. Testing standards have been developed to measure maximum exercise capacity (Wcap), but there are deficiencies in these standards at extremes of age and height. The accuracy of Wcap was reevaluated by examining the interaction between age and height on Wcap achieved and that predicted in 1,071 normal persons.

The 732 men and 339 women underwent incremental exercise testing on a cycle ergometer. Data for men and women were analyzed separately. The Wcap was predicted on the basis of age, sex, and height.

The Wcap predicted was not significantly different from that achieved in men. In women, predicted Wcap was underestimated by less than 5%. However, there were significant differences for individuals at the extremes of the population ranges for age and height. The influences of age and height were nonlinear and interactive. New equations were developed to correct the deficiencies: for men, $Wcap = 1,506 \cdot Ht^{2.7} \cdot Age^{-.46}$ ($r = .78$); for women: $Wcap = 969 \cdot Ht^{2.8} \cdot Age^{-.43}$ ($r = .77$).

When Wcap predicted by the new equations was compared with Wcap achieved in 100 persons who formed the basis of the original study from which the original normal standards had been derived, there were no significant differences (Fig 4–1). The interactive influences of age and height expressed by the new equations are more logical from a biologic standpoint than the previously used linear, additive relationships. These equations should be more reliable predictors than those that were developed earlier for patients referred for exercise testing.

▶ Jones and colleagues have had extensive experience in the clinical testing of exercise tolerance on the cycle ergometer. In setting normal standards, they were previously guided by their experience in the respiratory function laboratory, using equations that start from an individual's height and then subtract a standard age-related figure. However, they have found empirically that such a standard gives erroneous predictions at the extremes of the height and age dis-

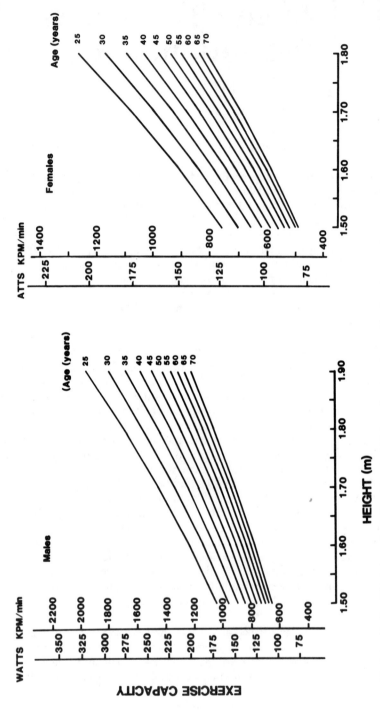

Fig 4–1.— Predicted Wcap for males (*left*) and females (*right*) as a function of age and height. (Courtesy of Jones NL, Summers E, Killian KJ: *Am Rev Respir Dis* 140:1373–1380, 1989.)

tributions. Apart from possible changes of height with age (e.g., as a result of vertebral collapse), it is easy to see that the age correction for a small person should be less than that for a large one; their original equations led to prediction of a 22% reduction of working capacity between the ages of 20 and 60 years for an individual whose height was 1.80 m, but a 30% reduction in one whose height was only 1.60 m. These problems are overcome by the use of interactive power functions of height and age in the new equations; the much larger sample also means that the numbers can be accepted with greater confidence, although one may question the use of data from a clinical laboratory to set norms. It would have been better if the subjects had been from somewhere other than a hospital setting. It is also interesting that the power function for height is 2.7–2.8, in line with some of our studies on growing children (1), but in disagreement with earlier theoretical predictions based on dimensional considerations (2).—R.J. Shephard, M.D., Ph.D.

References

1. Shephard RJ, et al: On the basis of data standardization in pre-pubescent children, in Ostyn M, et al (eds): *Kinanthropometry II.* Basel, Karger, 1980.
2. Von Döbeln W: Kroppstorlek, Energiomsattning och Kondition in Luthman G, et al (eds): *Handboki Ergonomi.* Stockholm, Almqvist & Wiksell, 1966.

Ergometric Characteristics of the Speedskating Simulator: Comparison of the Relationships Between Oxygen Consumption and Heart Rate, and Between Heart Rate and Power Developed on an Exercise Bicycle and on a Speedskating Simulator in 2 Groups of Athletes
Nielens H, Sturbois X (UCL, Louvain-la-Neuve, Belgium)
Médecine Sport 63:189–194, July 1989
4–2

The exercise bicycle and the treadmill are the most commonly used pieces of testing equipment in the sports physiology laboratory. The speedskating simulator is used by professional speedskaters to increase endurance (Fig 4–2). To determine whether the speedskating simulator can be used for measuring aerobic performance, studies were done in 6 top-ranked speedskaters aged 18–35 years and 10 students aged 22–25 years who were majoring in physical education and rehabilitation. Although all of the students were active in various sports, none was an experienced skater. Each study participant was tested on an exercise bicycle and on the speedskating simulator. Heart rate, oxygen consumption, and power (i.e., work performed per time unit) were measured.

During ergometric testing on both the exercise bicycle and the skating simulator, significantly greater maximal oxygen consumption was seen in the speedskaters. However, there was an important difference in how the test was carried out by each group. Experienced speedskaters were used to the skating simulator and took on a horizontal position as if skating on ice when exercising, swinging their arms and making sliding motions

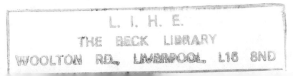

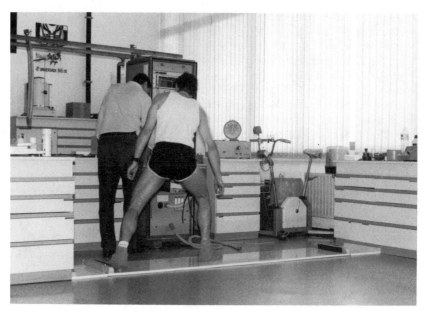

Fig 4–2.—Speedskating simulator in use. (Courtesy of Nielens H, Sturbois X: *Médecine Sport* 63:189–194, July 1989.)

as if skating, while putting out great effort. The students, who were not experienced skaters, were not used to the speedskating simulator and had to put forth great effort simply to stay in balance. Consequently, the speedskaters worked much harder than the students. However, the simulator was not equipped to measure external work. The speedskating simulator can be used to obtain ergometric measurements, but its primary value is as a training device.

▶ Athlete testing laboratories around the world are coming to recognize that it does not make a lot of sense to test a cyclist or a swimmer on a standard treadmill. Rather, the competitor should use a device on which the required exercise approximates closely that of the actual sport. One important characteristic of the top-level competitor relative to an average person is his or her ability to approach the treadmill maximal oxygen intake much more closely while using the sport-specific device. The present paper describes the use of a speedskating simulator. It notes the more effective technique of the experienced speedskaters relative to novices, but unfortunately the device gives no indication of the mechanical work that has been performed; also, because the subjects were not carried to a directly measured maximal oxygen intake, it is necessary to rely on rather unsatisfactory extrapolations of the heart rate/oxygen consumption line to a theoretical maximal heart rate. In fact, if maximal effort is not attained, it is very difficult to know what theoretical heart rate to suggest for extrapolation when using a sport-specific ergometer.—R.J. Shephard, M.D., Ph.D.

The Safety of Maximal Exercise Testing
Gibbons L, Blair SN, Kohl HW, Cooper K (Cooper Clinic, Dallas; Inst for Aerobics Research, Dallas)
Circulation 80:846–852, October 1989   4–3

Exercise testing is used extensively both by physicians and nonphysicians, but definitive data on the safety of exercise testing are more than 20 years old. More recent data concerning exercise tests performed by a large group of patients under uniform conditions were reviewed for the period 1971 through 1987, during which time 71,914 maximal exercise tests were conducted. The prevalence of known heart disease was low. Before exercise, subjects underwent physical examination, blood pressure (BP) testing, and resting ECG. Every 5 minutes during maximal treadmill testing, ECG recordings and BP measurements were taken.

There were 6 major cardiac complications, including 1 death, during maximal treadmill testing; however, in 45,000 maximal tests conducted in the past 10 years, there have been no complications. Complications included 2 ventricular fibrillations, 1 myocardial infarction during recovery, and 3 delayed infarctions. Five of 6 subjects with complications had known coronary disease, and 1 had a history of rheumatoid arthritis (table).

Maximal exercise testing appears to be safer than many had thought. The complication rate was less than 1 complication in 10,000 tests. Furthermore, testing seems to be getting safer with time.

▶ There have previously been many studies of the safety of maximal exercise testing, but in general these have suffered from technical problems. Often, the approach has been to circulate a questionnaire to major centers to ask how many persons were tested and to note any emergencies; however, the estimate of numbers tested is then imprecise, and centers with poor records could conceivably fail to respond to inquiries. The present data, from the Cooper Clinic, relate to a large sample of subjects but suffers from the problem that most of those tested were fit, health-oriented individuals and most were tested more than once; the study could thus underestimate the risk for the general population tested on a single occasion. The overall risk (95% confidence intervals of 0.3 to 1.9 complications per 10,000 tests) is not grossly dissimilar from that cited in earlier reports. However, because of the extensive experience of the Cooper group and superior laboratory facilities, there was only 1 death in more than 70,000 tests, this occurring relatively early in the 20 years of data collection. (Although the authors conclude that their tests are getting safer, cynics might argue that the most vulnerable subject had already died!) The lesson drawn from the early experience of the clinic was to insist on a warm-down, as most of the complications occurred during the warm-down phase. Given that McDonough's paper on warm-down was published in 1969(1), it is surprising that this recommendation was not implemented earlier.—R.J. Shephard, M.D., Ph.D.

Complications of Maximal Exercise Testing

Patient	Age (yr)/gender	History	Problem	Result	Max hr
1	67 F	Angina, previous myocardial infarction	Ventricular tachycardia, ventricular fibrillation	CPR successful	117
2	58M	Previous myocardial infarction	Ventricular tachycardia, ventricular fibrillation	Defibrillation successful	145
3	71M	Angina, Paroxysmal atrial tachycardia	Subendocardial myocardial infarction	Successful rehabilitation	130
4	34M	Rheumatoid arthritis	Inferior myocardial infarction	Successful rehabilitation	180
5	52M	Angina	Post-test myocardial infarction (24 hr)	Successful treatment	136
6	63M	Myocardial infarction	Post-test myocardial infarction (12 hr)	Deceased after 1 wk	138

(Courtesy of Gibbons L, Blair SN, Kohl HW, et al: *Circulation* 80:846–852, October 1989.)

Reference

1. McDonough JR: *J South Carolina Med Assoc* 65:26, 1969.

Failure of Target Heart Rate to Accurately Monitor Intensity During Aerobic Dance
Parker SB, Hurley BF, Hanlon DP, Vaccaro P (Univ of Maryland, College Park)
Med Sci Sports Exerc 21:230–234, April 1989 4–4

Based on the assumption that the heart rate increases proportionally to the increase in oxygen consumption, the target heart rate is often used to monitor exercise intensity in aerobic dance training. This relationship has been established in running and cycling but not in aerobic dance. The heart rate-oxygen consumption relationship during aerobic dance was compared with that of running performed at the same rate of oxygen consumption.

Before and after aerobic training maximal oxygen uptake was measured in 14 untrained women during a continuous treadmill test. Underwater weight was also recorded to determine body composition. A control group of 10 untrained women was also tested for maximal oxygen uptake and body composition. The women participated in a continuous 25-minute aerobic dance session 3 days per week for 8 weeks. Each woman was assigned a training heart rate representing 75% to 85% of maximal heart rate. Exercise heart rates were monitored by palpation at 10 minutes and 25 minutes during exercise.

After 8 weeks there were no significant differences in body weight, percentage of body fat, or fat-free weight between the aerobic dance group and controls. However, there was a significant difference between maximal oxygen uptake values in the aerobic dance group and controls. There was also a significant difference between pre- and posttraining values in the aerobic dance group. Aerobic dancing elicited a significantly lower oxygen pulse than did treadmill exercise.

The heart rate produced by aerobic dance represents a lower relative exercise intensity than that of running. The assumption that aerobic dance training produces the same cardiovascular changes as running training is probably unwarranted.

▶ The authors have concluded that aerobic dance training does not produce the same cardiovascular changes as running training. They believe that the ". . . smaller increase in $\dot{V}O_{2max}$ may be attributed to the low $\dot{V}O_2$ relative to heart rate during aerobic dance compared to running."—F.J. George, ATC, PT

The Self-Selected Walking Pace Test and Beta Blockade
Rechnitzer PA, Cunningham DA, Howard JH (Univ of Western Ontario, London, Ont)
Can J Appl Sport Sci 14:178–181, September 1989   4–5

The self-selected walking pace test is a method to determine an individual's perception of walking speed. This test is more closely related to maximal oxygen intake than to age. Whether β blockade, which often causes fatigue, affects test scores was investigated in 23 healthy men whose mean age was 43 years. A double-blind, crossover study was conducted in which the intervention was oxprenolol, a nonselective β blocker. The men walked at 3 self-selected speeds—rather slow, normal, and rather fast—for 80 m.

When the men were taking oxprenolol, there was a significant reduc-

Effect of β Blockade on Heart Rate, Choice of Walking Speed, and
Step Length in Self-Paced Walking Test

Variable	Condition	n	X	SD	p >
Slow heart rate	Drug	23	76.61	8.14	.023
	No drug	23	81.91	10.03	
Normal heart rate	Drug	23	81.52	7.44	<.001
	No drug	23	87.60	9.10	
Fast heart rate	Drug	22	87.69	7.88	<.001
	No drug	22	95.54	10.96	
Slow speed (ms⁻¹)	Drug	23	1.08	0.17	.754
	No drug	23	1.07	0.14	
Normal speed (ms⁻¹)	Drug	23	1.32	0.15	.778
	No drug	23	1.33	0.17	
Fast speed (ms⁻¹)	Drug	23	1.63	0.17	.747
	No drug	23	1.61	0.12	
Slow step length (m)	Drug	23	0.67	0.08	.584
	No Drug	23	0.67	0.07	
Normal step length (m)	Drug	23	0.74	0.06	.760
	No drug	23	0.74	0.06	
Fast step length (m)	Drug	23	0.83	0.08	.751
	No drug	23	0.83	0.06	

(Courtesy of Rechnitzer PA, Cunningham DA, Howard JH: *Can J Appl Sport Sci* 14:178–181, September 1989.)

tion in heart rate. However, there were no significant differences in walking speeds at any speed whether or not they were taking the drug (table). The stride length remained similar as well.

Apparently, β-blocking drugs do not interfere with the self-selected walking test. However, this study involved only a nonselective β-blocking agent given to persons not receiving chronic treatment with the drug.

▶ β-Blocking agents become ever more popular, creating problems in both exercise testing and the setting of exercise prescriptions. One simple option suggested for the testing of the frail elderly is the self-selected walking pace (1), it has been argued that this measure has a useful correlation with the individual's maximal oxygen intake, thus avoiding the dangers of a formal exercise test in the aged.

In theory, β blockade might be expected to influence the self-selected pace of working. The maximal heart rate is substantially reduced, and unless the subject is capable of a compensating increase in the stroke volume, there will be a corresponding drop in peak cardiac output and maximal oxygen transport. Also, there is a decrease in muscle blood flow as well as more direct local metabolic effects, particularly a blockade of free fatty acid release. The present paper does not entirely answer the question as to whether the test is applicable to elderly persons taking β blockers, because the test subjects were healthy and had a mean age of 43 years; such a group would be much more likely to have a compensatory increase in stroke volume.

A further issue is the practical value of self-paced walking as a measure of an individual's maximal oxygen intake. Although the correlation between these 2 measurements is statistically significant, it is very low (0.3–0.4), and even if the question of β blockade can be answered more satisfactorily, it is still unlikely that such a test will give more than a very crude categorization of working capacity in very old individuals.— R.J. Shephard, M.D., Ph.D.

Reference

1. Cunningham DA, et al: *J Gerontol* 37:560, 1982.

Estimating the Prevalence of Leisure-Time Physical Activity
Goodman RA, Baker DB, Powell KE, Sayre JW (Ctrs for Disease Control, Atlanta; Univ of California, Los Angeles)
J Sports Med Phys Fitness 28:360–366, December 1988   4–6

Because vigorous physical activity seems to provide health benefits, it is useful to have population-based estimates of physical activity levels. Data from a population survey were used to illustrate the way in which components and cutpoints of summary scores influence the estimates of the prevalence of leisure-time physical activity and to show that prevalence estimates are related to the definition used within a given population.

Data were obtained from a survey of physical activity patterns among 356 black, white, and Hispanic adult residents of Los Angeles County, Approximately 80% of blacks, 67% of Hispanics, and 46% of whites were younger than age 40 years. Two thirds of the whites, half of the blacks, and one third of the Hispanics had attended college. Definitions of physical activity level included participation only, frequency of participation, monthly hours of participation, and estimated energy expenditure. Four continuous measures of physical activity were used: times per month, hours per month, kcal/kg/d, and kcal/wk.

The frequency distribution for continuous measures of physical activity can be characterized by a χ-square distribution pattern with 1° of freedom. There was relatively poor correlation between times per month and kcal/kg/d, indicating that times per month is not a satisfactory determinant for energy expenditure. Hours per month correlated well with kcal/kg/d, suggesting that hours per month may be a better enumeration measure of the level of physical activity. There was a high correlation between kcal/wk and kcal/kg/d, thus body weight may not be a critical factor in measuring energy expenditure.

Estimates of the prevalence of activity vary with the definition used and with the cutpoint selected to define "active" persons. In this study, the prevalence of active persons was 77% when activity was defined as participation during the preceding 30 days; however, it was only 24% when activity was defined as the expenditure of at least 4 kcal/kg/d. Researchers are advised to be cautious when interpreting prevalence estimates of levels of physical activity in study populations.

▶ Fitness experts are constantly decrying the lack of physical activity in average members of the North American population. However, the objective evidence supporting such concern is very unsatisfactory. In the course of the past few years, various authors have sampled ostensibly similar populations, reporting the prevalence of regular physical activity among the adult population as 9% and 78% (1). Plainly, both numbers cannot be correct! A critical review of available reports suggests that the apparent prevalence of physical activity decreases as the rigidity of the definition is increased; the lower numbers have much greater credibility than the high numbers. The present report tests this same hypothesis on a single sample of adults in the Los Angeles area. Again, the prevalence of physical activity ranges from 24% to 77%, depending on the method of assessment that is adopted. It is doubtful if much better answers will ever be forthcoming, either from questionnaires or from instrumentation, although laboratories continue to search for cost-effective and reliable physiologic monitors of human activity.—R.J. Shephard, M.D., Ph.D.

Reference

1. Shephard RJ: *Fitness of a Nation.* Basel, Karger, 1986.

Exercise Training Bradycardia: The Role of Autonomic Balance
Smith ML, Hudson DL, Graitzer HM, Raven PB (Texas College of Osteopathic Medicine, Forth Worth)
Med Sci Sports Exerc 21:40–44, February 1989   4–7

Resting bradycardia in endurance exercise-trained individuals is a well-known phenomenon, but the mechanisms responsible for it have not been conclusively defined. Some studies attribute this type of bradycardia to decreased sympathetic influence, whereas others conclude that it results from an increase in parasympathetic influence, or that the resting bradycardia of training may be attributable, in part, to both an increase in parasympathetic influence and a decrease in sympathetic influence.

The role of the autonomic nervous system in exercise training-induced bradycardia was examined in 20 young men (median age, 25 years); 10 were endurance-trained and 10 were nontrained. All trained participants had been running competitively for several years and averaged more than 50 miles per week in their training routines. The nontrained participants led sedentary lives. Each participant was tested on a standard graded exercise protocol to determine maximal oxygen uptake. Metoprolol tartrate was given in titrated doses to produce complete blockade of any sympathetic influence on the heart and represented that heart rate attributable to the intact parasympathetic system and the intrinsic heart rate. On another day, atropine sulfate was administered to block all parasympathetic influence on the heart and measure the heart rate attributable to the intact sympathetic system and the intrinsic heart rate. An algebraic model was then used to determine the resting heart rate based on the measured values. The product of the parasympathetic influence times the sympathetic influence represented the autonomic balance.

In trained participants the parasympathetic influence on the intrinsic heart rate was greater and the sympathetic influence on heart rate was slightly less than in nontrained individuals. Consequently, the value of the autonomic balance was significantly less in the trained group, indicating that the resting parasympathetic predominance was significantly greater than in the nontrained group. Thus the trained men tested adapted to exercise training with a decrease in the intrinsic heart rate and increased predominance of parasympathetic autonomic control at rest.

▶ The mechanism whereby endurance-trained athletes have a resting bradycardia continues to fascinate physiologists and physicians. The slowing of the heart is sometimes so pronounced that the intrinsic discharge rate of the sinus node is even too great for other cardiac pacemaking tissue and a junctional pacemaker takes over, resulting in a junctional escape rhythm. The classic understanding of heart rate is that it is a balance between those factors tending to speed up the heart—predominantly sympathetic/catecholamine influences—and those that slow it down—predominantly the vagus. In endurance-trained athletes most authors have considered that the resting bradycardia is mainly caused by an increased vagal tone (1), but others have indicated that a reduction in sympathetic tone is important (2). However, with the introduction of double and pharmacologic autonomic blockade by Jose (3) using atropine to block the vagus and propranolol to block the cardiac sympathetic nerves, a resultant intrinsic heart rate bereft of any autonomic influences was obtained. It was subsequently demonstrated that endurance-trained athletes had a lower intrinsic heart rate than did sedentary individuals (4). Noteworthy in this paper is the application of a mathematical model to help apportion the contribution of all 3 factors to the resting bradycardia of the endurance-trained athlete, although the authors confirmed what has been previously observed, i.e., the intrinsic heart rate and parasympathetic influence dominate.—J.R. Sutton, M.D.

References

1. Donald DE, et al: *Am J Physiol* 212:901, 1967.
2. Ekblom B, et al: *Scand J Clin Lab Invest* 32:251, 1973.
3. Jose AD: *Am J Cardiol* 18:476, 1966.
4. Sutton JR, et al: *Lancet* 2:1398, 1967.

Trainability of the Prepubescent Child

Bar-Or O (McMaster Univ, Hamilton, Ont)
Phys Sportsmed 17:65–82, May 1989   4–8

The increase in children's participation in competitive sports has led to increased interest in their ability to respond to training. Although more studies are needed in which proper statistical and epidemiologic principles are used, some conclusions about training can be drawn from existing data.

In prepubescent girls and boys (those at the maturation level of Tanner stage 1) maximal aerobic power can be enhanced with training. However, the degree of trainability (the magnitude of physiologic changes that occur as a result of a training program) of muscle strength appears to be somewhat lower than in more mature athletes. Performance in middle- and long-distance running frequently improves when maximal aerobic power does not increase, suggesting that a decrease in the metabolic cost of running may be a major factor.

Trainability of muscle strength probably does not depend on a child's level of maturity. However, until more is known about the potential damage that may be incurred with strength training, this type of training should be used only when indicated for well-defined athletic or rehabilitation objectives. Strength training in prepubescent children should always be done under the supervision of a qualified instructor. Maximal weight lifting should not be done. Anaerobic muscle performance is trainable despite a child's level of maturity.

▶ A good overview of the pros and cons of training in children. Aerobic power is trainable, but prepubescent children seem less trainable than their more mature counterparts. Distance running, for example, may improve more from enhanced running economy than from aerobic gains. Anaerobic power is trainable regardless of maturation level. Muscle strength, too, is trainable in children, but caution is advised, and more research here is encouraged. Some of the interindividual differences in trainability among children are doubtless genetic. The cautious framework here for strength training of children seems right on the mark.—E.R. Eichner, M.D.

Cardiorespiratory Strain During Walking in Snow With Boots of Differing Weights

Smolander J, Louhevaara V, Hakola T, Ahonen E, Klen T (Inst of Occupational Health, Helsinki; Kuopio Regional Inst of Occupational Health, Finland)
Ergonomics 32:3–13, January 1989   4–9

Safety boots provide protection against lower-limb injuries, but they are often heavier than regular footwear. Walking in safety boots therefore requires a greater expenditure of energy. If safety boots are worn in snow, the increase in physiologic strain could be critically high.

Seven men and 3 women walked in snow and on a treadmill while

Mean Cardiorespiratory Data During Walking on Treadmill and in Snow With Boots of Differing Weights*

	$\dot{V}_E$ $(l\,min^{-1})$	$\dot{V}O_2$ $(l\,min^{-1})$	$\dot{V}CO_2$ $(l\,min^{-1})$	R	HR $(beats\,min^{-1})$
Walking on treadmill					
Winter jogging boots	23.2 ± 1.6	0.79 ± 0.05	0.64 ± 0.05	0.81 ± 0.02†	106 ± 4‡
Rubber boots	21.9 ± 1.3	0.81 ± 0.06	0.62 ± 0.05	0.77 ± 0.03	93 ± 5
Rubber safety boots	23.3 ± 1.3	0.83 ± 0.04	0.66 ± 0.04	0.79 ± 0.02	95 ± 5
Walking in snow					
Winter jogging boots	48.1 ± 3.9	2.24 ± 0.18	2.16 ± 0.22	0.94 ± 0.02	151 ± 11
Rubber boots	48.6 ± 3.4	2.34 ± 0.17§	2.18 ± 0.21	0.92 ± 0.02	150 ± 11
Rubber safety boots	50.0 ± 3.2	2.34 ± 0.19§	2.22 ± 0.21	0.94 ± 0.02	151 ± 12

*The values are the mean ± SE for 10 subjects except the heart rate (HR) in snow where n = 9, $\dot{V}_E$, pulmonary ventilation (BTPS); $\dot{V}O_2$, oxygen consumption (STPD); $\dot{V}CO_2$, carbon dioxide production (STPD); R, respiratory gas exchange ratio (STPD).
†$P < .01$ compared with the rubber boots.
‡$P < .05$ compared with the rubber boots and rubber safety boots.
§$P < .01$ compared to winter jogging boots.
(Courtesy of Smolander J, Louhevaara V, Hakola T, et al: *Ergonomics* 32:3–13, January 1989.)

wearing 3 types of boots: winter jogging boots, rubber boots, and rubber safety boots. The boots weighed .9, 1.9, and 2.5 kg, respectively. The subjects wore the same clothing and walked at the same speed for each 10-minute trial.

Self-selected walking speeds did not correlate significantly with oxygen consumption, but walking in snow significantly increased the heart rate, pulmonary ventilation, oxygen consumption, carbon dioxide production, and respiratory gas exchange ratio compared with walking on a treadmill (table). The type of boot did not significantly affect pulmonary ventilation regardless of the surface; however, on both surfaces, oxygen consumption was slightly but systematically higher with the 2 heavier boots. In snow the difference was statistically significant. The mean heart rate was about 50 beats per minute greater when walking in snow than on the treadmill, but the type of boot worn was not significant. Overall, perceived exertion in snow varied from very very light to heavy. Safety boots are recommended for wear while performing potentially dangerous work because they provide greater protection.

▶ Walking is increasingly suggested as the most effective and practical endurance component of an exercise prescription, both for older individuals and for postcoronary patients. It is thus important to recognize that the energy cost and cardiac work-rate associated with a given walking speed is substantially influenced both by ground conditions and the type of footwear worn. Although snow boots may weigh only 2 kg, because they are on the legs rather than on the back they are lifted through a substantial distance at each stride, thus causing a disproportionate increase in the heart rate. If there has been a heavy fall of snow, the energy consumption may be 2 or 3 times greater than when walk ing in normal shoes on a dry sidewalk. Careful account must thus be taken of such changes when setting exercise prescriptions for winter conditions.—R.J. Shephard, M.D., Ph.D.

Exercise and Self-Esteem: Rationale and Model
Sonstroem RJ, Morgan WP (Univ of Rhode Island, Kingston; Univ of Wisconsin)
Med Sci Sports Exerc 21:329–337, June 1989   4–10

Self-esteem may be the feature most closely reflecting psychological benefit from regular exercise. A proposed model for examining mechanisms of change in self-esteem through exercise (Fig 4–3) is arranged in degrees of increasing situational generality, from physical self-efficacy to global self-esteem. As individuals engage in more activity and become more familiar with their responses to exercise, they become better able to make personal self-efficacy judgments. Physical competence refers to a general assessment of the self as possessing overall fitness. Acceptance reflects the degree of satisfaction with one's bodily processes.

It is hoped that weighting specific self-evaluations at all levels of self-conception by their perceived importance will yield greater associations with higher levels in this model than will ability ratings alone. For exam-

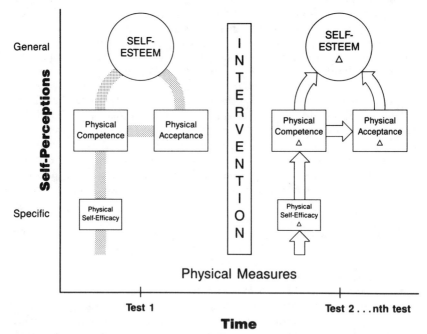

Fig 4–3.—Proposed model for examining exercise and self-esteem interactions. (Courtesy of Sonstroem RJ, Morgan WP: *Med Sci Sports Exercise* 21:329–337, June 1989.)

ple, it may be hypothesized that fitness is related more closely to physical self-efficacy than to physical competence, acceptance, or global self-esteem. Similarly, physical competence could relate closely to global self-esteem than physical self-efficacy or fitness. This model seems especially useful for studying the physically impaired. It is possible that changes in fitness directly influence self-esteem through an improved sense of health and well-being.

▶ When people are asked why they exercise, a common response is, "Because I feel better." Part of this sensation arises from an elevation of mood, associated with arousal (an increased proprioceptive input, a change of environment, and secretion of mood-altering chemicals). However, another important element is a change in perception of the self. A person may feel better able to carry out physical tasks, or proud of a slimmer waistline, and there is a narrowing of the gap between the perceived and the desired body image. All of these things add up to greater self-esteem. If exercise is to improve self-esteem, it is important that the objectives set for the individual are realistic. With an older person, a young exercise class leader who is very athletic and makes unrealistic demands on participants can have a negative effect on the older person's body image and self-esteem, particularly if the suggested training targets are not realized. There are thus advantages to matching the age of exercise class leaders with those of the average class member, and it is also helpful to match individual class members in terms of their initial levels of physical ability.—R.J. Shephard, M.D., Ph.D.

Added-Purpose Versus Rote Exercise in Female Nursing Home Residents
Yoder RM, Nelson DL, Smith DA (Inst of Physical Medicine and Rehabilitation, Peoria, Ill; Western Michigan Univ, Kalamazoo)
Am J Occup Ther 43:581–586, September 1989   4–11

Several recent studies have compared nonpurposeful exercise with exercise when individuals are told to pursue an added goal. Elderly female nursing home residents performed rotary arm exercise either alone or with the added purpose of stirring cookie dough. The 30 women had a mean age of 81.5 years. Functional capacity was assessed using the Parachek Geriatric Rating Scale.

The added-purpose, "occupationally embedded" exercise elicited significantly more repetitions than did rote exercise. Women performing rote exercise tended to stop more often than did those doing added-purpose exercise. These findings support the traditional view that it is a good idea to embed exercise within an occupational context.

▶ The real challenge of any exercise prescription is sustaining motivation, and activity that is built into the structure of the normal day is much less readily forgotten than exercise that requires special facilities. Although the conditions of the present study were somewhat artificial for both experimental and control groups, the results suggest that the idea that "cookies taste best when stirred for a long time" was enough to motivate a group of elderly women to engage in significantly longer periods of exercise before they stopped from "tiredness."—R.J. Shephard, M.D., Ph.D.

Effects of Resistive Training on Left Ventricular Function
Effron MB (Sinai Hosp of Baltimore)
Med Sci Sports Exerc 21:694–697, December 1989   4–12

Resistive training programs are popular, both among healthy adults and cardiac patients. Left ventricular (LV) function was assessed after acute resistive exercise and chronic resistive training.

Acute isometric exercise increases blood pressure but has little effect on LV function. In normal persons, dynamic exercise increases the stroke volume index to a greater extent and causes a greater decrease in systemic vascular resistance than acute isometric exercise. Resistive training effects on LV function appear to be related to training intensity. One training study of 10–12 weeks showed that LV mass index increased by 20% and LV wall thickness by 10%. Most resistive training studies, however, reveal no increase in LV volume and no changes in indices of LV systolic and diastolic function.

Hypertensive and cardiac patients who have normal LV function at rest have an increased LV mass index with resistive training and experience no adverse effects on LV systolic and diastolic function. There can be undesirable effects in patients with abnormal resting LV function. Although moderate levels of resistive training may be appropriate in cardiac rehabilitation, this type of training should be monitored closely in patients with abnormal LV function at rest. Resistive exercise in such patients may cause further dysfunction to develop.

▶ Although it is well recognized that certain types of endurance athletes have very large hearts (1), there is little evidence that such hypertrophy can result from the usual short-term laboratory training experiment. Ventricular hypertrophy undoubtedly arises from heavy afterloading (as in aortic or pulmonary stenosis), but such loads are imposed 24 hours per day rather than for the few minutes of exercise involved in a typical exercise program. It may thus be that certain athletes have inherited rather than earned a large heart, although there have also been suggestions that if these athletes retire from competition there is eventual regression to a more normal ventricular size.

If there is to be an effect from training, then a larger response might be anticipated in groups such as weight lifters, in whom the rise in blood pressure is much greater than in endurance activity. Only a limited amount of data (mostly cross-sectional) was available to Effron for this review, but it does seem to suggest that ventricular hypertrophy does develop in national and international level weight lifters. One issue not discussed here is the possible contribution of anabolic steroid abuse to this hypertrophy.

If hypertrophy is detected clinically, for example, on echocardiography, the question arises as to whether this is a healthy or an abnormal finding; if healthy, both systolic and diastolic function should remain within normal limits. If the patient has established coronary vascular disease, it may also be asked whether circuit training has acute adverse effects on myocardial performance. However, observations by Butler et al. (2) suggest that moderate isometric exercise does not increase wall motion abnormalities and is thus unlikely to cause severe myocardial ischemia.— R.J. Shephard, M.D., Ph.D.

References

1. Grimby G, Saltin B: *Acta Med Scand* 179:513, 1970.
2. Butler RM, et al: *J Cardiopulmonary Rehabil* 7:402, 1987.

Physiological Changes in Skeletal Muscle as a Result of Strength Training
Jones DA, Rutherford OM, Parker DF (Univ College London; Rayne Inst, London)
Q J Exp Physiol 74:233–256, 1989   4–13

All physical activities—sports and more usual everyday activities—require skill, strength, speed, and endurance. The goal of training is to match the mixture of these components to the particular needs of an activity and to a subject's deficiencies. The physiologic changes accompanying training for "explosive" events such as sprinting, jumping, and throwing, in which the chief aim is to maximize power output, were reviewed. An increase in power output of a muscle requires an increase in either the velocity of shortening or muscle strength, or both. The results of training are more evident in the training exercise itself than in objective measures of muscle size or strength.

In the initial phase of training the ability to perform the training exercise improves rapidly when the correct sequence of contractions is established as a motor pattern in the CNS. This process is highly specific. A phase of increased strength of individual muscles follows, with no concomitant increase in cross-sectional area. Increased neural activation or alterations in fiber arrangement or connective tissue content might be responsible. If training continues past about 12 weeks, both muscle size and strength increase slowly but steadily. This phase probably reflects some form of damage that leads to division of satellite cells and their incorporation into existing muscle fibers. The optimal combination of exercise type, intensity, and frequency remains a matter of individual choice for the athlete or patient who wishes to increase muscle size by weight training.

▶ This article provides a useful review of current knowledge of strength training, emphasizing the current orthodoxy that early gains of strength reflect improvement of muscular function rather than hypertrophy, although in a longer term perspective an appropriate regimen can induce true hypertrophy. To induce true hypertrophy, training must be pursued to the point of increased protein turnover, and possibly also disruption of the Z disks, with fiber splitting.

The margin between an effective training stimulus and an overload causing muscle damage is thus quite critical, calling for careful monitoring of the response to a given exercise prescription.—R.J. Shephard, M.D., Ph.D.

Effect of Running versus Isometric Training Programs on Healthy Elderly at Rest

Sagiv M, Fisher N, Yaniv A, Rudoy J (Zinman College at the Wingate Inst, Wingate, Israel)
Gerontology 35:72–77, March–June 1989   4–14

Although the effects of running exercise (REX) programs in elderly persons are well established, little information has been gathered on the cardiovascular effects of isometric exercise (IEX) programs using large muscle mass. Left ventricular and hemodynamic changes between IEX and REX training programs were compared in 40 healthy elderly persons at rest.

The study volunteers had taken part in a supervised aerobic program for at least 1 year, 3 times a week. They were randomly assigned to either an IEX group or an REX group. Training in the 12-week program was held 3 times a week for 30-minute periods. Five tests were administered—at baseline and at 3, 6, 9, and 12 weeks. The IEX program included weight lifting using large muscle mass at 30% of maximal voluntary contraction; the REX group had an aerobic exercise conditioning program at 70% of the maximum oxygen uptake.

Members of the REX group had a significant increase in maximal oxygen uptake at 12 weeks when compared with the IEX group (table). Body fat was significantly decreased in the REX group; lean body mass and total body mass did not change significantly in either group. The REX group had achieved significantly lower end-systolic volume values at posttraining measurement, whereas values were unchanged in the IEX group.

This comparison of the effects of REX and IEX training indicates than the maximum oxygen uptake can be improved in a healthy elderly popu-

	Physical Characteristics (Mean ± SD)			
	REX		IEX	
	pre	post	pre	post
Weight, kg	69.5 ± 7.6	68.0 ± 3.5	70.0 ± 10.2	70.5 ± 9.7
Fat, %	19.6 ± 6.1	15.1 ± 5.6*	20.3 ± 8	19.1 ± 5.6
LBM, kg	55.9 ± 7.4	58.3 ± 4.2	55.8 ± 5.8	56.5 ± 5.4
VO_2max, l/min	2.08 ± 0.37	2.36 ± 0.41*	2.12 ± 0.44	2.15 ± 0.35

Note: There were 20 persons in each of the 2 groups. *LBM,* lean body mass.
*$P < .05$.
(Courtesy of Sagiv M, Fisher N, Yaniv A, et al: *Gerontology* 35:72–77, March–June 1989.)

lation only through endurance exercise training programs. Nevertheless, weight-lifting programs are recommended for the healthy elderly at an intensity not to exceed 30% of the maximal voluntary contraction.

▶ Several recent reports have suggested that patients can undertake muscle-building exercise both after myocardial infarction and also in extreme old age. Evans of Tufts University has successfully used such a regimen in subjects older than 80 years. The big argument in favor of adding a muscle-building component to an exercise prescription is that aerobic training alone sometimes leads to loss of lean tissue from the inactive muscles.

The present report contains a number of surprises. Given that the subjects had been involved in a training program for at least 1 year before the experiment, it is remarkable that those undergoing aerobic training had about a 14% gain of maximal oxygen intake and a 2.4-kg increment in lean mass over a further 12 weeks of training. Further, it is puzzling that although various simple measurements of strength were made, the findings are not reported; one must presume that there were no changes, which leads one to question the effectiveness of the muscle-building regimen. The authors conclude ". . . we recommend the usage of [a] weight lifting program for [the] healthy elderly . . ."; however, they give no indication of how they leap from their results (which seem rather against muscle training) to this conclusion (which is more in line with much recent research).—R.J. Shephard, M.D., Ph.D.

5 Nutrition and Obesity

Sports Nutrition: Approaching the Nineties
Burke LM, Read RSD (Deakin Univ, Geelong, Victoria, Australia)
Sports Med 8:80–100, 1989   5–1

A relationship between diet and sports performance has long been recognized. An athlete's basic nutritional needs are determined largely by the training regimen. The concept of the "healthy," varied diet is basic, although the importance of a "balanced" diet for athletes in training remains controversial. The energy needs of individual athletes vary with their sex, age, body mass, and body composition. The most important variables are the type, intensity, frequency, and duration of activity.

Adequate stores of glycogen in muscle are a key performance factor in many sports. Longer-lasting activities raise the question of whether fuel stores can be increased beyond the normal maximum. Carbohydrate loading is an example. Carbohydrate intake during prolonged exercise enhances performance, but the mechanisms involved are not clear. Caffeine has been used before endurance exercise to stimulate the utilization of free fatty acids.

Many compounds, so-called ergogenic aids, reportedly enhance performance when taken just before exercise. Controlled trials have provided little evidence confirming the efficacy of such nonnutrients as ginseng, comfrey, and chlorophyll. Lacking direct physiologic banefit, the placebo effect or psychological stimulation of performance is worth considering.

▶ This is an excellent review of the subject matter. The interested reader is referred to the original article.—J.S. Torg, M.D.

Effect of Chronic Endurance Exercise on Retention of Dietary Protein
Friedman JE, Lemon PWR (Kent State Univ, Kent, Ohio)
Int J Sports Med 10:118–123, April 1989   5–2

During acute prolonged exercise there is an increase in amino acid oxidation that appears to be proportional to metabolic rate. Sedentary individuals embarking on an endurance training program require protein exceeding the recommended dietary allowance (RDA) to maintain a positive nitrogen balance. However, it has been observed that over the course of longer endurance training, nitrogen retention increases, which suggests that protein requirements might actually decrease with endurance training.

Five healthy, highly trained men who were long-distance runners had been in training for more than 5 years. Exchange values for 150 foods were calculated and organized into 6 meat-free groups: milk, vegetables, bread, protein, fruit, and fat. In 1 dietary trial the men consumed the

Daily Nitrogen Intake, Nitrogen Excretion, and Nitrogen Status*

Subject (#)	Nitrogen Intake (g/d)	Nitrogen Excretion (g/d)	Nitrogen Retention[†] (g/d)	Corrected Nitrogen Retention[‡] (g/d)
HI-PRO				
1	15.49 ± 2.22	5.70 ± 1.80	9.79 ± 2.27	5.11 ± 2.27
2	13.64 ± 1.06	6.37 ± 1.30	7.27 ± 2.88	4.77 ± 2.88
3	12.95 ± 1.31	7.70 ± 1.56	5.25 ± 2.49	0.79 ± 2.49
4	15.07 ± 2.19	8.62 ± 2.20	6.45 ± 1.53	1.29 ± 1.53
5	14.08 ± 1.57	10.80 ± 2.44	3.28 ± 3.93	0.07 ± 3.93
x̄ ± SE	14.25 ± 1.11	7.84 ± 1.34	6.41 ± 1.77	2.41 ± 1.99
REC-PRO				
1	5.17 ± 0.48	6.23 ± 0.72	−1.06 ± 1.06	−3.56 ± 1.06
2	8.04 ± 1.09	6.34 ± 0.22	1.70 ± 0.88	−0.80 ± 0.88
3	8.45 ± 0.98	8.21 ± 0.94	0.24 ± 0.42	−2.26 ± 0.42
4	9.17 ± 1.24	14.12 ± 1.18	−4.95 ± 2.41	−7.45 ± 2.41
5	8.26 ± 0.82	18.05 ± 1.03	−9.79 ± 1.31	−12.29 ± 1.31
w ± SE	7.82 ± 0.78 §	10.61 ± 2.53	−2.79 ± 2.58 §	−5.27 ± 2.58 §

*Values are means ± SE.
†Based on sweat and urinary urea nitrogen excretion.
‡Based on fecal nitrogen loss (2 g/day), miscellaneous nitrogen loss (0.5 g/day), and nitrogen retention because of excess energy consumption (0.72 mg nitrogen/kJ).
§$P < .005$ between dietary treatments.
(Courtesy of Friedman JE, Lemon PWR: *Int J Sports Med* 10:118–123, April 1989.)

Recommended Daily Allowance (RDA) of protein; in the other, the protein intake was 1.7 times higher. Each trial lasted for 6 days, with 2 weeks between trials. The men followed their regular exercise training programs, and on day 5 of each trial they completed a treadmill run of similar duration and intensity. Measurements were obtained for 72-hour urinary urea nitrogen loss on days 4, 5, and 6, and for exercise sweat urea nitrogen excretion on day 5.

With both diets, serum urea nitrogen and creatinine levels increased significantly during the treadmill run. There were no significant differences in sweat or urinary urea nitrogen excretion between the diets, although excretion of both tended to be higher with the RDA diet. However, combining nitrogen-excretion values and differences in protein intake yielded significant differences in estimated whole-body nitrogen retention between the 2 diets. Nitrogen retention remained positive during the high-protein trial but was significantly reduced during the RDA trial (table).

It is not possible to determine specific protein requirements for endurance athletes on the basis of this study, but findings show that high-intensity endurance training may call for more protein than that currently recommended. Further studies are needed to validate this observation.

▶ Exercise physiologists and nutritionists have for some years attacked the concept that the RDA of protein (originally designed for a sedentary individual) is adequate for the high-performance competitor. One major source of increased protein need during training is the synthesis of additional muscle, particularly in power athletes such as weight lifters and wrestlers (1). A second factor is the metabolism of amino acids for the purposes of gluconeogenesis, particularly in the long-distance competitor. The present report, unfortunately, was not able to correct data for fecal or miscellaneous nitrogen losses, but it did suggest a trend to greater nitrogen retention in endurance runners who consumed a high-protein diet relative to those who were consuming only the RDA. There thus seems some justification for allowing athletes extra protein, although this should not be pursued to the point of causing hypercholesterolemia.—R.J. Shephard, M.D., Ph.D.

Reference

1. Celejowa I, Homa M: *Nutr Metab* 12:259, 1970.

Protein and Energy Metabolism During Prolonged Exercise in Trained Athletes
Stein TP, Hoyt RW, O'Toole M, Leskiw MJ, Schluter MD, Wolfe RR, Hiller WDB (Univ of Medicine & Dentistry of New Jersey-School of Osteopathic Medicine, Camden; US Army Research Inst of Environmental Medicine, Natick, Mass; Healthplex, Memphis; Univ of Texas, Galveston)
Int J Sports Med 10:311–316, October 1989   5–3

Studies of animals subjected to exhaustive exercise showed a net breakdown of protein. The effect of strenuous exercise on protein metabolism in humans, however, is not clear. Previous studies did not use highly trained persons. Four male and 4 female triathlon athletes took part in endurance exercise under laboratory conditions to determine the effects on protein, glucose, and energy metabolism.

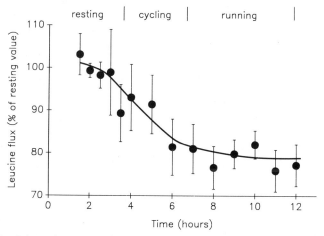

Fig 5–1.—Relative change in the plasma leucine flux with exercise (n = 8). The mean of the preexercise values = 100%. Data are mean and SEM. (Courtesy of Stein TP, Hoyt RW, O'Toole M, et al: *Int J Sports Med* 10:311–316, October 1989.)

During the exercise sessions 3 hours of bicycling were followed by 5 hours of level treadmill running. Before the session a primed constant infusion of $1\text{-}^{13}C$ leucine and $6,6\text{-}^2H$ glucose was started. Serial blood samples were obtained during rest and exercise for isotopic analysis. Oxygen consumption and carbon dioxide production were measured at half-hour intervals for 5 minutes.

All study participants completed the 8 hours of exercise. Some were extremely fatigued, but the level of exhaustion was probably less than that experienced at the end of a triathlon. The individuals exercised at an average of 53% × 3% of peak $\dot{V}O_2$ and expended about 5,100 kcal. During the 8-hour period glucose utilization declined and lipid oxidation increased. Most of the glucose oxidized during the first part of the exercise was of muscle origin. Hepatic glucose production rose from 20 g/hr to a maximum of 60 g/hr after 4 hours of exercise, then decreased toward the preexercise rate. No changes were seen in the plasma urea concentration.

After 3 to 4 hours of exercise the leucine flux decreased and then attained a new plateau (Fig 5–1). The final plateau leucine flux was about 20% less than baseline (preexercise) values. Although no major changes in protein balance were observed, an adaptive reduction occurred in protein turnover.

▶ Protein metabolism has classically been excluded from consideration as an important source of energy during exercise. However, in the past decade this has changed, largely because of the influence of 2 groups, i.e., Wolfe and colleagues from Galveston and Rennie and colleagues from Dundee, Scotland. Both groups have brought the modern technology of stable isotopes to the study of exercise largely by use of $1\text{-}^{13}C$ leucine.

In the present study of 8 hours of exercise—3 hours of cycling and 5 hours of treadmill running—there was a decline in glucose utilization and a progressive increase in lipid oxidation (Fig 5–1).

One area of controversy is the apparent conflict between the results of leucine metabolism in this study with those of Rennie et al., who found no change in leucine flux (1); in the present study there was a decrease to a new steady state after about 4 hours. There are several notable differences in the studies, not the least of which is the fitness of the subjects and the intensity of exercise used.—J.R. Sutton, M.D.

Reference

1. Rennie MJ, et al: *Clin Sci* 61:627, 1981.

Effect of Glucose Polymer Ingestion on Glycogen Depletion During a Soccer Match
Leatt PB, Jacobs I (Defence and Civil Inst of Environmental Medicine, Toronto)
Can J Sports Sci 14:112–116, June 1989   5–4

It is well established that depletion of muscle glycogen is related to impaired performance in both endurance and short-term, high-intensity exercise. To determine whether glucose feeding before or during exercise, or

Mean Muscle Concentration of Glycogen Before and After Soccer Match in Glucose-Treated (Experimental) and Placebo-Treated (Control) Players*

Group	n	Pre-game	Post-game	Change
Control	5	394±88	213±77	181±23
Experimental	5	351±71	240±56	111±24 †

Abbreviation: n, numbers.
*Millimoles of glucose units per kilogram of dry weight. Values are means ± SD.
†Significant between group difference: $P = .002$.
(Courtesy of Leatt PB, Jacobs I: *Can J Sports Sci* 14:112–116, June 1989.)

both, may delay or inhibit impaired performance, 2 soccer teams of 8 players each participated in an intrasquad exhibition match that consisted of 45-minute halves separated by a 10-minute half-time break. The study team received a 7% glucose polymer solution in a noncaloric orange drink; the control team received the same orange drink but with water added. Both teams had .5 L of their drink no more than 10 minutes before the game began and again at half-time. No other food or drinks were permitted.

Percutaneous needle biopsy specimens were obtained from the vastus lateralis muscle of 5 players from each team prior to the game before the drink was consumed and again within 45 minutes of the end of the game. The second biopsy specimen was obtained from the contralateral extremity. Venous blood was sampled from all players before the game and the prematch drink and within 20 minutes of the end of the game.

There was no difference in the concentration of glycogen between the teams before the match. After the match all players had decreased concentrations of glycogen, but the decrease was greater in the placebo group than in the study group (table). The blood level of glucose increased during the game, but there was no difference between the teams. Body mass decreased significantly during the game and the absolute and relative change in body mass was similar in both groups.

Ingestion of glucose reduces net utilization of muscle glycogen during performance of endurance sport and high-intensity exercise, does not harm performance, and may delay the onset of fatigue.

▶ Glycogen levels are important in games such as soccer and ice hockey in which repeated sprints are required. If muscle glycogen reserves fall toward the end of the game, a player feels tired and sprinting ability flags. Administration of a glucose/polymer preparation immediately before a game and at half-time should help to slow the rate of glycogen loss. The present data support this assumption. Blood glucose is also important to cerebral function, and there has been some suggestion that boosting the blood glucose can improve scoring performance through an action on the brain. On the other hand, if glucose is given too long before competition, it can provoke a large secretion of insulin, so that by the time the game begins the blood glucose levels may be lower in the treated than in the untreated player. The present results suggest that the potential handicap of hyperinsulinemia is avoided if the glucose/polymer solution is administered within 10 minutes of commencement of a game.— R.J. Shephard, M.D., Ph.D.

Oxidation of Corn Starch, Glucose, and Fructose Ingested Before Exercise

Guezennec CY, Satabin P, Duforez F, Merino D, Peronnet F, Koziet J (Centre d'Etudes et de Recherches de Médecine Aérospatiale, Paris; Univ of Montreal; Centre de Recherche Pernod Ricard, France)
Med Sci Sports Exerc 21:45–50, February 1989   5–5

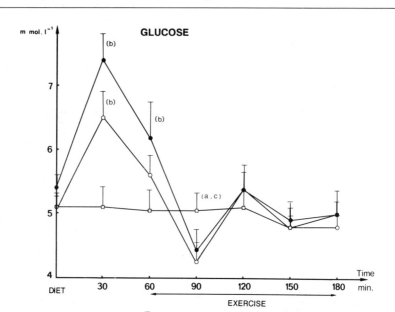

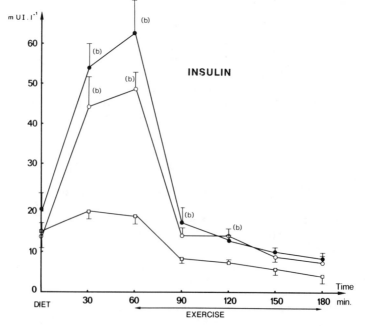

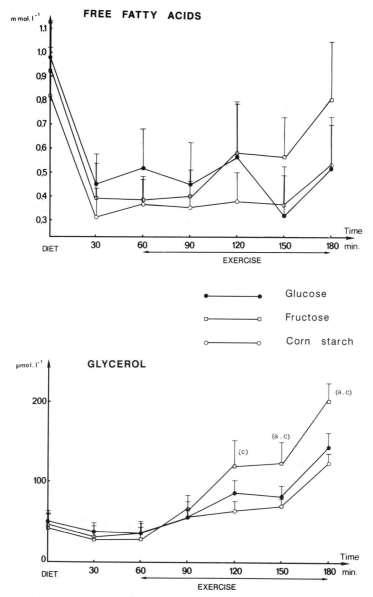

Fig 5–2.—Plasma insulin and blood metabolites for 3 hours (1 hour rest + 2 hours exercise at 60% of V̇O₂max) after ingestion of glucose, fructose, or pure corn starch. Results are means ± SEM of 6 determinations. $a = P < .05$ from glucose; $b = P < .05$ from fructose; $c = P < .05$ from starch. (Courtesy of Guezennec CY, Satabin P, Duforez F, et al: *Med Sci Sports Exerc* 21:45–50, February 1989.)

Endurance time to exhaustion during prolonged exercise can be increased by carbohydrate feeding. The inclusion of complex carbohydrates in preexercise meals may offer some advantages. The endocrine and metabolic responses and amounts of exogenous carbohydrate oxidized during prolonged moderate exercise when isoenergetic amounts of pure corn starch, glucose, or fructose were ingested 1 hour before exercise were investigated in 6 male physical education students. The men performed a series of 2-hour exercise bouts 3 times on a cycle ergometer at 1-week intervals. One hour before exercise, they ingested either 100 g of glucose or fructose diluted in water or 90 g of pure cornstarch in cake form, taken with water. Plasma glucose, expiratory gas, and blood glucose and glycerol were measured immediately before and at 30-minute intervals during exercise.

Plasma glucose and insulin concentrations increased significantly with glucose and cornstarch feedings. During the first hour of exercise the high plasma insulin values with these feedings caused a significant transient reduction in the plasma glucose concentration and blunted the response of plasma free fatty acid and glycerol concentrations (Fig 5–2). In contrast, fructose ingestion did not modify plasma glucose or insulin concentrations. During the 2-hour exercise period the percentages of exogenous glucose and starch oxidized were not significantly different but were significantly higher than the percentage of exogenous fructose oxidized.

Exogenous fructose is less available for oxidation than glucose or starch. As a preexercise meal, pure cornstarch offers no advantages over glucose.

▶ Athletes who ingest a large quantity of glucose shortly before a competition stimulate an outpouring of insulin. The blood glucose level falls as a result and their performance may be poorer than if they had refrained from taking carbohydrate. There are thus theoretical attractions to a meal containing complex carbohydrates (e.g., rice, corn, bread, lentils, or potatoes). It is argued that the increase in blood glucose develops more slowly, and there is less provocation of insulin secretion (1–3). The present experiment, with pure cornstarch, failed to confirm such expectations. The course of both blood glucose and insulin secretion was very similar whether the pregame diet contained glucose or cornstarch.

The authors' experiments also included fructose feeding. This avoids insulin secretion, but most of the carbohydrate then seems to pass to the liver, and there may also be gastrointestinal symptoms

As the authors point out, the physical properties of the food (e.g., the presence of fibers, particle size, and nature of the cuticule) may explain the discrepancy from earlier work. There thus is a need to repeat these studies using natural rather than prepared forms of complex carbohydrate.—R.J. Shephard, M.D., Ph.D.

References

1. Reaven GM: *Am J Clin Nutr* 32:2568, 1979.
2. O'Dea K, et al: *Am J Clin Nutr* 33:760, 1980.
3. Goddard MS, et al: *Am J Clin Nutr* 39:388, 1984.

Effects of 4 H Preexercise Carbohydrate Feedings on Cycling Performance
Sherman WM, Brodowicz G, Wright DA, Allen WK, Simonsen J, Dernbach A
(Ohio State Univ)
Med Sci Sports Exerc 21:598–604, October 1989   5–6

Carbohydrate consumption up to 4 hours before exercise causes increased carbohydrate combustion that may contribute to premature fatigue. Carbohydrate oxidation during exercise may be variable, depending on the amount of carbohydrate and the degree of insulinemia produced.

Nine men and 1 woman participated in experiment 1, and 8 men and 2 women participated in experiment 2. All were young adult recreational cyclists. Each cyclist completed 3 exercise trials on a cycle ergometer 1 to 2 weeks apart. Four hours before exercise, those in experiment 1 consumed either 45 (L) or 156 (M) of carbohydrate in isoenergetic liquid form. In experiment 2, the group consumed either a noncarbohydrate placebo or 312 (H) g of carbohydrate in liquid form.

One hour after all feedings the blood glucose level had reached baseline. The blood insulin concentration reached baseline 3 hours after ingestion of placebo, L, and M; however, after ingestion of H, blood insulin was still 84% higher at the start of exercise than after ingestion of

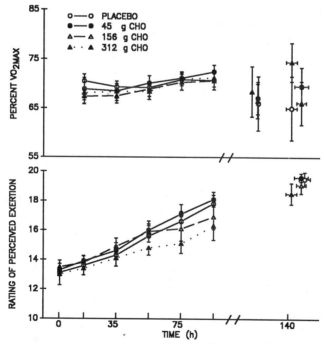

Fig 5–3.—Oxygen consumption and perceived exertion during exercise. Research subjects consumed various amounts of carbohydrate 4 hours before exercise. (Courtesy of Sherman WM, Brodowicz G, Wright DA, et al: *Med Sci Sports Exerc* 21:598–604, October 1989.)

placebo. During exercise, insulin averaged 48% higher with H than with placebo.

With placebo, L, and M, the blood glucose concentration decreased by 16% during exercise. With H there was a transient drop during the first 15 minutes of exercise, after which glucose increased and remained constant throughout exercise. More carbohydrate oxidation occurred during exercise when H was ingested than when placebo was ingested. Results for L and M were similar. The ingestion of H improved performance by 15% as compared with placebo; however, performance was similar whether L or M was ingested. There was a trend toward a lower rating of perceived exertion beginning at 55 minutes of exercise after ingestion of H (Fig 5−3).

Individuals who consume 312 g of carbohydrate 4 hours before prolonged, moderately intense exercise may improve their performance, although insulin levels may be elevated. Improved performance may be caused by enhanced carbohydrate oxidation.

▶ The timing of carbohydrate supplements before competition seems very critical. The worst time to give carbohydrate seems to be about 45 minutes before competing; the scenario of hyperinsulinemia and declining blood glucose levels is then unleashed (1). If carbohydrate is given 5–10 minutes before an event, the plasma insulin level rises, but there is an increase in the blood glucose level and enhancement of performance (2). The present report also shows a useful influence of high doses of carbohydrate (312 g) if taken 4 hours before exercise; on a cycle ergometer the rating of perceived exertion was appreciably lower, and the time required to complete a given task was shorter. There is now a need to take these concepts from the exercise physiology laboratory to the track.—R.J. Shephard, M.D., Ph.D.

References

1. Costill DL, et al: *J Appl Physiol* 43:695, 1977.
2. Snyder AC, et al: *Med Sci Sports Exerc* 15:S126, 1983.

Muscle Glycogen Storage Postexercise: Effect of Mode of Carbohydrate Administration
Reed MJ, Brozinick JT Jr, Lee MC, Ivy JL (Univ of Texas, Austin)
J Appl Physiol 66:720–726, February 1989   5−7

Adequate muscle glycogen reserves are necessary for optimum performance during prolonged exercise of at least moderate intensity. Carbohydrate supplements given at 2-hour intervals during the first 6 hours after exercise result in a relatively consistent rate of muscle glycogen storage. However, increasing the amount of supplement does not increase the rate of storage. To determine whether gastric emptying limits the rate of glycogen storage during the first 4 hours after exercise when a carbohydrate supplement is provided and to determine whether liquid and solid carbo-

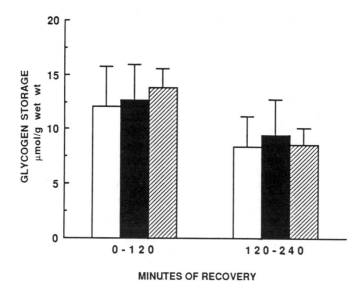

MINUTES OF RECOVERY

Fig 5–4.—Glycogen storage rates during each 120 minutes of recovery for liquid treatment *(open bars)*, solid treatment *(filled bars)*, and infusion treatment *(hatched bars)*. (Courtesy of Reed MJ, Brozinick JT Jr, Lee MC, et al: *J Appl Physiol* 66:720–726, February 1989.)

hydrate feedings result in different storage rates after exercise, 8 male college students (average age, 20 years) exercised for 2 hours on cycle ergometer on 3 separate occasions to deplete muscle glycogen stores.

After each session they received either a liquid or solid carbohydrate feeding or an intravenous glucose infusion. The liquid and solid feedings, divided into 2 equal doses, were given immediately after and 2 hours after exercise. In the infusion trial glucose was infused at a constant rate for all but 5 minutes of the 4-hour recovery period. Blood samples were drawn before and during exercise and throughout recovery, and muscle biopsy specimens were taken immediately after and at 2 and 4 hours after exercise.

With all treatments blood levels of glucose and insulin declined during exercise and increased significantly above preexercise levels during recovery. However, the increase in the blood level of glucose was 3 times greater with infusion than with the other 2 treatments. The average insulin response with the liquid feeding was significantly greater than with the solid feeding, but it was not significantly greater than with the infusion treatment. During the first 2 hours of recovery there were no significant differences in muscle glycogen storage rates regardless of the treatment (Fig 5–4).

The rate of muscle glycogen storage is similar whether carbohydrate supplements administered after exercise are in liquid or solid form. The rate of storage under these conditions is not limited by the gastric emptying rate of the supplement.

▶ Athletes who must compete in a series of heats of glycogen-depleting exercise (e.g., players in a soccer competition) gain a significant advantage if they are able to replenish muscle glycogen reserves rapidly. With the usual diet it may take as long as 48 hours for muscle glycogen reserves to reach a plateau value.

The initial rate of resynthesis noted here, about 1 mmol/min, is generally comparable with previous reports regarding glycogen-depleted subjects, although occasionally early resynthesis rates as high as 25 mmol/kg wet weight/hr (up to 10 mmol/min) have been reported (1,2).

The main objective of the present experiment was to determine whether gastric emptying of glucose-containing meals limits early glycogen replenishment. Because the rate of resynthesis was not greater with carbohydrate infusion, it was concluded that gastric emptying was not a limiting factor. However, one puzzling feature of the report is that more than half of the infused glucose failed to enter the depleted muscles. Possibly, much of the early intake of carbohydrate, whether infused or ingested, is used to replenish liver glycogen reserves.—R.J. Shephard, M.D., Ph.D.

References

1. Bergstrom J, Hultman E: *Acta Med Scand* 182:93, 1967.
2. Roch-Norland AE, et al: *Scand J Lab Clin Invest* 30:77, 1972.

Exercise Reverses Depressed Metabolic Rate Produced by Severe Caloric Restriction
Molé PA, Stern JS, Schultz CL, Bernauer EM, Holcomb BJ (Univ of California, Davis)
Med Sci Sports Exerc 21:29–33, February 1989   5–8

The rate of weight loss declines as the restriction of energy intake is prolonged, but the metabolic adaptations involved are uncertain. Restriction of food intake does lower energy expenditure, which could partly explain the decreased loss of body mass. If exercise increases the resting metabolic rate, it could help obese persons to lose body fat. A study was designed to show whether the decline in metabolic rate attending dietary restriction can be reserved by daily exercise.

Five obese patients with up to 42% body fat were studied during weight maintenance, after dietary restriction to 2 megajoules (500 kcal) daily, after dietary restriction with exercise added, and after a brief period of increased food intake without exercise. The exercise required an expenditure of about 600–800 kJ (150–200) kcal) daily.

The patients lost 5.5% of initial body mass in the first 2 weeks of dietary restriction and another 3.3% during the exercise period. The metabolic rate declined initially but increased during the exercise period (table). The respiratory quotient decreased with diet and exercise, and the rate of fat oxidation of resting metabolism increased progressively.

Daily exercise can reverse the depression in resting metabolic rate associated with severe dietary restriction. Energy expenditure and fat oxidation are stimulated, leading to a reduction in body fat.

Metabolic Responses During Predietary Control Period (Period 1),
Week 2 of 500-kcal Diet Without Exercise (Period 2), and Week 4
of 500-kcal Diet With Daily Exercise (Period 3)*

| | Resting Metabolic Rate | | | Resting Fat Oxidation |
Period	(ml $O_2 \cdot min^{-1} \cdot M^{-0.67}$)	(kcal $\cdot h^{-1} \cdot M^{-0.67}$)	R	(kcal $\cdot h^{-1} \cdot M^{-0.67}$)
1	12.7 ± 0.25^a	3.68 ± 0.067^a	0.82 ± 0.015^a	2.22 ± 0.204^a
2	11.1 ± 0.25^b	3.16 ± 0.069^b	0.75 ± 0.013^b	2.64 ± 0.169^b
3	13.0 ± 0.33^a	3.67 ± 0.083^a	0.73 ± 0.013^b	3.38 ± 0.216^c

*Values are means $\pm$ SEM for the group (n = 5) computed from each person's average for 10, 7, and 7 days during periods 1, 2, and 3, respectively. The F-ratios of analysis of variance were significant ($P < .05$) for all metabolic variables. Means with different superscripts are significantly different from each other ($P < .05$). R is the respiratory quotient at rest.

(Courtesy of Molé PA, Stern JS, Schultz CL, et al: *Med Sci Sports Exerc* 21:29–33, February 1989.)

▶ One of the excuses available to those who have difficulty in losing excess fat is that dietary restriction induces a decrease of resting metabolism that completely negates any sacrifices that are made at the dinner table. The impact of dieting on metabolic rate varies from one person to another. It is more marked in those who have a tendency to obesity, but it usually does not exceed a 15% decrease of resting metabolism—about 900 megajoules or 220 calories per day. If a person adheres to a stringent diet, loss of what the Germans have termed the "Luxuskonsumption" cannot therefore avert the resultant decrease in body fat. Nevertheless, it is encouraging to find the present paper confirming the idea that one of the many benefits of exercise as a treatment of obesity is that it reverses the tendency for the resting metabolic rate to fall during periods of negative energy balance. As in many other studies, there were also dramatic differences in the composition of the metabolized tissue. Diet alone leads to a 5.5% decrease of mass, but 3.0% of the loss is lean tissue. In contrast, diet plus exercise leads to an 8.8% loss, with 7.3% of this being fat and only 1.5% lean tissue. It is encouraging that the amount of exercise needed to increase resting metabolism, 600–800 kJ/day, is very modest and well within the compass of most obese patients.—R.J. Shephard, M.D., Ph.D.

Diet-Induced Thermogenesis in Well-Trained Subjects

Thörne A, Wahren J (Karolinska Inst; Huddinge Univ Hosp, Stockholm)
Clin Physiol 9:295–305, June 1989   5–9

The possible relationship between the thermogenic response to a mixed meal and aerobic power in healthy subjects was examined in 7 well-trained and 7 sedentary young men aged 18–30 years. Maximum oxygen uptake was determined on a cycle ergometer.

The average maximum oxygen intake in the well-trained group was 58 mL/kg · min; in the sedentary group it was 39 mL/kg · min. Respiratory gas exchange was measured at baseline for 1 hour and for 3 hours after the meal. All subjects ingested a liquid meal consisting of 17% kJ of pro-

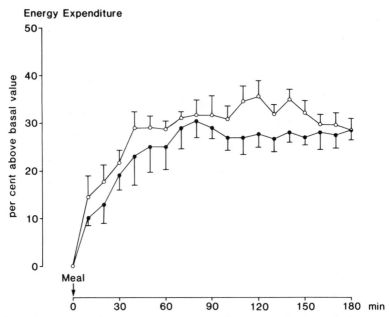

Fig 5–5.—Energy expenditure after mixed meal in well-trained *(filled circles)* and sedentary *(open circles)* subjects. Data are expressed as percent above basal value. (Courtesy of Thörne A, Wahren J: *Clin Physiol* 9:295–305, June 1989.)

tein, 28% kJ of lipids, and 55% kJ of carbohydrates in amounts corresponding to 60% of their individual 24-hour basal energy expenditure.

Basal oxygen uptake and energy expenditure were comparable in the 2 groups. After the meal energy expenditure and pulmonary oxygen uptake rose rapidly, reaching a plateau after 1 hour. There was no significant difference between the groups. The average rise in pulmonary oxygen uptake above baseline during the study was 24% in well-trained subjects and 26.7% in sedentary subjects. Similarly, energy expenditure rose by 25% and 29%, respectively (Fig 5–5). There was no apparent relationship between an individual thermogenic response and maximal oxygen intake in these healthy young men.

▶ A lack of dietary and/or exercise-induced thermogenesis has become a popular excuse for those patients who have difficulty in losing excess body fat. The present report suggests that when individuals are classified in terms of their aerobic power (mL/kg . min), there is little difference in dietary thermogenesis between the "fit" and the "unfit." Unfortunately, no information is given on differences of obesity between the 2 groups, but the sedentary subjects were much heavier (81 vs 69 kg). Another criticism of the paper is that data are compared in terms of percentages above basal values. However, the resting metabolism is substantially higher in the fit subjects, so that the *absolute* increase of metabolism in response to a meal is indeed greater in those who are fit than in those who are not.—R.J. Shephard, M.D., Ph.D.

6 Environmental and Psychological Factors

Effects of 100% Oxygen on Performance of Professional Soccer Players
Winter FD Jr, Snell PG, Stray-Gunderson J (Baylor Univ, Dallas; Univ of Texas, Dallas)
JAMA 262:227–229, July 14, 1989
6–1

A number of studies have analyzed the effects of oxygen administered during exercise, but few have addressed the effects of oxygen given after exercise is completed or administered between periods of exercise. Bouts of exhaustive exercise coupled with the random use of supplemental oxygen or room air immediately afterward were studied in 12 members of a professional indoor soccer team when they were in peak physical condition.

Before exercise blood samples were drawn to determine the baseline concentration or lactate. Each athlete warmed up for 3 minutes, rested briefly, then ran on a treadmill at 8.5 mph. The grade was increased by 2% per minute; the athletes ran to exhaustion. During exercise they ventilated through a mouthpiece open to room air. At exhaustion they were seated while a venous blood sample was drawn; then they breathed either compressed humidified air or 100% humidified oxygen. A randomized crossover design was used. Oxygen uptake was measured and reported every 30 seconds. After 4 minutes the concentration of lactate was again measured in blood samples. Subjects repeated the treadmill exercise before another blood sample was drawn at exhaustion. The entire procedure was repeated after 3 to 4 hours, with the subject receiving the opposite unidentified gas.

Administration of enriched oxygen during the recovery period had no effect on plasma level of lactate or performance on the second exercise test. The athletes could not identify which gas they had received at either session. The short-term use of 100% oxygen during recovery from exhaustive exercise offers no recovery benefits, nor does it improve subsequent exercise performance.

▶ The authors theorize that oxygen on the sideline will not improve performance or recovery rate because ". . . hemoglobin's strong affinity for oxygen leaves little room for improvement in extracting oxygen from inhaled gas."—F.J. George, ATC, PT

An Outbreak of Nitrogen Dioxide-Induced Respiratory Illness Among Ice Hockey Players

Hedberg K, Hedberg CW, Iber C, White KE, Osterholm MT, Jones DBW, Flink JR, MacDonald KL (Centers for Disease Control, Atlanta; Minnesota Dept of Health, Minneapolis; Hennepin County Med Ctr, Minneapolis; Pulmonary Health Associates, St Paul)
JAMA 262:3014–3017, Dec 1, 1989   6–2

Outbreaks of nitrogen dioxide-induced respiratory illness are rare. In February 1987 such an outbreak occurred among players and spectators at 2 high school hockey games played at an indoor ice arena. Malfunctioning of a Zamboni ice resurfacer's engine was identified as the source of the nitrogen dioxide. Several team members experienced the acute onset of cough, hemoptysis, or chest pain during or immediately after the games.

Questionnaires were administered to all hockey team members, cheerleaders, and band members who attended the games. Information was collected on symptoms, onset and duration of each symptom, general health status, length of time in the arena, and location in the arena during the games. All interviews were completed within 10 days after the participants had attended a game at the arena. Spirometry was performed within 10 days of exposure and again 2 months afterward on all members of a hockey team with a single exposure and those of a team with multiple exposures. Control data were obtained from members of an unexposed basketball team.

Questionnaires were completed on 92 hockey players with a single exposure, 34 hockey players with multiple exposures, 16 cheerleaders, and 25 band members. Overall, 116 patients were identified. Cough was reported by 97% of those having a single exposure. The mean duration of cough was 16 days in those with a single acute exposure and 41 days in those with multiple exposures. However, no differences in lung function were seen between the 2 exposed hockey teams and the control basketball team. Ten patients had follow-up physician visits, but none had ongoing signs or symptoms.

The problem of nitrogen dioxide exposure in indoor ice arenas may be more common than has been recognized, because respiratory symptoms caused by such exposure are generally mild and nonspecific and are thus easily misdiagnosed. Only 3 states currently monitor air quality in ice arenas on a routine basis.

▶ Carbon monoxide intoxication in ice arenas has been reported previously (1,2). Presumably, such occurrences are caused by exhaust from the gasoline internal combustion engine. In this important case, the ice resurfacer was powered by a propane internal combustion engine. If these engines are not properly tuned and the fuel mix in the carburetor receives too little oxygen, elevated levels of carbon monoxide may be produced. However, if the mixture has too much oxygen, elevated levels of nitrogen oxide may be produced. In any event, the potential problems presented by both the gasoline and propane internal combustion engines in an indoor arena have been documented. However, although there are somewhere on the order of 800 indoor ice arenas in the United States, only 3 states presently monitor the air quality on a routine basis. As the authors point out, respiratory symptoms associated with nitrogen dioxide may be relatively mild, nonspecific, and unrecognized. The suggestion that ice resurfacing equipment be properly maintained, ice arenas adequately ventilated, and regulations be implemented requiring routine exhaust emission checks of ice resurfacers are well taken.—J.S. Torg, M.D.

References

1. Centers for Disease Control: *MMWR* 33:49, 1984.
2. Kwok PW: *Can Gen Public Health* 74:261, 1983.

Radio Frequency (13.56 MHz) Energy Enhances Recovery From Mild Hypothermia
Hesslink RL Jr, Pepper S, Olsen RG, Lewis SB, Homer LD (Naval Med Research Inst, Bethesda, Md; Naval Aerospace Med Research Lab, Pensacola, Fla)
J Appl Physiol 67:1208–1212, September 1989   6–3

The rate of warming after hypothermia depends on what is used as a rewarming source. Hot water immersion is a standard method for actively rewarming hypothermic individuals, but this method has limited applications in field use. The insulated sleeping bags currently used to rewarm victims of hypothermia require the individual's own limited body heat for rewarming. Recent advances in radiofrequency (RF) energy (13.56 MHz) delivery systems have shown great promise in animal studies; therefore, the effectiveness of RF energy as a rewarming source was assessed in 6 healthy volunteers.

After fasting overnight, 6 men (median age, 25 years) wearing bathing trunks were instrumented with esophageal, rectal, and surface skin temperature probes. Each study participant was immersed to nipple level in a well-stirred cold water tank until their rectal temperatures had dropped by .5° C. Each man was then removed from the tank, lightly towel dried, and rewarmed for 60 minutes using either RF energy, immersion in hot water at 41° C, or wrapping in an insulated cocoon. Blood samples were collected 30 minutes after insertion of an indwelling catheter into the antecubital vein, just before removal from cold water, and at 5, 10, 30, and 60 minutes into the rewarming period. Each man served as his own control for 3 rewarming trials, which were also recorded on video cassette for determination of a shivering response.

Radiofrequency energy warmed the thoracic cavity faster than either hot water or an insulated cocoon. Thus the potential for cardiac arrhythmias associated with low core temperature may be diminished when RF rewarming is used after hypothermia. Rectal temperatures did not increase as rapidly as did esophageal temperatures. Each man immediately stopped shivering upon entry into hot water tank. When RF warming was used, moderate intermittent shivering was observed during the first

30 minutes but not during the last 30 minutes of the rewarming period. With use of the insulated cocoon, all men were observed to shiver throughout the entire 60-minute rewarming period. Radio frequency rewarming appears to be a promising alternative for rewarming victims of hypothermia in the field.

▶ A novel way to rewarm the hypothermic patient that conceivably could have application in the field.—J.R. Sutton, M.D.

Responses to Dehydration and Rehydration During Heat Exposure in Young and Older Men

Miescher E, Fortney SM (Johns Hopkins Univ)
Am J Physiol 257:R1050–R1056, 1989   6–4

Elderly persons often have a diminished capacity to respond effectively to environmental stress and to maintain homeostasis. Increasing age might influence heat tolerance because of an inability to maintain adequate hydration. The effect of moderate dehydration and rehydration on body fluid responses was examined in younger and older men subject to passive heat stress.

Five men aged 61–67 years and 6 men aged 21–29 years were matched for height, weight, body surface area, and moderate level of aerobic fitness. They were outfitted with a heart rate monitor and a thermistor rectal probe connected to a portable monitor. The men drank 200 mL of water and rested for 30 minutes before beginning experiments. They then rested in a hot dry chamber for 180 minutes without water; cool water was allowed ad libitum for the final 60 minutes, after which final measurements were taken.

Before heat exposure and after 30 minutes of rest, the older men had significantly lower rectal temperatures than younger men. Rectal temperatures increased significantly in both groups during the period of dehydration. During the first 30 minutes of heat exposure, younger men maintained body temperature, but older men immediately began to store heat. Both the rate and magnitude of increase in rectal temperatures was greater in older men than in younger men (Fig 6–1). The total body sweat rate did not differ between groups, however. After 180 minutes of heat exposure, both groups had similar mild dehydration rates. Before heat exposure plasma osmolality values were greater in older men, but after exposure the plasma volume decreased and plasma osmolality increased to a greater extent in older men (Fig 6–2). Water debt was similarly replaced in both groups on rehydration, but in younger men plasma volume and plasma osmolality were restored within 30 minutes, whereas in older men 60 minutes were required to restore plasma osmolality and 90 minutes to restore plasma volume. Despite higher rectal temperatures and greater change in plasma volume and plasma osmolality in older men, they rated themselves less thirsty and not significantly warmer than their younger counterparts.

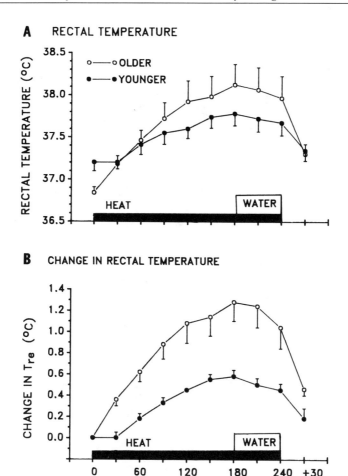

A RECTAL TEMPERATURE

B CHANGE IN RECTAL TEMPERATURE

Fig 6–1.—Absolute and relative changes in rectal temperature during heat exposure. **A,** except for initial preheat-exposure temperature ($P < .05$), there were no differences in rectal temperatures between older and younger men at any time during heat exposure. **B,** rectal temperatures increased more rapidly and to a significantly greater degree in older than in younger men ($P < .01$). (Courtesy of Miescher E, Fortney SM: *Am J Physiol* 257:R1050–R1056, 1989.)

Aging results in a diminished capacity to maintain rectal temperature during exposure to heat. Under conditions of thermal dehydration and rehydration, physiologic responses are poorly controlled and perceptual responses are altered. Older persons exposed to prolonged heat may be more susceptible to heat stress because of direct impairment of heat loss mechanisms, compounded by an inability to adequately maintain plasma volume and osmolality.

▶ If young men have to contend with "fine down below," older men have to contend with "fire within." This study shows that older men are more vulnerable to heat stress: Their rectal temperature climbs faster, their plasma

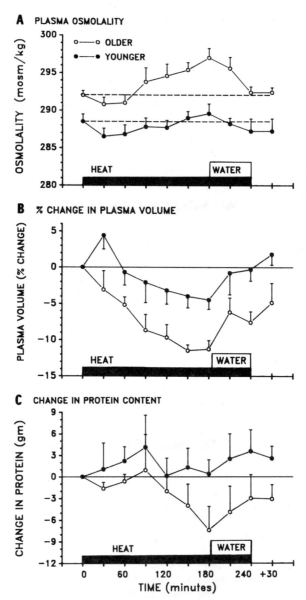

Fig 6–2.—Changes in plasma osmolality, relative plasma volume, and plasma protein content during course of heat exposure. **A,** increase in plasma osmolality was greater in older than in younger men ($P <$ .01). **B,** plasma volume decreased to a greater extent in older than in younger men ($P <$ .02). **C,** plasma protein content did not change significantly in younger men and decreased significantly in older men only after 150 minutes in heat ($P <$ .05). (Courtesy of Miescher E, Fortney SM: *Am J Physiol* 257:R1050–R1056, 1989.)

volume falls faster, and their plasma osmolality rises faster. Despite this, older men rate themselves as less thirsty and no hotter than their younger counterparts. As we age, it seems, homeostasis comes harder. This study has clinical implications for older men who exercise in the heat.—E.R. Eichner, M.D.

Evidence of Prolonged Myocardial Dysfunction in Heat Stroke
Zahger D, Moses A, Weiss AT (Hadassah Univ Hosp, Mt Scopus, Jerusalem)
Chest 95:1089–1091, May 1989   6–5

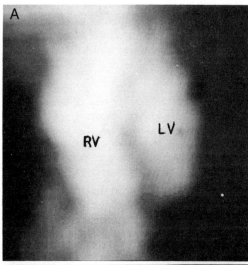

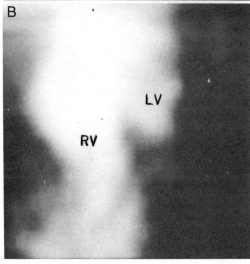

Fig 6–3.—The RVG in described patient; left anterior oblique projection, showing end-diastolic (**A**) and end-systolic (**B**) views. There is dilatation and diffuse hypocontractility of the right ventricle. (Courtesy of Zahger D, Moses A, Weiss AT: *Chest* 95:1089–1091, May 1989.)

Heat stroke is a potentially fatal condition that affects mostly military recruits, athletes, laborers, alcoholics, and elderly persons on exposure to high temperature. Cardiac failure is rare, but the heart may be involved in multiorgan damage, which has been shown pathologically and enzymatically, as well as by ECG. Two patients sustained heat stroke that was complicated by heart failure. Prolonged myocardial dysfunction, mainly right-sided, was demonstrated by right ventriculography (RVG).

Case 1.—Man, 18, military recruit, had been exercising in ambient temperature of 40° C on the morning of admission. He had 2 episodes of diarrhea that morning and complained of extreme fatigue. The ECG revealed only sinus tachycardia, and pulmonary edema developed. He was treated for heat stroke complicated by pulmonary edema. Ten hours after admission, RVG showed a left ventricular ejection fraction (LVEF) of 72%, the right ventricular ejection fraction (RVEF) was 32% (Fig 6–3). After discharge and an uneventful recovery, the patient underwent a repeat RVG 16 days later that showed an LVEF of 61%; the RVEF was 43%, and the right ventricle was still dilated. Twelve weeks later, findings on RVG and the LVEF were normal.

Case 2.—Male soldier, admitted to the hospital after having collapsed during physical training on a hot day, was given the diagnosis of heat exhaustion. The ECG showed only sinus tachycardia. Peripheral edema developed. Right ventriculography performed 1 month later showed an RVEF of 43%. The right ventricle was dilated.

These 2 cases illustrate the possibility of subclinical myocardial depression persisting for weeks after the onset of heat stroke. The more severe injury to the right ventricle, combined with other pathologic data, may indicate that it is more vulnerable than the left in heat stroke. Hemodynamically compromised victims of heat stroke should be evaluated by echocardiography or RVG. If impaired myocardial contractility is found, the patient should be followed until the abnormality resolves.

▶ These 2 cases represent physiologic cardiac impairment in heat stroke. Although pathologic studies in fatal heat stroke have demonstrated cardiac pathology such as subendocardial hemorrhages with myocyte necrosis, there have been few studies such as this one of cardiac pathophysiology in the survivors.—J.R. Sutton, M.D.

Ergonomic Aspects of Cold Stress and Cold Adaptation
Budd GM (Natl Inst of Occupational Health and Safety, Univ of Sydney, Australia)
Scand J Work Environ Health 15(suppl 1):15–26, August 1989   6–6

Problems of clothing and adaptation continue to compromise the safety of persons who live and work in cold regions. Although laboratory simulations of cold stress and adaptation are relatively simple, the real world of

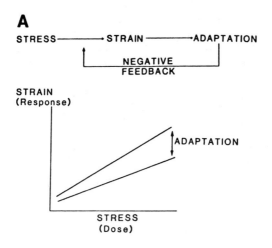

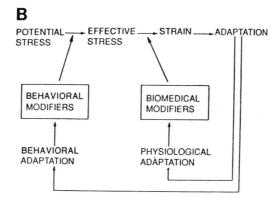

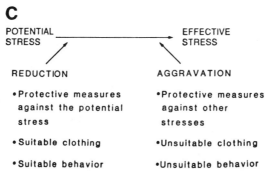

Fig 6–4.—Stress, strain, and adaptation, the basic idea (**A**), possible complications (**B**), and behavioral modifiers (**C**). (Courtesy of Budd GM: *Scand J Work Environ Health* 15(suppl 1):15–26, August 1989.)

individual behavior is much more complex (Fig 6–4). The most direct way of obtaining evidence of acquired general acclimatization is to expose subjects to controlled cold stress at different times and compare the responses.

Some believe that cold is not a problem even in the Antarctic when persons are given adequate fur clothing, but others—such as those in Scott's ill-fated expedition—would disagree. Thermal discomfort tends to be exaggerated during strenuous activities such as dog sledging and backpacking. Modern Antarctic clothing greatly reduces cold stress but does not eliminate it.

All 8 Antarctic field studies reviewed showed significant changes in the responses to cold that were consistent with increased tissue insulation. The changes differ from those that accompany physical training. The metabolic rate and the metabolic response to cold do not increase, and there is no evidence of nonshivering thermogenesis. Studies that provide more precise data on changes in tissue insulation and the peripheral circulation will be helpful.

▶ Environmental physiologists, the adventurous, and all those with an appreciation of classic physiology will find this review by Grahame Budd rewarding. The author has been a member of no fewer than 8 scientific expeditions to the Antarctic, including making the first ascent of Big Ben on Heard Island in 1963, and is thus well qualified to review this topic.

A number of salient points emerged, some of which are not obvious to the armchair explorer or physiologist. Travelers and workers in the Antarctic must rely on clothing and shelter for their thermal protection, and the physiologic adaptations, while potentially important, are of far less significance. However, the very nature of the clothing and the shelter must ensure that what provides thermal comfort at rest will guarantee thermal discomfort on exercise. Behavioral regulation, by adjusting clothing and seeking shelter, is the only way of surviving in the Antarctic environment.

Budd has concluded that more than half the time persons will experience thermal discomfort, but that it is attributable equally to heat and cold. During a summer dog sledge trip persons felt too hot more than 50% of the time, with rectal temperatures up to 38.7°C. *Ironically, in the subzero Antarctic cold they became acclimatized to heat!*

Other important conclusions are that acclimatization to cold does occur in the Antarctic, and that the process of this acclimatization is through increased physiologic insulation caused by vasoconstriction, unlike many animal adaptations of increasing insulation by fat and increasing their metabolic rate.—J.R. Sutton, M.D.

Thermoregulation During Cold Water Immersion Is Unimpaired by Low Muscle Glycogen Levels
Young AJ, Sawka MN, Neufer PD, Muza SR, Askew EW, Pandolf KB (US Army Research Inst of Environmental Medicine, Natick, Mass)
J Appl Physiol 66:1809–1816, April 1989   6–7

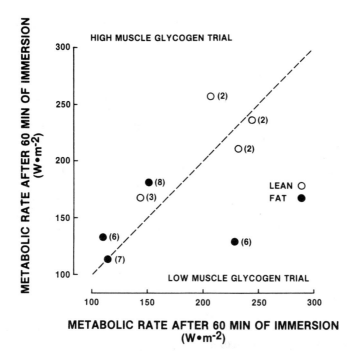

Fig 6–5.—Comparison of individual metabolic rates after 60 minutes of cold water immersion in low muscle glycogen and high muscle glycogen trials. Dashed line indicates line of identity. Lean subjects *(light circles)* have ≤ 12% body fat, and fat subjects *(dark circles)* have ≥ 17% body fat. Value in parentheses beside each symbol is mean thickness of subcutaneous fat for the subject. (Courtesy of Young AJ, Sawka MN, Neufer PD, et al: *J Appl Physiol* 66:1809–1816, April 1989.)

In significant cold stress increased metabolic heat production is required to maintain body temperature. Shivering thermogenesis depends on an adequate supply of energy substrates, including glucose. The importance of muscle glycogen for body temperature regulation during acute cold stress was investigated.

Thermoregulatory and metabolic responses were measured in 8 men during cold water immersion. Some studies were preceded by 3 days of a 15% carbohydrate diet, as well as exercise for 3 hours each day at 75% of maximal heart rate. Four of the men were relatively lean and 4 had more than 17% body fat.

Baseline vastus lateralis glycogen levels were lower after the restricted carbohydrate diet with exercise. Shivering and body cooling during immersion at 18° C were similar in the 2 trials (Fig 6–5), and postimmersion muscle glycogen levels were unchanged. There were small but significant increases in plasma glucose and lactate levels in both trials, as well as in free fatty acid levels. Plasma glycerol increased only in the low-glycogen trials.

A substantial reduction in muscle glycogen does not impair thermoregulatory responses to cold stress in normal persons. Presumably, other metabolic substrates are used, sparing muscle glycogen.

▶ The classic view has been that the victim of accidental hypothermia faces impairment of cerebral function (because of a low blood level of glucose) and restriction of shivering (because intramuscular stores of glycogen have been depleted). Shivering involves an intense contraction of agonist and antagonist muscles in a manner likely to impair local blood flow, and a heavy reliance upon glycogen as a source of fuel might thus be anticipated. However, attempts to demonstrate such a dependence in the laboratory have not been very convincing. Martineau and Jacobs (1) found that heat conservation in subjects immersed in cold water was not improved by boosting local glycogen reserves, although cooling did proceed somewhat more rapidly after glycogen depletion. The present paper also reports essentially negative findings. One problem in both experiments is that cooling was (quite properly) stopped when core temperature dropped to 35.5° C. However, in accidental hypothermia exposure is much longer and more severe, so that a person is more likely to reach a state in which glycogen reserves are exhausted. The issue cannot really be resolved unless opportunity presents to make measurements of muscle glycogen and blood glucose in hypothermia victims.—R.J. Shephard, M.D., Ph.D.

Reference

1. Martineau L, Jacobs I: *J Appl Physiol* 66:72, 1989.

Electrocardiographic Aspects of Skin Diving
Bonneau A, Friemel F, Lapierre D (CHU Henri Mondor, Creteil, France)
Eur J Appl Physiol 58:487–493, 1989   6–8

Little research has been done on the long-term effects of repeated underwater activity on the body in general and on the heart in particular. Electrocardiographic changes were analyzed in sports divers who dove holding their breath.

Nine men and 1 woman aged 24–45 years performed in a swimming pool 15 m deep at a water temperature of 28° C. An ECG recording was begun 1 hour before the dive. Holding the breath, each subject dove to depths of 6, 9, and 12 or 15 meters. Divers rested for 10 minutes between dives.

All 10 skin divers experienced bradycardia during the ascending parts of the dives. The minimal heart rate was negatively correlated with the diver's experience. Six divers had cardiac arrhythmias. In some cases, atrial arrhythmias were isolated occurrences but, more commonly, there were multiple occurrences. Other arrhythmias encountered were ventricular premature beats that were sometimes single and sometimes double. Other than during dives, 24-hour ECG recordings revealed no arrhythmias.

Bradycardia is a constant phenomenon during snorkeling. Forced expiration through the snorkel when surfacing seems to induce the appearance of cardiac arrhythmias. Further research should be undertaken to evaluate the role of disorders of rhythm and conduction in cases of sudden death during skin diving.

▶ Diving bradycardia at immersion is a well-recognized phenomenon related to the coldness of the water and mechanical stimulation of the face, as well as to breath-holding. The associated release of catecholamines can sometimes provoke abnormalities of cardiac rhythm at this stage. Toward the end of a dive, the usual cause of difficulty is that the alveolar oxygen pressure has dropped to a low value, which is further reduced by the decompression of ascent.

The present experiments are unusual in that the water temperature was relatively high. Bradycardia was apparently provoked by the increasing intrapulmonary pressure during the ascent, with resultant right atrial distention, and stimulation of stretch receptors, although the hypoxia of ascent may also have been a contributing factor. In 6 of 10 divers there were associated abnormalities of rhythm, possibly because the bradycardia allowed the emergence of aberrant signals. Plainly, this paper reinforces the argument for careful evaluation of the stability of electrical rhythms in divers.—R.J. Shephard, M.D., Ph.D.

Prolonged Whole-Body Cold Water Immersion: Fluid and Ion Shifts

Deuster PA, Smith DJ, Smoak BL, Montgomery LC, Singh A, Doubt TJ (Naval Med Research Inst, Bethesda, Md)
J Appl Physiol 66:34–41, January 1989   6–9

Previous studies found that head-out immersions in thermoneutral water for long periods and in cold water for short periods cause fluid and ion shifts, diuresis, an increase in urinary solute excretion, and a reduction in plasma volume. Fluid and ion shifts were assessed during whole-body immersion in cold water for prolonged periods in persons equipped with thermal protection attire who exercised intermittently.

Sixteen male divers wearing dry suits completed 4 whole body immersions in 5° C water as part of two 5-day air saturation dives (ASD) in a hyperbaric chamber that was being maintained at 6.1 msw. To assess diurnal variations, 1 immersion was started at 10 AM and 1 at 10 PM. The immersions were separated by 54 hours and lasted for up to 6 hours each. All divers were lean and in above-average physical condition. Compressed air for breathing was provided by a surface-supplied demand regulator system. Blood samples were obtained in the fasting state before the divers entered the hyperbaric chamber, 30 minutes before the start of each immersion, and 15 minutes after completion of each immersion. Urine samples were also collected. All participants were given special high-caloric diets. No fluids were provided during the immersion period. Each diver exercised on a cycle ergometer for 3 minutes at predetermined times and loads.

All divers experienced marked diuresis, associated with a reduction in plasma volume and an increase in urinary sodium, potassium, calcium, magnesium, and zinc excretion (table). Urine flow and potassium excretion were significantly greater during the morning than during the evening immersions. Thus the responses to prolonged whole-body immersion in cold water with thermal protection, intermittent exercise, and no fluid replacement are similar to those occurring with head-out, long-

Serum/Plasma Concentrations of Selected Ions and Protein Before and After Cold Water Immersions Lasting 3–6 Hours

	AM Immersion		PM Immersion	
	Before	After	Before	After
Serum K, meq/l	4.50±0.05	4.21±0.06*	4.43±0.06	4.29±0.05*
Serum Na, meq/l	143.4±0.5	145.4±0.5	143.8±0.7	145.3±0.7
Serum Osm, mosmol/l	288.4±1.5	296.4±5.4	294.4±2.1	296.1±2.4
Plasma Ca, mg/dl	10.7±0.2	11.0±0.3	11.0±0.3	11.0±0.3
Plasma Mg, meq/l	1.58±0.02	1.61±0.02	1.65±0.02	1.62±0.03
Plasma Zn, μg/dl	74.0±1.7	84.3±2.1*	68.1±1.6†	80.3±1.8*
Serum Alb, g/dl	4.88±0.13	5.54±0.16*	4.92±0.17	5.26±0.15*
Plasma α_2-MG, mg/dl	217.4±8.8	256.3±9.4*	223.9±8.5	257.7±9.4*

Abbreviations: Osm, osmolality; *Alb,* albumin; α_2-MG, α_2-macroglobulin.
Values are means ± SE. AM, 10:00; PM, 10:00.
*Significant difference between before and after immersion values within respective time period ($P < .01$).
†Significant difference between AM and PM values ($P < .05$).
(Courtesy of Deuster PA, Smith DJ, Smoak BL, et al: *J Appl Physiol* 66:34–41, January 1989.)

duration immersion in thermoneutral water and head-out, short-duration immersion in cold water without thermal protection.

▶ Diuresis is a well recognized, and sometimes embarassing, accompaniment of diving. Both cold exposure and the pressure of water on the peripheral veins contribute to the phenomenon. The present paper draws attention to the associated loss of minerals. If a subject dives repeatedly, the fluid loss will be made good in the evenings, but unless the intake of minerals is also boosted, there might seem to be a potential for a cumulative mineral loss. In fact, however, the body reserves of minerals such as sodium are considerable, and because the kidneys are sufficiently efficient in adjusting excretion rates, problems rarely arise.—R.J. Shephard, M.D., Ph.D.

Patent Foramen Ovale and Decompression Sickness in Divers
Moon RE, Camporesi EM, Kisslo JA (Duke Univ)
Lancet 1:513–514, March 11, 1989   6–10

It has been postulated that a patent foramen ovale may be a risk factor for the development of neurologic decompression sickness by allowing the passage of venous gas emboli into the systemic circulation. Thirty sports scuba and professional divers with a history of decompression sickness were examined for the presence of patent foramen ovale by bubble-contrast, 2-dimensional echocardiography and by color flow Doppler imaging.

During bubble-contrast echocardiography 11 patients (37%) had right-to-left shunting through a patent foramen ovale during spontaneous breathing. Eleven of 18 patients (61%) with serious signs and symptoms of decompression sickness had shunting. In contrast, none of the 12 patients with mild symptoms and only 5 of 167 healthy controls (5%) had shunting. None of the patients with decompression sickness had detectable shunting with color flow Doppler imaging.

The presence of a patent foramen ovale is a risk factor for the development of decompression sickness in divers. Bubble-contrast echocardiography seems to be a more sensitive method of detecting a patent foramen ovale in this population than color flow Doppler imaging.

▶ Neurologic forms of decompression sickness carry an adverse prognosis, and it is disturbing to find that as many as 122 recreational SCUBA divers in the United States experienced the neurologic form of sickness during 1987 alone. To date, the reasons for the neurologic manifestations have been obscure, and it is useful to find that a high proportion are attributable to a patent foramen ovale. Various factors tend to increase right atrial pressures during diving (1), and it may well be that the resultant distention of the atrial septum increases the likelihood of a right to left intracardiac shunt of bubbles. The use of a Valsalva maneuver may help to identify those patients at risk of such a shunt (2).—R.J. Shephard, M.D., Ph.D., D.P.E.

References

1. Arborelius M, et al: *Aerospace Med* 43:592, 1972.
2. Lynch JJ, et al: *Am J Cardiol* 53:1478, 1984.

Ocular Fundus Lesions in Divers
Polkinghorne PJ, Sehmi K, Cross MR, Minassian D, Bird AC (Univ of London; Diving Diseases Research Ctr, Plymouth, England)
Lancet 2:1381–1383, Dec 17, 1988   6–11

Many disorders related to decompression are caused by the formation of bubbles that occurs where the partial pressure of the dissolved gas exceeds the ambient pressure. Occasional reports of unilateral transient visual loss, fundus hemorrhages, and bubbles within retinal blood vessels suggest occular ischemia. Retinal fluorescein angiography was used to determine whether changes in blood vessels are common in the ocular fundi of divers. (Such lesions may be indicative of vascular obstruction elsewhere, especially in the CNS.)

The study group included 69 men and 15 women divers aged 20–55 years. Twelve had experienced decompression sickness, and 9 of the 12 had neurologic sequelae but no visual symptoms. Three had a history of joint pain. Eighteen men and 5 women nondivers enrolled in a diving course served as controls. No participants had general disorders likely to cause vascular changes.

All 84 divers had a visual acuity of 6/9 or better with each eye. One nondiver had pigment epithelial changes, as did approximately half of the divers. The prevalence of pigment epithelial changes increased with the duration of diving experience, and the prevalence of these lesions was significantly higher in divers who had decompression sickness. The pigment epithelial lesions were largely confined to the posterior pole and were usually multifocal. Some defects were visible only on angiography, but others were visible clinically. In divers, but not in nondivers, the capillary bed at the posterior pole had undergone changes consisting of dilated arteriolar terminals and microaneurysms.

There may be a causal association between diving and abnormalities of the fundus. All fundus changes were explainable in terms of vascular obstruction. The abnormalities are similar to those seen in other disorders that involve vascular obstruction. Although the prevalence of ocular abnormalities was high, no diver had visual loss as a consequence of diving. However, these lesions may be relevant to retinal disorders that arise later in life.

Cold-Induced Pulmonary Oedema in Scuba Divers and Swimmers and Subsequent Development of Hypertension
Wilmshurst PT, Nuri M, Crowther A, Webb-Peploe MM (St Thomas' Hosp, London)
Lancet 1:62–65, Jan 14, 1989   6–12

There is evidence that cardiogenic pulmonary edema may occur in persons with normal hearts if preload and afterload rise acutely. Findings in 11 divers who had up to 7 episodes of pulmonary edema when in the water were compared with findings in 10 divers who had no cardiorespiratory symptoms.

All divers who had pulmonary edema had dived for years before the first episode. Two divers also had episodes while surface swimming. On land these patients were free of cardiorespiratory symptoms and had good exercise tolerance. All episodes occurred in cold water.

Subjects were measured before and after testing, which included exercise with isometric left handgrips up to 75% of maximum exertion for 2 minutes. The second intervention involved packing the head and neck in ice-water-soaked towels for 5 minutes. Subjects then breathed a gas mixture of 67% oxygen and 33% nitrogen, with measurements made after 7 minutes. They next underwent a combination of the latter 2 tests for 5 minutes. An interval of at least 15 minutes was allowed between interventions.

At baseline there was no significant difference between heart rates in normal and abnormal divers. The rise in heart rate was similar in both groups in response to isometric exercise. Heart rates did not rise significantly in either group during other interventions. At baseline the blood pressure was slightly, but not significantly, higher in abnormal divers; however, it was significantly higher in abnormal divers after each intervention. In the control state, forearm blood flow was significantly lower in abnormal divers, and the difference widened during each intervention. Nine abnormal divers had evidence of cardiac decompensation during the cold pressor test or the combination of ice and oxygen, or both. The combination of ice and oxygen had no greater effect in either group than cold alone.

The effect of cold or a raised partial pressure of oxygen, or both; induced pathologic vasoconstriction in subjects who had pulmonary edema while scuba diving. Nine of 11 patients also had evidence of cardiac decompensation. On follow-up, 7 of these patients had become hypertensive, but there had been no cardiac events and no deaths.

▶ Two intriguing new syndromes in divers. The first article (Abstract 6–11) makes a strong case for ocular fundal lesions as an occupational hazard. These retinal lesions, which resemble those of the sickling diseases, seem to stem from microvascular obstruction of the retinal and choroidal circulations. Likely causes: intravascular bubbles from decompression, or hyperviscosity of the blood from hyperbaric conditions. No diver here had visual loss; the implications for vision in later life are unclear but worrisome.

The second article (Abstract 6–12) teaches us that water inhalation, i.e., drowning, is not the only immersion injury that produces wet lungs. Basically, it describes a "total-body cold-pressor test." Certain persons—those with abnormally high resting peripheral vascular resistance—can sustain acute heart failure and pulmonary edema when they dive or swim in cold water. The reason: Sharp rises in both preload and afterload. The pathophysiology: Immersion itself increases preload, and the cold-induced vasoconstriction increases both preload and afterload. As might be expected, essential hypertension tends to develop in these persons later in life.—E.R. Eichner, M.D.

Avalanche Trauma

Grossman MD, Saffle JR, Thomas F, Tremper B (Univ of Utah)
J Trauma 29:1705–1709, December 1989   6–13

Avalanches cause approximately 25 deaths each year in the United States and injure many other persons. In 149 avalanches involving 188 persons reported to a Utah center between 1982 and 1987, 91 persons were caught; 70 were able to save themselves and required no medical attention. Of the 21 requiring attention, 9 were injured and 12 died. Fifteen of these 21 persons were totally buried in direct contact with the snow. Seven were pronounced dead after attempted resuscitation and rewarming, and in 3 of them, perfusing cardiac rhythms were obtained. The deaths were chiefly the result of asphyxia and blunt trauma. The survivors underwent passive external rewarming before arrival in the emergency unit, but they were only slightly hypothermic.

Ten of those who died were expert skiers, as were most of the survivors. Most accidents occurred in the back country, as was true in European and Canadian avalanches. Several of the victims were involved in nonrecreational activities such as driving or working on a highway, and some were not buried in direct contact with the snow.

Most avalanches are preventable. Asphyxia and multiple injuries are the most serious problems. Patients should be assessed aggressively and treated for blunt trauma. The trend is toward active core rewarming for arrested, markedly hypothermic patients. In stable patients who are hypothermic, external rewarming probably is adequate.

▶ Back country skiing is exciting but, as this report indicates, it carries with it a significant risk of avalanche accidents. Naturally, most of these skiers were experts who were knowledgeable of snowpack hazards and aware of the high avalanche danger present at the time of the accident.

The authors conclude that most deaths result from multiple trauma and asphyxia and discount the importance of hypothermia in causing cardiac arrest. Nevertheless, the nonsurvivors had the lowest rectal temperature (the lowest in this series being 28.7° C) and were buried for the longest time (up to 3 hours). This experience should be contrasted with the report of Althaus et al. (1), who were able to resuscitate 3 victims of avalanche or crevasse falls whose temperatures were below 25° C.

The most remarkable case reported by Althaus et al. was a patient trapped for 5 hours in a crevasse before rescue and declared dead on site. After evacuation by helicopter to a nearby hospital, a core temperature of 19° C was noted and cardiopulmonary resuscitation commenced more than 6 hours after the accident. Partial bypass was begun 3 hours after the rescue (8 hours after the accident), and the patient's heart was warmed directly by mediastinal irrigation. After a further 30 minutes he had warmed to 36° C and was succesfully defibrillated. The patient subsequently made a full recovery without any neurologic defects. It must be noted that he was not asphyxiated.

These cases emphasize the importance of the initial hypothermia, which may well be the neurologic salvation of many by producing a "metabolic ice box" for the brain and other vital organs. It also brings out the old adage that, "No one is dead until they are warm dead."—J.R. Sutton, M.D.

Reference

1. Althaus U, et al: *Ann Surg* 195, 492, 1982.

Helicopter Rescues and Deaths Among Trekkers in Nepal
Shlim DR, Houston R (Himalayan Rescue Assoc, Kathmandu; US Peace Corps, Kathmandu, Nepal)
JAMA 261:1017–1019, Feb 17, 1989   6–14

Trekking in Nepal is becoming increasingly popular; in 1986 nearly 50,000 foreigners obtained a permit to trek. A trek involves an average of 11 days of hiking over mountainous terrain that may be more than 5,500 high.

A review of helicopter evacuations and deaths in a 3.5-year period revealed 23 deaths and 111 helicopter rescues. The risk of dying was 15 deaths per 100,000 permits, and the frequency of rescue was 75 per 100,000 permits. Eleven deaths were traumatic, 8 were caused by illness, and 3 were attributed to acute mountain sickness. (The cause of death in 1 climber is unknown.) Deaths did not differ markedly by altitude (Fig

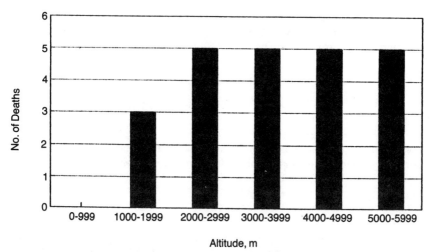

Fig 6-6.—Number of deaths in relation to altitude. (Courtesy of Shlim DR, Houston R: *JAMA* 261:1017–1019, Feb 17, 1989.)

6–6). Trekkers aged 50 and older were not more likely than younger persons to die, but they were rescued more often.

Trekking in Nepal may be relatively safe, but the decision to engage in this activity should imply an acquaintance with the problems related to high altitude, being in a remote place, and becoming ill where medical facilities are not available. The terrain can be hazardous at any altitude because of falls and rockfall.

▶ With the increasing popularity of trekking in the Himalayas, this timely article puts to rest some common misconceptions regarding the safety and extent of serious altitude maladies. The estimated trekking population was 148,000 persons in a 3.5-year period. Of the 23 deaths recorded, only 3 (13%) were directly attributable to altitude illness, although altitude illness was responsible for 38, or 34%, of the rescues.

The deaths occurred nearly equally at all altitudes, but the altitude at which those who died of altitude illness and the altitude at which those who were evacuated because of altitude illness were not recorded, although presumably the authors have these data.

Another interesting point the authors make is that no trekker died because of heart disease. Two trekkers in their late 50s with known severe cardiac disease who had been advised not to trek were evacuated. A 27-year-old man with frequent ectopic beats and 3 others aged 39, 41, and 55 with chest pains of undiagnosed etiology also were evacuated. The authors speculate that these latter 3 cases may have sustained the substernal chest pain often associated with high-altitude pulmonary edema that is difficult to distinguish from angina at altitude.

This paper did not address the issue of whether traveling to altitude posed an unacceptable risk to patients with known heart disease, in light of recent controversies (1). They were quick to point out that there have been no published reports demonstrating an increased risk of cardiac problems in trekkers. Furthermore, they reiterated the obvious—if a person has a cardiac limitation to exercise at sea level, it would be unwise to trek at altitude where it can be predicted that the limitation will occur with even less effort and where evacuation and medical help may be a minimum of 24 hours away.—J.R. Sutton, M.D.

Reference

1. Froelicher VF, West JB: *JAMA* 259:3184, 1988.

Hemodynamic Responses to Acute Hypoxia, Hypobaria, and Exercise in Subjects Susceptible to High-Altitude Pulmonary Edema

Kawashima A, Kubo K, Kobayashi T, Sekiguchi M (Shinshu Univ, Matsumoto, Japan)
J Appl Physiol 67:1982–1989, November 1989   6–15

High-altitude pulmonary edema (HAPE) is a severe form of acute mountain sickness. Individuals who have previously experienced HAPE are more likely to experience it again. High-altitude pulmonary edema-susceptible (HAPE-S) subjects may have certain constitutional abnormalities that are implicated in the pathogenesis of HAPE.

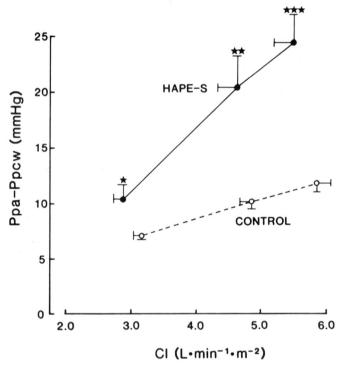

Fig 6–7.—Relationship between pulmonary driving pressure (Ppa-Ppcw) and cardiac index (pulmonary vascular pressure-flow curve) during exercise. $*P < .05$, $**P < .01$, $***P < .001$, compared with controls. (Courtesy of Kawashima A, Kubo K, Kobayashi T, et al: *J Appl Physiol* 67:1982–1989, November 1989.)

Five HAPE-S and 5 controls underwent physical examination, routine laboratory tests, chest roentgenography, ECG, and lung function tests. The hemodynamic responses to hypoxia, hypobaria, and exercise in all subjects were evaluated.

The HAPE-S group had a much greater increase in the pulmonary vascular resistance index than did controls. This increase resulted in a much higher level of pulmonary arterial pressure under acute hypoxia of 15% O_2 and also under acute hypobaria of 515 torr. In addition, the pulmonary vascular resistance index in HAPE-S subjects had a tendency to increase even during light exercise on a supine bicycle ergometer (Fig 6–7). In contrast, the pulmonary vascular resistance index in controls significantly decreased. The HAPE-S subjects had a greater increase in pulmonary arterial pressure and a greater decrease in arterial oxygen tension than did controls.

Susceptibility to HAPE may be attributable in part to constitutional abnormalities in hemodynamic responses to causative factors of HAPE (e.g., hypoxia, hypobaria, and exercise). These variables can be evaluated at low altitude in those thought to be susceptible to HAPE.

▶ From a predictive standpoint it would be very desirable to know before embarking on a high-altitude expedition, or trekking at altitude, who in a group is most likely to experience acute mountain sickness and HAPE. The latter entity can be fatal, but to date no practical means of predicting such persons has been developed.

In the studies of victims of HAPE, ventilatory and circulatory peculiarities have been demonstrated. In the present article by Kawashima and co-workers, HAPE-S persons appeared to have much greater pulmonary artery sensitivity to alveola hypoxia and exercise. These findings are very reminiscent of those of Hultgren and Marticorena (1) presented some years ago. What is especially interesting about the Hultgren et al. observation is that his group went on to hypothesize that HAPE is a "vasogenic" edema and the result of uneven pulmonary vasoconstriction, leaving areas of lung overperfused and susceptible to edema formation (2). Such a theory was given further support by the observation of Hackett and colleagues (3) who reported HAPE in several patients with an absent pulmonary artery. Thus the whole cardiac output perfused 1 lung, and it was in this lung that HAPE developed.—J.R. Sutton, M.D.

References

1. Hultgren HN, Marticorena EA: *Chest* 74:372, 1978.
2. Hultgren HN, et al: *Circulation* 34(suppl III):132, 1966.
3. Hackett PH, et al: *N Engl J Med* 302:1070, 1980.

Blunted Hypoxic Ventilatory Drive in Subjects Susceptible to High-Altitude Pulmonary Edema

Matsuzawa Y, Fujimoto K, Kobayashi T, Namushi NR, Harada K, Kohno H, Fukushima M, Kusama S (Shinshu Univ, Matsumoto, Japan)

J Appl Physiol 66:1152–1157, March 1989   6–16

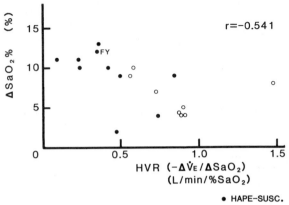

Fig 6−8.—Relationship between magnitude of fall in arterial O_2 saturation (Δ Sao_2%) at 3 hours after ascent to an altitude of 2,763 m on day 1 and hypoxic ventilatory response (Δ VE/Δ Sao_2) at low altitude (610 m) in HAPE-susceptible individuals and controls. The mean value for Δ Sao_2% was relatively high in HAPE-susceptible individuals (9%) compared with controls (6%). High-altitude pulmonary edema recurred in 1 of HAPE-susceptible individuals *(FY)* on day 4. (Courtesy of Matsuzawa Y, Fujimoto K, Kobayashi T, et al: *J Appl Physiol* 66:1152−1157, March 1989.)

High-altitude pulmonary edema (HAPE) develops in some individuals after rapid exposure to altitude. Perhaps HAPE-susceptible individuals have exaggerated hypoxemia with relative hypoventilation during early exposure to high altitude. A relationship has been shown between a blunted hypoxic ventilatory response (HVR) and HAPE.

The standard pulmonary function test and its relationship to HVR and to hypercapnia was evaluated in 9 HAPE-susceptible men and 1 woman. Their responses were assessed at low altitude and compared with responses in 8 controls with no histories of high-altitude dysfunction. Pulmonary function was tested approximately 1 hour before ventilatory responses were tested. Both HVR and hypercapnia were measured with a rebreathing circuit. Ventilation was recorded using a bag-in-box system.

All HAPE-susceptible patients had normal pulmonary function, but they had a significantly lower HVR than controls. Thus patients who are HAPE-susceptible may have lower HVR at low altitude (Fig 6−8). However, because 2 of 10 HAPE-susceptible patients had HVR values within the normal range, apparently low HVR alone may not be a critical factor for HAPE. Low HVR may be only 1 of several factors contributing to HAPE.

▶ High-altitude pulmonary edema is one of the most serious and potentially fatal of all altitude maladies. Its formal recognition as a specific high-altitude illness is of relatively recent origin, being first described by Charles Houston in 1960 (1). In that instance a young skier was rescued from the mountains around Aspen, Colorado, one New Year's Eve. His chest x-ray appearance was bizarre, showing what seemed to be pneumonia. After he was put into an oxygen tent, he rapidly improved. The lungs cleared rapidly, too quickly for his condition to have been pneumonia, and an alternate diagnosis of pulmonary edema was made, the most common cause of which is heart failure. However, the clinical findings were not of heart failure. Later, a friend of Houston's cardiologist Paul Dudley White, visited and confirmed that the pulmonary edema was most likely of noncardiac origin.

In retrospect, many episodes of the high-altitude "pneumonia," known to be rapidly fatal, may have been HAPE. But how can we predict who is susceptible to HAPE?

In the present paper, 9 HAPE-susceptible men and 1 woman had ventilatory response hypoxia and hypercapnia measured at sea level. All hypercapnic ventilatory responses (HVR) were normal, as were 2 of the 10 hypoxic ventilatory responses, although as a group HVR tended to be lower in the HAPE-susceptible subjects. Furthermore, the interlaboratory variation and normal ranges of HVR mean that measurement of ventilatory responsiveness is of limited predictive value for identifying HAPE-susceptible individuals. These tests would therefore not be recommended as screening tests to select climbers for mountaineering expeditions.

One of the early clues that persons who hypoventilate at altitude may be susceptible to the development of HAPE came from a study of acute mountain sickness (2). In that study the hypoventilators, on arrival at 5,360 m (17,580 ft), subsequently experience the most severe acute mountain sickness (headache, anorexia, nausea, vomiting, insomnia, ataxia). These same individuals had marked widening of their (A-a) gradients and increases in venous admixture, all consistent with the development of subclinical pulmonary edema. About that time, Lakshminarayan and Pierson (3) reported a patient with recurrent HAPE who had blunted chemosensitivity. We therefore wondered if it might be possible to predict at sea level who might be susceptible to HAPE by examining ventilatory responsiveness. However, further studies on Mt. Logan were to no avail as too few persons experienced HAPE.—J.R. Sutton, M.D.

References

1. Houston CS: *N Engl J Med* 263:478, 1960.
2. Sutton JR, et al: *Aviat Space Environ Med* 47:1032, 1976.
3. Lakshminarayan S, Pierson DJ: *Am Rev Respir Dis* 111:869, 1975.

Chronic Mountain Sickness in Tibet
Pei SX, Chen XJ, Si Ren BZ, Liu YH, Cheng XS, Harris EM, Enand IS, Harris PC (Workers' Hosp of the Tibet Autonomous Region of the People's Republic of China, Lhasa, Tibet; Chinese Academy of Med Sciences, Beijing; Postgrad Inst of Med Education and Research, Chandigarh, India; Natl Heart and Lung Inst, London)
Q J Med 71:555–574, June 1989   6–17

The chronic mountain sickness first identified in the Peruvian Andes also occurs in the Tibetan Himalayas, where men of Han origin who have moved to a high altitude from the lowlands are particularly susceptible to the syndrome. Sixteen of 17 patients treated at the Workers' Hospital in Lhasa for chronic mountain sickness were Han immigrants. All were cigarette smokers. The other patient was a Tibetan woman who took snuff and had lived most of her life in higher altitudes.

Common symptoms included dyspnea, cough, swelling of the face and feet, headache, memory loss, fatigue, and a tendency to bleed, which affected a number of organs. In 9 patients the jugular venous pressure was raised at admission. In 10 patients chest radiographs showed cardiac enlargement. All patients had polycythemia, the cause of early symptoms of chronic mountain sickness. In 6 patients proteinuria was found in urine tests. The patients began to notice symptoms at an average of 15 years after moving to a higher altitude. Symptoms usually worsened over time. One patient who returned to a low altitude for 2 months experienced temporary relief of symptoms and a fall in the hemoglobin level from 20 g/dL to 11 g/dL.

In 5 men who underwent studies of pulmonary hemodynamics and respiratory gas exchange, as well as assessment of the effects of inhalation of oxygen on those measurements, findings included pulmonary hypertension, with a normal cardiac output and dilatation of the right ventricle. Evidence of alveolar underventilation and ventilation:perfusion inhomogeneity also was found. Inhalation of oxygen led to only partial restoration of the pulmonary arterial resistance.

Epidemiologic studies in a Tibetan hospital population showed the disease to occur most often in Han men who smoke. Women rarely have the disease, although they are as susceptible as men to acute mountain sickness. Tibetans appear to have become resistant to the harmful effects of chronic hypoxia. Polycythemia dominates in the earlier stages of the disease, and cardiopulmonary involvement increases over the years.

▶ Monge's disease, as chronic mountain sickness (CMS) is also called, was first described in the Peruvian Andes by the physician whose name it bears (1). Most reports of CMS have come from the Andes, and therefore it has been assumed that the Andean Indians may be more susceptible to CMS than other mountain dwellers, although no data exist to support such an idea. Occasional reports of CMS have come from the continental United States and a few from the Himalayas. In the present paper several points emerge that have not been the published experience elsewhere: The condition appeared infrequently in women, the Han seemed more susceptible than native Tibetans, and cigarette smoking may be an additional risk factor. The authors also performed hemodynamic measurements on a subset of this group (5 persons) and found universal pulmonary hypertension, which has been previously reported from the Andes (2), but expressed surprise at the failure of oxygen breathing to completely return the pulmonary artery pressure to normal (1). However, even short-term exposure to high altitude for several weeks results in pulmonary hypertension that is not totally reversible even after oxygen administration (3). Of 5 patients with CMS who had arterial and Swan-Ganz catheterization, 3 had unequivocal systemic hypertension with blood pressures ranging from 168/110 to 187/130 mm Hg.—J.R. Sutton, M.D.

References

1. Monge C: *An Fac Med Lima* 11:314, 1928.
2. Penaloza D, Sime F: *Am J Med* 50:728, 1971.
3. Groves BM, et al: *J Appl Physiol* 63:521, 1987.

Persistent Cognitive Impairment in Climbers After Repeated Exposure to Extreme Altitude
Regard M, Oelz O, Brugger P, Landis T (Univ Hosp, Zurich)
Neurology 39:210–213, February 1989   6–18

Persons exposed to extreme high altitude experience a variety of neurologic problems, but little is known about persisting effects on the CNS. Neuropsychological tests were performed on 8 persons who had climbed higher than 8,500 m without supplementary oxygen. Subjects were compared with matched controls, who were rock climbers at moderate altitudes. The study group underwent electroencephalography, took the digit-span test from the Wechsler Adult Intelligence Scale, a concentration test, and had assessment of short-term memory. Cognitive flexibility and visuospatial perception were evaluated.

Performance was generally high in both the study group and in controls on most tests, but study subjects fluctuated more in performance on the concentration test. On complex Rey figure recall, they displaced more elements, their figural fluency was lower, and they made more errors. They also took longer to suppress interference in the Stroop task. In a test to assess cognitive flexibility, they made more errors and matched fewer concepts correctly, compared with controls.

Summary of Cognitive Impairments for Each Subject

Functions	1	2	3	4	5	6	7	8
				Subjects				
Attention span	—	—	—	x	—	—	x	—
Concentration	—	xx	—	xx	x	x	x	x
Memory & learning								
Verbal	—	x	—	xx	xx	—	x	x
Figural	xx	x	—	xx	xx	—	xx	xx
Cognitive flexibility	x	xx	xx	xx	xx	xx	x	xx
Visuospatial perception	—	—	—	—	x	x	—	—
Motor performance	—	—	—	—	—	—	x	x
Laterality	—	—	—	—	—	—	—	—

x Performance below or above 1 SD of the mean of the control group.
xx Two SD beyond mean of the control group.

(Courtesy of Regard M, Oelz O, Brugger P, et al: *Neurology* 39:210–213, February 1989.)

Intragroup variability was also much higher in the study group than in controls (table). The pattern of impairment suggests malfunctioning of bifronto-temporo-limbic structures. Repeated extreme-altitude exposure may cause mild but persistent cognitive impairment.

▶ There have been previous reports that claims above 8,500 m without oxygen lead to at least temporary deficits of memory and psychomotor disorders (1,2). The earlier studies had the advantage of being longitudinal in nature, but the disadvantage was that the climbers had other problems (e.g., head injuries, food and water deprivation that could have contributed to their symptoms. The present report suggests more persistent changes in brain function, but the study is cross-sectional in type—we do not really know whether the climbers were "normal" before they began climbing. Nevertheless, we noted similar symptoms in a colleague who had been a Spitfire pilot in World War II; in an attempt to gain an advantage over his German adversaries, he had frequently exceeded the ceiling for unpressurized flying while using a simple oxygen mask. Given the intersubject variation in response, it seems wise to caution mountaineers of these dangers. Whether they will heed medical advice is another matter!—R.J. Shephard, M.D., Ph.D.

References

1. Ryn Z: *Acta Med Pol* 12:453, 1971.
2. West JB: *Lancet* 2:387, 1986.

Exercise Performance of Hemodialysis Patients During Short-Term and Prolonged Exposure to Altitude
Mairbäurl H, Schobersberger W, Hasibeder W, Knapp E, Hopferwieser T, Humpeler E, Loeffler HD, Wetzels E, Wybitul K, Baumgartl P, Dittrich P (Univ Innsbruck, Austria; Universitätsklinik für Innere Medizin, Innsbruck; Dialyse-Trainingszentren-Verein e V, Emmendingen, West Germany; Städtisch Krankenanstalten, Rosenheim, West Germany; Benedikt-Kreutz Rehabilitationszentrum e V, Bad Krozingen, West Germany; et al)
Clin Nephrol 32:39, July 1989   6–19

In healthy persons an increase in pulmonary ventilation and cardiac output can compensate for the reduced inspiratory oxygen pressure experienced at exposure to high altitude. Prolonged exposure and increasing altitude, however, result in a reduction of work capacity. This effect is exaggerated in patients undergoing maintenance hemodialysis, as most of the compensatory mechanisms required to adjust to high altitude are impaired or absent. Yet, these patients appear to have good exercise tolerance when exposed to altitude hypoxia. The tolerance of hemodialysis patients was tested hypoxia and the results were compared with prealtitude or control values.

Patients were tested during short-term exposure to altitudes of 2,000 m and 3,000 m and during 2 weeks of exposure to an altitude of 2,000 m. They were encouraged to exercise to their subjective limit on a bicycle ergometer. During prealtitude tests, patients in the short-term experiment reached workloads that were about 66% of age- and sex-matched standard values. Comparable workloads were achieved after 3 hours of exposure to an altitude of 2,000 m. After similar exposure to 3,000 m, however, workloads were reduced significantly (12%).

Patients taken to 2,000 m for 2 weeks showed no change in maximal performance 1 day after ascent. By the end of the 2-week stay, workloads at completion of exercise were significantly improved (17%). In these patients diastolic pressure was comparable to prealtitude values, but peak oxygen intake, blood lactate, heart rate, and systolic blood pressure all increased. Neither the reduction of performance at 3,000 m nor the improvement after 2 weeks at 2,000 m could be related to the degree of anemia or other clinical data. It appears that exercise is performed more economically after long-term exposure, probably a result of more efficient work of the heart and muscles.

▶ This paper is included primarily to illustrate that yet another group of patients with a disability are able to enjoy exercise in the invigorating mountain environment. These patients were in a chronic dialysis program and their exercise performance was well correlated to their degree of anemia. In principle, the responses to altitude are similar to those of normal subjects—but allow for the lower starting point.—J.R. Sutton, M.D.

Suprachiasmatic Nucleus: Phase-Dependent Activation During the Hibernation Cycle
Kilduff TS, Radeke CM, Randall TL, Sharp FR, Heller HC (Stanford Univ; VA Med Ctr, San Francisco)
Am J Physiol 257:R605–R612, September 1989   6–20

There is considerable evidence that the suprachiasmatic nucleus (SCN) of the hypothalamus serves as a circadian oscillator in mammals. The uptake of ^{14}C-labeled 2-deoxyglucose (2-DG) in the SCN of the ground squirrel was examined through the hibernation cycle because high levels have been found at this site relative to other brain structures. Studies were done at an ambient temperature of 5° C. Animals were injected with 2-DG in darkness during entrance to hibernation, stable deep hibernation, and arousal.

Relative 2-DG uptake in the SCN (Fig 6–9) was greatest during entrance into hibernation and during deep hibernation. No circadian changes were noted in euthermic ground squirrels, but photic stimulation during the day increased relative to 2-DG uptake in the SCN. An increase also occurred in the paraventricular nucleus during entrance to hibernation but not after photic stimulation during euthermia.

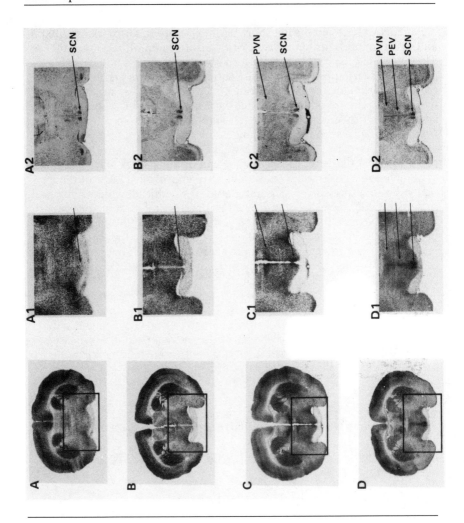

The findings support an important functional role for the SCN in the initiation and maintenance of hibernation in the ground squirrel. Within the preoptic-anterior hypothalamic region, the critical sites of action for regulation of hibernation may be the suprachiasmatic, paraventricular, and periventricular nuclei.

► Some fascinating insights into the metabolic accompaniment of hibernation have come from these authors.

Electrophysiologic studies have demonstrated a circadian rhythm within the SCN of the hypothalamus of mammals. Furthermore, if the SCN is isolated from other nuclei, those nuclei also lose their circadian rhythmicity. In addition to the electrophysiologic rhythmicity there is a concomitant, but metabolic,

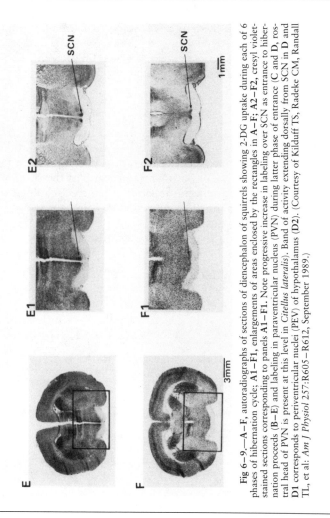

Fig 6–9.—A–F, autoradiographs of sections of diencephalon of squirrels showing 2-DG uptake during each of 6 phases of hibernation cycle; **A1–F1**, enlargements of areas enclosed by the rectangles in **A–F**; **A2–F2**, cresyl violet-stained sections corresponding to panels **A1–F1**. Note progressive increase in labeling over SCN as entrance to hibernation proceeds (**B–E**) and labeling in paraventricular nucleus (PVN) during latter phase of entrance (C and D, rostral head of PVN is present at this level in *Citellus lateralis*). Band of activity extending dorsally from SCN in D and **D1** corresponds to periventricular nuclei (PEV) of hypothalamus (**D2**). (Courtesy of Kilduff TS, Radeke CM, Randall TL, et al: *Am J Physiol* 257:R605–R612, September 1989.)

rhythmicity when studied as the metabolism of 2[^{14}C] deoxy-D-glucose (2-DG). The authors have now applied their 2-DG techniques to the study of hibernation in ground squirrels and found quite significant increases as hypothermia develops during the onset of hibernation and especially as deep hibernation occurs. Whether this is characteristic of the hibernating state or can also be found in nonhibernating hypothermia is now an important issue still to be addressed.

When changes in SCN labeling are considered alongside the pineal and plasma melatonin rhythms, there is a 12-hour phase lag, with the 2-DG uptake in the SCN peaking during the night. Yet the pineal's endogenous rhythm is regulated by the SCN. However, during hibernation a dramatic change occurs and the rhythmicity ceases with the plasma concentration of melatonin remaining at the low daytime levels.—J.R. Sutton, M.D.

The Cost to the Central Nervous System of Climbing to Extremely High Altitude

Hornbein TF, Townes BD, Schoene RB, Sutton JR, Houston CS (Univ of Washington; McMaster Univ, Hamilton, Ont; Univ of Vermont)
N Engl J Med 321:1714–1719, Dec 21, 1989   6–21

Mountaineers may exhibit both transient and long-lasting neurobehavioral deficits. Neurobehavioral changes were evaluated in 35 mountaineers who ascended to more than 5,488 m and in 6 members (study group) of Operation Everest II who underwent gradual decompression in an altitude chamber to the equivalent barometric pressure of the summit of Mount Everest. The 6 study subjects underwent neuropsychological testing before and after entering the altitude chamber. Climbers also underwent testing before and after their climbs.

In the 6 members of Operation Everest II no significant differences in

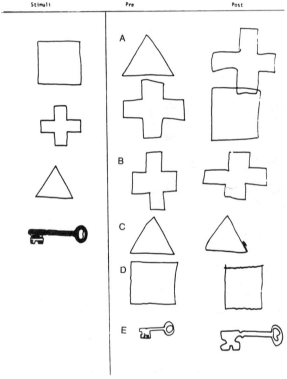

Fig 6–10.—Selected drawings by the subjects of Operation Everest II at testing before and after exposure to hypoxia. After exposure the subjects had difficulty planning ahead and organizing the figures correctly on the page (note overlap, panel **A**), reproducing the proportions of the cross accurately (panel **B**), and obtaining accurate closure of the triangle (panel **C**). One subject had a pronounced hand tremor after the expedition, as well as difficulty with closure (panel **D**), and another subject could not maintain the spatial organization of the notches on the key (panel **E**). (Courtesy of Hornbein TF, Townes BD, Schoene RB, et al: *N Engl J Med* 321:1714–1719, Dec 21, 1989.)

performance on vocabulary tests, attention, paired-associate learning task, digit-span test, or efficient problem-solving before and after exposure to hypoxia were observed. They needed the same number of trials to learn a list of 10 words, but their recall of the words 20 minutes later was poorer after recompression. Operation Everest II members, but not mountaineers, had decrements in visual motor performance after hypoxic exposure (Fig 6–10). Mountaineers only had a statistically significant decrement in motor speed of the right and left hands after decompression; these decrements persisted a year later. Mountaineers also had deficits in verbal expression after their expeditions. Among Operation Everest II members, a higher hypoxic ventilatory response was significantly correlated with increased impairment on the Selective Reminder Test, the Wechsler Memory Scale, and aphasic errors. Improved arterial oxygenation and lower $PaCO_2$ at 8,100 m and 8,848 m were also associated with poorer neurobehavioral outcomes. Poorer oxygenation during sleep was associated with poorer subsequent neurobehavioral functioning. In 11 mountaineers, higher values for the hypoxic ventilatory response were correlated with increased aphasic errors (Fig 6–11).

Impairments were identified in neurobehavioral performance after exposure to hypoxia of extremely high altitudes. Persons with a high hypoxic ventilatory response who appear more impaired after exposure to extremely high altitudes nevertheless perform best physically at great

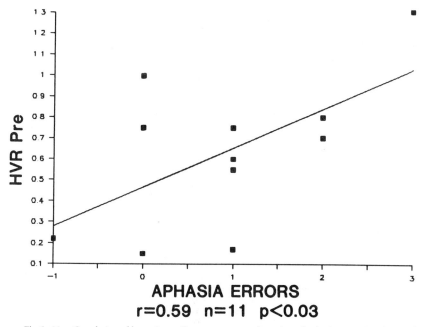

APHASIA ERRORS
r=0.59 n=11 p<0.03

Fig 6–11.—Correlation of hypoxic ventilatory response and number of aphasic errors in subjects of the American Medical Research Expedition to Everest. Persons with a higher hypoxic ventilatory response had more aphasic errors as measured on the aphasia screening test. (Courtesy of Hornbein TF, Townes BD, Schoene RB, et al: *N Engl J Med* 321:1714–1719, Dec 21, 1989.)

heights. Higher levels of resting arterial oxygenation consequent to a brisk ventilatory response to hypoxia were correlated with poorer neurobehavioral outcomes. This unexpected finding may be explained by decreases in cerebral blood flow and oxygen delivery to the brain resulting from hypocapnia at rest, exercise, or moments of severe arterial hypoxemia associated with greater periodicity of breathing during sleep in persons with higher hypoxic ventilatory responses.

Dexamethasone in the Treatment of Acute Mountain Sickness
Levine BD, Yoshimura K, Kobayashi T, Fukushima M, Shibamoto T, Ueda G (Shinshu Univ, Matsumoto, Japan)
N Engl J Med 321:1707–1713, Dec 21, 1989   6–22

Travelers who rapidly ascend to high altitudes often experience acute mountain sickness. The illness is usually self-limited, but it occasionally progresses to life-threatening, high-altitude cerebral edema. Early swelling of the brain may be the cause of even mild mountain sickness. De-

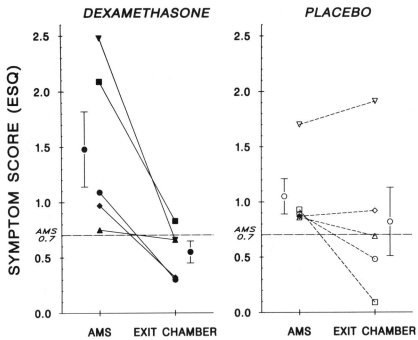

Fig 6–12.—Results on cerebral component of environmental symptoms questionnaire in the 6 subjects. Acute mountain sickness (AMS) was considered present when the factor score was more than 0.7. The score was derived from answers to questions regarding symptoms of headache, nausea, dizziness, faintness, lack of coordination, dimness of vision, weakness, anorexia, and general sensations of being "hung over" and "feeling sick." *I-bars* denote means ± SE. (Courtesy of Sampson JB, Cymerman A, Burse RL, et al: *Aviat Space Environ Med* 54:1063–1073, 1983, and Chapuis F: Verlag Hans Huber, 1959. From Levine BD, Yoshimura K, Kobayashi T, et al: *N Engl J Med* 321:1707–1713, Dec 21, 1989.)

scent is the definitive cure, but because this is not always immediately possible, the role of dexamethasone in the treatment of acute mountain sickness was studied.

Six healthy men aged 18–23 years were studied at baseline at an altitude of 600 m and then in a hypobaric chamber at a simulated altitude of 3,700 m. They remained in the chamber for 48 hours; during this time they engaged in leisure activities and exercised to 70% maximal predicted heart rate on a bicycle ergometer for 20 minutes daily. Acute mountain sickness was diagnosed by a symptoms questionnaire. After the diagnosis was established, the men were randomized to a dexamethasone

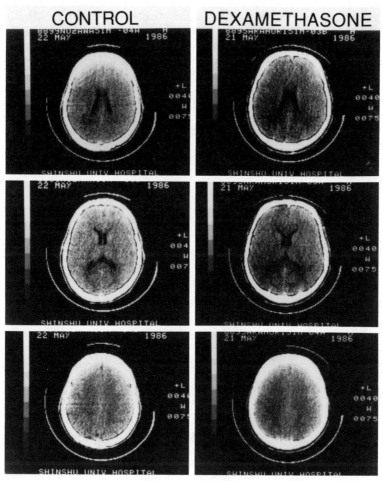

Fig 6–13.—Brain CT scan in sickest subject after 48 hours at simulated high altitude and treatment with dexamethasone. The *right panel* shows mild cerebral edema, evident in the decreased density *(darker area)* of the white matter. For comparison, the *left panel* shows a normal scan produced on the same machine in the 1 subject in whom acute mountain sickness did not develop after exposure to simulated high altitude. (Courtesy of Levine BD, Yoshimura K, Kobayashi T, et al: *N Engl J Med* 321:1707–1713, Dec 21, 1989.)

group (4 mg every 6 hours for the duration of exposure) or a placebo group. The trial was repeated 4 weeks later with the treatments crossed over. The men were evaluated by psychometric testing, cardiopulmonary monitoring, chest radiography, lung perfusion scanning, brain CT, and sleep monitoring with impedance plethysmography of the chest wall.

Five of the 6 men became sick during both trials and therefore received both placebo and dexamethasone. After receiving dexamethasone, all had rapid improvement in symptoms (Fig 6–12). Two improved with placebo but at a slower rate than with dexamethasone. On cardiopulmonary testing there was no difference among any variables between treatment and placebo. Five of the 6 men had no abnormalities on imaging, but in 1 a pattern consistent with cerebral edema was noted (Fig 6–13). Dexamethasone caused a small reduction in the percentage of sleep time spent in periodic breathing. Psychometric testing revealed no differences between treated and control subjects. All of those given dexamethasone had significantly elevated fasting blood glucose levels.

Dexamethasone effectively relieves the symptoms of acute mountain sickness, but the mechanism by which the drug works in the setting is unclear. There was no evidence that the drug brought objective improvement in pathophysiologic changes induced by high-altitude exposure. Considering its potential for serious side effects, dexamethasone should be reserved for use when descent is impossible or when the patient's cooperation is required for descent.

▶ These 2 articles (Abstracts 6–21 and 6–22) illustrate the price we pay for standing atop our world. The first article shows that mountaineers can sustain long-lasting neurobehavioral impairments, e.g., declines in visual and verbal long-term memory, increases in aphasia, and decrements in motor speed of the hands. Such impairments are attributed to brain dysfunction caused by lack of oxygen at altitude. Ironically, climbers with the strongest ventilatory response to hypoxia, who consequently climb best at great heights, seem to end up with the most neurobehavioral impairment.

The second article shows that dexamethasone reduces the symptoms of acute mountain sickness. How it does so, however, remains unclear. It may shore up capillary membranes in the brain and/or somehow relieve cerebral edema, but proof here is lacking. Rapid descent, of course, is the definitive treatment for acute mountain sickness. When rapid descent is impossible, dexamethasone may help.—E.R. Eichner, M.D.

Physical and Psychological Effects of Aerobic Exercise in Delinquent Adolescent Males
MacMahon JR, Gross RT (Stanford Univ)
Am J Dis Child 142:1361–1366, December 1988   6–23

Aerobic exercise in adults is associated with improved psychological status and physical fitness. The affects of aerobic exercise on self-concept, depression level, and physical fitness were assessed in 98 incarcerated boys. They were assigned in blind fashion to either of 2 similarly structured exercise programs that differed only in physical intensity. One program emphasized aerobic exercise and the other, limited exertion; both programs lasted for 3 months. Self-concept was assessed by the Piers-Harris Children's Self-Concept Scale, mood was measured by the Beck Depression Inventory, and cardiovascular fitness by submaximal exercise testing.

Persons who participated in the aerobic exercise had significantly greater improvements in mood and physical fitness than those who participated in less vigorous activity. Improvement in self-concept was also greater for the aerobic group members. Improvements in self-concept and mood were not correlated and occurred independently of changes in physical fitness.

Participation in an aerobic exercise program is associated with improvement in self-concept, depression, and physical fitness in delinquent boys. Aerobic exercise may play a role in the rehabilitation programs for delinquent adolescents.

▶ This groundbreaking study holds promise of benefits for troubled individuals and for society. In only 3 months a program of aerobic exercise for juvenile delinquents improved not only their physical fitness but also their self-concept and mood. These youths felt better about themselves and learned something about self-discipline. Further research along these lines would be welcome.—E.R. Eichner, M.D.

Predictors of Competitive Trait Anxiety in Male Young Sport Participants
Lewthwaite R, Scanlan TK (Univ of Wisconsin, Milwaukee; Univ of California, Los Angeles)
Med Sci Sports Exerc 21:221–229, April 1989   6–24

Most young people enjoy sports, but some experience chronic stress in the sports environment. Competitive trait anxiety (CTA) reflects a tendency to perceive threat and experience stress during sports competition. The intrapersonal and significant adult factors related to the levels of dispositional anxiety or CTA were examined in a field study of 76 boys aged 9–14 years who completed 2 qualifying rounds of a season-end wrestling tournament.

Participants completed questionnaires before the tournament, after weigh-in, and before the first match. The children's form of Martens' Sport Competition Anxiety Text (SCAT) was used to assess pretournament somatic CTA. Cognitive aspects of CTA were assessed after weigh-in. The 14-item Washington Self-Description Questionnaire was used to evaluate self-esteem. The post-weigh-in questionnaire also assessed generalized expectations for wrestling success and participants' perceptions of characteristic influences of parents and coaches. On the prematch questionnaire each wrestler was asked whether he would prefer to wrestle his assigned opponent, draw a bye, or receive an automatic win in that tournament round.

On the somatic anxiety subscale of SCAT scores were correlated with worries about failure and with worries about adult expectations and social evaluation. Wrestlers with higher somatic CTA scores had lower self-esteem, were more upset if they performed poorly, and were more likely to prefer a bye to a match. Wrestlers who had more frequent adult-related worries were more upset when they performed poorly, perceived greater parental and coach shame and upset with poor performance, perceived more negative adult evaluations and interactions, and felt greater parental pressure to wrestle.

These findings corroborate reported connections between chronic CTA and children's decisions to drop sports competition or avoid it in the first place. Future research should explore actual adult expectations and interactions that high-anxiety children encounter in the competitive sports context, as well as the match between these behaviors and children's perceptions thereof.

▶ Our society says this about sports: Winning is everything. This study is a good start at probing how and why parents and coaches team up to ruin the sports experience for children. What price victory?—E.R. Eichner, M.D.

Young Long Distance Runners: Physiological and Psychological Characteristics
Nudel DB, Hassett I, Gurian A, Diamant S, Weinhouse E, Gootman N (Long Island Jewish Med Ctr, New Hyde Park, NY; Med College of Wisconsin, Milwaukee; Ichilov Hosp, Tel-Aviv)
Clin Pediatr 28:500–505, November 1989   6–25

The advisability of long-distance running at an early age has been questioned. Objections are based on potential risk of injuries, growth retardation, questions about the beneficial effects of aerobic training, and the psychological effects of intense physical training at this age.

The physiologic and psychological characteristics and long-term running histories were examined in 10 boys and 6 girls who began long-distance running at ages 4–12 years and who ran for at least 30 miles/wk year-round. Participants had been running for a mean of 8.4 years at the time of evaluation; athletes were evaluated at a mean of 15.4 years. Athletes trained at 30–105 miles/wk. Medical assessment included history, cardiovascular examination, ECG, M-mode, 2-D echocardiography, x-ray examinations of the hand and wrist, and maximal exercise testing. Results were compared with those in 20 matched controls. Thirteen athletes also received psychological evaluation. One legally blind participant and 2 with diagnoses of anorexia nervosa were excluded from psychological testing.

All ECGs were normal. Athletes had larger left ventricular diastolic dimensions, higher maximal O_2 uptake, and delayed onset of anaerobic metabolism than controls. The mean IQ of athletes was 121; 4 athletes had grade point averages of 3.0 or less, 4 had averages of 3.6–3.9, and 5 had

4.0 averages. Seven participants ranked above the 85th percentile in boldness, warmth, conformity, sensitivity, and high drive with tension and dominance. Eight runners scored above the 93rd percentile in self-discipline and emotional stability. Seven human-figure drawings indicated immaturity and an underdeveloped body image.

During follow-up, athletes experienced 2 stress fractures, 1 back sprain, and 1 knee injury. Two sisters, both of whom had anorexia nervosa 18 months after beginning long-distance running, were still under psychiatric care at the time of evaluation. Another girl committed suicide 2 years after beginning running and 8 months after an evaluation that showed a distorted body image, high drive with tension, and frustration. Psychiatric care had been recommended at evaluation.

Athletes demonstrated high physical fitness without growth retardation; however, runners shared distinct positive and negative personality characteristics. The relatively high incidence of severe psychological disorders suggests that young children entering strenuous training programs should undergo psychological screening and long-term psychological monitoring.

▶ Some young runners may be on unhealthy courses. These 16 children, who in grade school began running heroic mileage—30–105 miles a week, tended to have major psychological disorders, including high drive with tension, frustration, and underdeveloped or distorted body images. Two girls had anorexia nervosa, and another girl committed suicide. These athletes, recruited mainly by word-of-mouth, probably constitute a skewed sample, but this report implies that we should screen or at least monitor the psychological health of young distance runners.—E.R. Eichner, M.D.

Predicting Injury in Young Cross Country Runners With the Self-Motivation Inventory

McClay MH, Appleby DC, Plascak FD (Indiana Univ, Indianapolis; Marian College, Indianapolis)

Sports Training Med Rehabil 1:191–195, 1989   6–26

The level of self-motivation may affect athletic performance and injury, but whether high levels of self-motivation can have as negative effects as external stressors is not known. To study the relationship between self-motivation and performance and injury, the full-scale Self-Motivation Inventory (SMI) was applied in 28 high school cross-country runners. The SMI, which contains 40 questions with multiple-choice answers, was administered just before the beginning of the competitive season; test scores were tabulated after the season had ended.

Test scores were highest for those with severe injury, with a significant difference between those with severe injury and with no injury. The difference between boys and girls with severe injury was marginally significant. There were weak negative correlations between the Inventory score and the best individual performance and team position.

The SMI provides a good prediction of the potential for injury, especially severe injury in girls, but not performance, in adolescent cross-country runners. The psychological processes that underlie this relationship are not known, but high self-motivation may be a component of type A behavior. Whether the relationship between susceptibility to injury and self-motivation applies to other sports warrants investigation.

▶ This article suggests that, among high-school runners at least, self-motivation, i.e., hard-driving discipline, does not predict for victory, but, especially among girls, seems to predict for injury. Female runners who score high on the SMI tend to push their bodies through overload to injury. A 1990 review of the epidemiology of running injuries finds that such injuries generally stem from a complex interplay of (1) training errors, especially excessive mileage; (2) anatomical variations that might be tolerated in other sports; (3) shoes and surfaces; (4) previous injuries and/or arthritis; (5) hormonal milieu, especially in women; and (6) psychological makeup(1).— E.R. Eichner, M.D.

Reference

1. Eichner ER: *Techniques in Orthopaedics.* In press, 1990.

7 Doping

Physiological Responses to Caffeine During Endurance Running in Habitual Caffeine Users
Tarnopolsky MA, Atkinson SA, MacDougall JD, Sale DG, Sutton JR (McMaster Univ, Hamilton, Ont)
Med Sci Sports Exerc 21:418–424, August 1989   7–1

To determine the ergogenic benefit of caffeine in exercise performance, the effects of caffeine on neuromuscular and metabolic responses to endurance running were studied in 6 variety-level male runners who habitually had a low-to-moderate caffeine intake. Exercise testing was performed on a cycle dynamometer 1 hour after caffeine, 6 mg/kg, was taken in sweetened lemonade or a placebo solution.

Caffeine administration significantly increased plasma free fatty acid levels before and during the 90-minute bout of exercise (Fig 7–1). It did not alter any of the other parameters, which included oxygen consumption, respiratory exchange ratio, perceived exertional level, neuromuscular function, or plasma levels of glucose, lactate, and catecholamines. Plasma dopamine responses to exercise were similar with and without caffeine ingestion.

In this study, caffeine ingestion by low-to-moderate caffeine consumers was not associated with ergogenic metabolic or neuromuscular changes. The lack of effect may reflect tolerance related to habitual caffeine use.

▶ Many long-distance athletes consume as large quantities of caffeine as are permitted by the rules of their particular competition on the basis that it enhances their performance. There have been many suggestions as to the site of any ergogenic action of caffeine. It may depress fatigue and reduce the perception of exertion by its stimulant effect on the brain (1). There have also been reports of an impact on neuromuscular function (2,3). Finally, at the cellular level, there may be mobilization of free fatty acids, stimulation of intramuscular triglyceride utilization, and inhibition of glycogenolysis (4,5). The present report suggests that in practice the effects of caffeine are much more limited. There are several possible explanations of the discrepancy between theory and practice. First, some laboratory experiments have been based on large doses of caffeine that would now be regarded as doping. Second, many endurance competitors regularly ingest large amounts of caffeine; it may thus be that they have developed a tolerance to permitted doses, so that the effects seen in naive subjects no longer occur (6). Finally, it is necessary to simulate the carbohydrate loading that precedes endurance competition if the data are to be applicable to actual athletic events.—R.J. Shephard, M.D., Ph.D.

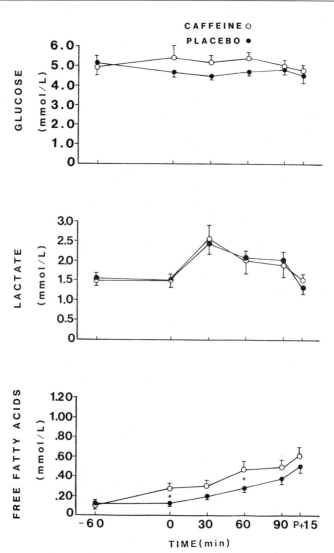

Fig 7–1.—*Upper panel,* plasma glucose concentration; *middle panel,* plasma lactate concentration; *lower panel,* plasma free fatty acid concentration. Values are mean ± SEM. *Asterisk* indicates P < .05. (Courtesy of Tarnopolsky MA, Atkinson SA, MacDougall JD, et al: *Med Sci Sports Exerc* 21:418–424, August 1989.)

References

1. Giles D, MacLaren D: *J Sports Sci* 2:35, 1984.
2. Costill DL, et al: *Med Sci Sports* 10:155, 1978.
3. Ivy JL, et al: *Med Sci Sports Exerc* 11:6, 1979.
4. Erickson MA, et al: *Med Sci Sports Exerc* 19:579, 1987.
5. Essig D, et al: *Int J Sports Med* 1:86, 1980.
6. Robertson D, et al: *J Clin Invest* 67:1111, 1981.

Mechanism of Enhanced Cold Tolerance by an Ephedrine-Caffeine Mixture in Humans
Vallerand AL, Jacobs I, Kavanagh MF (Defence and Civil Inst of Environmental Medicine, Downsview, Ont)
J Appl Physiol 67:438–444, July 1989   7–2

Once body insulation and peripheral vasoconstriction have been maximized, human beings rely on their ability to elevate heat production to avoid deep body hypothermia. The value of an ephedrine-caffeine mixture in improving cold tolerance was examined in 9 healthy young men exposed to cold air for 3 hours at 10° C and a wind speed of 1 m/sec while wearing only a bathing suit. Before the 2 trials, subjects ingested a mixture of ephedrine, 1 mg/kg, and caffeine, 2.5 mg/kg.

Drug ingestion limited the final fall in core, mean skin, and mean body temperatures. Total 3-hour energy expenditure increased by more than 18% compared with placebo ingestion (Fig 7–2). Carbohydrate oxidation increased by as much as 42% above the control level when the drugs were ingested. There were no significant effects on lipid or protein metabolism.

Ingestion of ephedrine and caffeine significantly improved cold tolerance in these subjects by promoting heat production. The latter change appears dependent on enhanced carbohydrate oxidation.

▶ The main conclusion of the paper—that subjects cool less when given the ephedrine/caffeine mixture—is well established. The precise mechanism is less certain, as detailed records of shivering activity were not obtained. One source of heat production in the cold is "futile cycling," or the breakdown of triglycerides to fatty acids and their subsequent resynthesis. The intriguing suggestion of Vallerand and associates is that the ephedrine/caffeine mixture may stimulate this process, with a resultant increase in carbohydrate usage. The practical application to sports medicine is less clear. An event such as a swim across the cold waters of Lake Ontario is not regulated by international agencies; it might then be permissible to take such a mixture, but even if this were the case, it is not certain that an increased rate of carbohydrate depletion would help performance. Again, in a hypothermic emergency situation (when

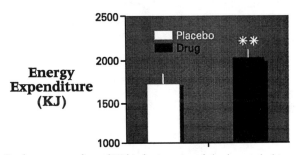

Fig 7–2.—Total energy expenditure (kJ/3 h) after ingestion of placebo or ephedrine-caffeine mixture in the same persons exposed to cold. Significant difference from placebo condition: *asterisks* indicate $P < .01$. (Courtesy of Vallerand AL, Jacobs I, Kavanagh MF: *J Appl Physiol* 67:438–444, July 1989.)

there is no committee of Human Ethics to call a halt to the experiment), I am not sure that faster usage of carbohydrate would increase survival.—R.J. Shephard, M.D., Ph.D.

The Effect of Citrate Loading on Exercise Performance, Acid-Base Balance, and Metabolism
Kowalchuk JM, Maltais SA, Yamaji K, Hughson RL (Univ of Waterloo, Ont)
Eur J Appl Physiol 58:858–864, 1989   7–3

The increased anaerobic glycolysis occurring at exercise power outputs of more than 70% to 80% of maximal aerobic capacity lowers the plasma pH and causes fatigue. The beneficial effect of sodium bicarbonate ingestion on exercise performance is well established. Similar beneficial effects have been reported with ingestion of fruit juices high in potassium citrate or of alkaline salts of citric acids. However, other studies have found no such benefit from citrate-based alkalinizing agents.

The effects of citrate ingestion on acid-base balance, metabolism, and exercise performance were assessed in 9 active university students (mean age, 23 years). Each student performed a progressive exercise test to exhaustion to determine individual maximal aerobic capacity. The student then performed 2 experimental exercise sessions, 1 of submaximal aerobic power and 1 up to near-maximal intensity after oral ingestion of 500 mL of a glucose-free, orange-flavored drink containing either sodium chloride as a placebo or sodium citrate. All exercise tests were done on a cycle ergometer.

Although sodium citrate loading had a significant alkalinizing effect in plasma when compared with placebo, it did not improve endurance performance during exercise at 95% of maximal aerobic capacity. Sodium citrate loading reduced plasma glycerol levels but did not affect the plasma concentrations of free fatty acids, glucose, or lactate. Plasma hemoglobin and hematocrit levels increased with increasing exercise intensity, but increased less in the citrate-induced alkalosis state.

The alkalinizing effect in plasma after citrate loading was clearly demonstrated, but no improvement in endurance time during exercise at 95% of maximal aerobic capacity was observed.

▶ The concept of increasing the body's ability to buffer the additional [H+] generated during exercise as a means of enhancing performance has been debated since the early part of this century. Implicit in the assumption that such a state would enhance performance is, of course, that the extra [H+] in some way limits performance. Many studies aiming to demonstrate such an effect have used exercise models that were inappropriate. Such is not the case with this paper, in which both the addition of citrate, sufficient to have the same alkalinizing effects as bicarbonate administration previously used, and the exercise model had an effective track record (1, 2). Although the endurance times were not enhanced by citrate, an even more physiologically interesting observation was that plasma lactate also was not different between the alkaline and control states unlike the previous work; this observation, unfortunately, is not addressed by the authors.—J.R. Sutton, M.D.

References

1. Sutton JR et al: *Clin Sci Mol Med* 50:241, 1976.
2. Jones NL, et al: *J Appl Physiol* 43:959, 1977.

The Effect of Nicotine on Energy Expenditure During Light Physical Activity

Perkins KA, Epstein LH, Marks BL, Stiller RL, Jacob RG (Univ of Pittsburgh)
N Engl J Med 320:898–903, Apr 6, 1989   7–4

Metabolic effects of nicotine are implicated in the demonstrable relationship between smoking and lower body weight, but the exact nature

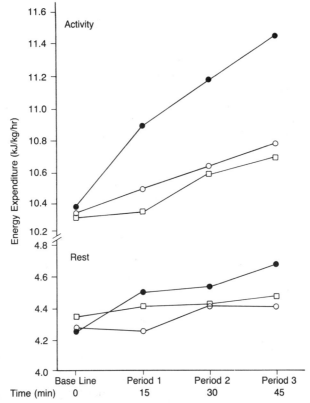

Fig 7–3.—Mean energy expenditure during baseline activity or baseline rest and periods 1–3 during activity and rest sessions in smokers receiving nicotine *(solid circles)*, smokers receiving placebo *(open circles)*, and nonsmokers receiving placebo *(open squares)*. Nicotine or placebo was administered before each period. (Courtesy of Perkins KA, Epstein LH, Marks BL, et al: *N Engl J Med* 320:898–903, Apr 6, 1989.)

of the relationship is not understood. Energy expenditure was measured during cycle ergometer work simulating light daily activity in 10 male smokers given nicotine, 15 μg/kg, and in 10 others given placebo. Nicotine was administered using a measured-dose, nasal spray pump in a double-blind design.

The excess energy expenditure ascribed to nicotine was more than twice as great during exercise than at rest (Fig 7–3). Placebo spray did not influence energy expenditure at rest or on exercise in either the smokers or in a comparison group of nonsmokers. Respiratory quotient values did not differ significantly in the various groups. There also were no group differences in distance pedaled, confirming standardization of activity. Both groups of smokers had higher levels of perceived exertion than nonsmokers had.

Light exercise enhances the metabolic effects of nicotine, but the metabolic effects of smoking appear to be transient. The decrease in metabolic rate after cessation of smoking may be complete within 24 hours, leading to an immediate gain of body mass.

▶ The authors note that nicotine has previously been shown to increase the basal metabolic rate in both animals and humans, but they do not speculate as to the cause of this phenomenon. One contributory factor that deserves further exploration is the impact of nicotine on the cardiac and respiratory work rate (1). Cardiac and respiratory work is a small component of total metabolism at rest, but it rises to between 5% and 10% of the total energy expenditure during vigorous exercise, even in a nonsmoker. The higher heart rate and the bronchospasm that develop with smoking would produce the exercise-dependent increase of metabolism observed here. It would also explain why smoking makes a larger contribution to the control of body mass in people who are physically active than in those who are inactive.—R.J. Shephard, M.D., Ph.D.

Reference

1. Rode A, et al: *Arch Environ Health* 24:27, 1971.

Epidemiological and Policy Issues in the Measurement of the Long Term Health Effects of Anabolic-Androgenic Steroids
Yesalis CE III, Wright JE, Bahrke MS (Pennsylvania State Univ, University Park; Sports Science Consultants, Plattsburgh, NY; US Army Physical Fitness School, Fort Benjamin Harrison, Ind)
Sports Med 8:129–138, 1989   7–5

Probably more than a million persons in the United States alone use anabolic-androgenic steroids. The role of steroid use in various diseases remains uncertain, but therapeutic and laboratory studies have shown that they produce adverse changes in risk factors and in the physiologic state of many organs and body systems. In particular, risk factors for cardiovascular disease are adversely affected and liver structure and function are altered.

A potential study population must have a significant incidence of steroid use; the leading candidates are power lifters, football players, and bodybuilders. A retrospective study would circumvent the reluctance of many athletes to acknowledge steroid use. Outcomes should include diseases for which risk factors are known to be affected in the short term as well as those involving known target tissues of androgens, such as prostatic cancer.

Long-term studies of the health effects of anabolic-androgenic steroids still are unavailable. Some may be concerned that, if no adverse long-term effects are found, steroid use will increase while the moral issue of fair play persists. It is hoped that a middle ground between definitive studies and anectodal evidence will be found.

▶ This is an excellent review of the subject matter. The interested reader is referred to the original article.—J.S. Torg, M.D.

Anabolic Steroid Use by Male Adolescents
Johnson MD, Jay MS, Shoup B, Rickert VI (Univ of Arkansas for Med Sciences; Arkansas Children's Hosp, Little Rock)
Pediatrics 83:921–924, June 1989   7–6

Steroid use among intercollegiate male athletes has been estimated to range from 2% to 20%. In a more recent study, anabolic steroid use among male high school seniors was reported to be 6.6%. Although this study was intended to be nationally representative, the fewest number of participants were from the south. Anabolic steroid use by male adolescents in a southern state was evaluated in 6 high schools in Arkansas.

Of 853 boys surveyed, 95 reported past or current use of anabolic steroids. The range of use among the high schools was 9% to 19.4% (table). Of the steroid users, 80% correctly identified increase in muscle mass and 65% mentioned increase in strength as possible effects; 12% said incorrectly that steroids produced an increase in height, and 18% thought steroids improved aerobic performance. Of the users, 30% knew that steroids can stunt growth and 38% knew that steroids can cause

---

Male Adolescents Using Anabolic Steroids

	High Schools					
	A	B	C	D	E	F
No. of male adolescents surveyed	144	85	148	223	97	156
No. (%) of users	28 (19.4)	9 (10.5)	14 (9.5)	21 (9.4)	9 (9.3)	14 (9.0)
% involved in sports	96	89	86	76	78	79

Note: Of 853 male adolescents surveyed, 95 (11%) reported using anabolic steroids; 84% were involved in competitive or noncompetitive sports.
(Courtesy of Johnson MD, Jay MS, Shoup B, et al: *Pediatrics* 83:921–924, June 1989.)

liver disease; 38%, cancer of the liver; and 18%, acne. Of the users, 22% were unaware that steroid use had any side effects. Whereas 64% took steroids to increase strength and 50% to increase size, 27% took steroids to improve their physical appearance and 10% because their friends were taking them.

This survey reveals that there is a segment of adolescent boys using anabolic steroids without appropriate knowledge of their effects and adverse complications. The use of steroids may be more widespread than previously thought, or at least distributed differently than thought by geographic region. Health care providers must be more knowledgeable about anabolic steroids so that they can provide guidance, particularly during the preparticipation sports assessment, to reduce unnecessary risk taking.

The Use of Anabolic Steroids in High School Students
Terney R, McLain LG (Loyola Univ, Chicago and Maywood, Ill)
Am J Dis Child 144:99–103, January 1990   7–7

The lay press has publicized anabolic steroid use by athletes. However, scientific literature contains little documentation about the incidence of

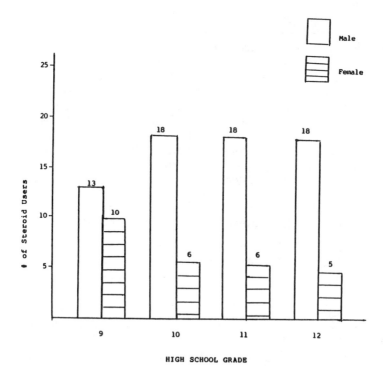

Fig 7–4.—High school grades of steroid users. (Courtesy of Terney R, McLain LG: *Am J Dis Child* 144:99–103, January 1990.)

anabolic steroid use among adolescents. On a single day in May 1988, 2,113 high school students in a suburban Chicago high school were surveyed. Participants included 1,028 boys and 1,085 girls.

Ninety-four students (67 boys, 27 girls) reported using anabolic steroids. Of 1,436 students who participated in sports, 79 (55 boys, 24 girls) used anabolic steroids. Analysis of steroid use by grade showed that 13 boys and 10 girls were in grade 9, 18 boys and 6 girls were in grade 10, 18 boys and 6 girls were in grade 11, and 18 boys and 5 girls were in grade 12 (Fig 7–4). Twenty-three students received steroids from coaches, 31 from physicians, 43 from friends, and 24 from others (Fig 7–5).

Steroid use was higher among athletes (5.5%) than nonathletes (2.4%). The reason for using steroids was not questioned, so it can only be presumed that nonathletes used steroids to improve their appearance. Steroid use was almost equally distributed among grade levels. Football players (9.3%) and wrestlers (12.2%) had the highest percentage of steroid use. This finding is not surprising because strength is thought to be a major asset in these sports. If the incidence of anabolic steroid use in this population is reflective of the national population, approximately 700,000 high school students use anabolic steroids. If this estimate is accurate, anabolic steroids are a serious drug problem in adolescents.

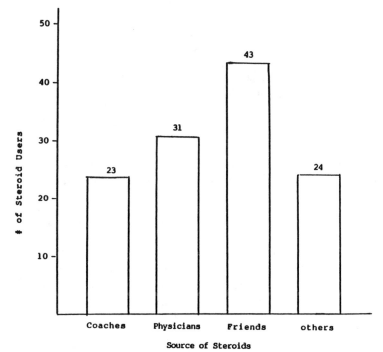

Fig 7–5.—Sources of steroids. (Courtesy of Terney R, McLain LG: *Am J Dis Child* 144:99–103, January 1990.)

Contrasting Effects of Testosterone and Stanozolol on Serum Lipoprotein Levels

Thompson PD, Cullinane EM, Sady SP, Chenevert C, Saritelli AL, Sady MA, Herbert PN (Miriam Hosp, Providence, RI; Brown Univ)
JAMA 261:1165–1168, Feb 24, 1989   7–8

Orally administered anabolic steroids reduce serum concentrations of high-density lipoprotein (HDL)-cholesterol and the HDL_2 subfraction. It is possible that these effects might depend on the route of administration and be unrelated to the androgenic effect of the steroids. To test this hypothesis, oral stanozolol (6 mg/d) or a supraphysiologic dose of intramuscular testosterone enanthate (200 mg/wk) was administered to 11 male weight lifters for a 6-week period, using an unblinded crossover design. Concentrations of lipids, lipoproteins, apolipoproteins, postheparin hepatic triglyceride lipase activity, and gonadotropic hormones were measured weekly.

Stanozolol produced mean reductions of 33% in serum HDL-cholesterol levels, 71% in HDL_2 cholesterol levels, and 32% in apolipoprotein A-1 levels; testosterone resulted in more modest reductions of 9%, 0%, and 8%, respectively (Fig 7–6). Stanozolol administration resulted in a mean 29% increase in the low-density lipoprotein-cholesterol concentration and a mean 35% increase in apolipoprotein B values, whereas testosterone administration produced a mean 16% decrease in low-density lipoprotein-cholesterol and no significant change in apolipoprotein B levels. Stanozolol administration more than doubled (+123%) hepatic triglyceride lipase activity, which was unaffected by testosterone administration. Both drugs led to similar weight gains, but testosterone resulted in more effective suppression of serum levels of follicle-stimulating hormone and luteinizing hormone.

The undesirable alterations in lipoprotein levels produced by orally administered anabolic steroids are more severe than those resulting from testosterone. This finding implies that such effects are not directly related to the androgenic potency of the steroids. Intramuscularly administered testosterone may be preferable to orally administered anabolic steroids for long-term use, although definite conclusions on this issue require appropriate clinical trials.

▶ These 3 articles (Abstracts 7–6—7–8) continue the focus on anabolic steroid use by young persons (see the 1989 YEAR BOOK OF SPORTS MEDICINE, pp 306–308). Now we know that, in Arkansas 11% of high-school boys are using or have used steroids; 84% of the users are athletes; and rampant are misconceptions as to what these drugs do. In a suburban Chicago high school, 6.5% of the boys and 2.5% of the girls use steroids; steroid use is evenly distributed among all 4 grades; and some students get the drug from coaches or physicians. Results similar to these come from a survey in San Antonio, where 10% of the male athletes in the more affluent high schools use anabolic steroids (1). The third article shows us that not all anabolic steroids are alike; that oral forms of steroids (e.g., stanozolol) are more apt than parenteral forms (e.g., testoster-

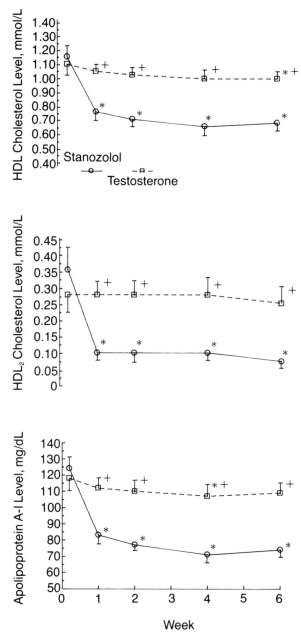

Fig 7–6.—Serum concentrations of HDL-cholesterol, HDL$_2$ cholesterol, and apolipoprotein A-1 before (week 0) and during treatment with stanozolol or testosterone. Multiplying by 38.7 converts cholesterol value from mmol/L to mg/dL. *Asterisks* indicate significant difference from week 0 value, and plus signs, significant difference between 2 treatment groups. *Vertical bars* indicate standard error of the mean. (Courtesy of Thompson PD, Cullinane EM, Sady SP, et al: *JAMA* 261:1165–1168, Feb 24, 1989.)

one) to alter lipoproteins unfavorably, i.e., to raise the low-density lipoprotein-cholesterol and lower HDL-cholesterol. Probably, however, most young persons taking anabolic steroids use 1 or more oral forms. A recent review highlights the many clinical side effects of anabolic steroids (2).—E.R. Eichner, M.D.

References

1. Windsor RE, Dumitru D: *Int J Sports Med* 4:37, 1988.
2. Siegel AJ, Eichner ER: *Your Patient & Fitness* 2:10–17, 1990.

Anabolic-Androgenic Steroids: A Guide for the Physician
Frankle MA (Univ of South Florida, Tampa)
J Musculoskel Med 6:69–88, November 1989   7–9

It has been estimated that 40% of all athletes who train regularly in weight rooms use anabolic-androgenic steroids. Furthermore, about 500,000 or more adolescent boys use these drugs. Knowledge of the pharmacologic properties of anabolic-androgenic steroids is essential to understanding the problems associated with their use by athletes.

An anabolic steroid promotes tissue growth or repair, or both. An androgenic steroid enhances secondary male sex characteristics. Anabolic agents may increase muscle mass, but may not enhance strength and performance as well as androgenic agents do. However, drugs in both groups are testosterone derivatives that stimulate cellular protein synthesis.

All anabolic-androgenic steroids are metabolized in the liver and excreted by the kidney. Oral agents are metabolized rapidly and have a short half-life, whereas injected steroids are metabolized at a lower rate. Consequently, the drug concentration in the liver at any time is less if injected than if ingested. The adverse effects of steroid use also differ depending on whether the oral or the injectable form is taken. Adverse hepatic effects associated with orally administered steroids include increased liver enzymes activity, cholestatic jaundice, peliosis hepatitis, and hepatic carcinoma. Although the last is extremely rare, it has occurred in 2 athletes taking steroids. Adverse effects associated with injected anabolic steroids are related more to the injection itself than to the preparation; AIDS resulting from the use of contaminated needles has been reported. Localized infections and sciatic nerve injury are not uncommon. Side effects related to the dose and the ratio of anabolic to androgenic drugs include virilization, gonadotropic effects, gestagenic effects, estrogenic effects, and changes in lipoprotein distribution. Premature closure of growth plates in skeletally immature persons, acne, changes in libido, and increased aggressiveness are all known side effects of chronic steroid use.

To avoid catastrophic side effects, regular checkups of athletes involved with anabolic-androgenic steroids is imperative. At the time of examination, the physician should explain the potential side effects of steroids and encourage the patient to diminish and ultimately stop the use of these drugs.

▶ The author presents an excellent review of the subject matter. The original article is suggested reading for the interested clinician.—J.S. Torg, M.D.

One- and Two-Dimensional Echocardiography in Bodybuilders Using Anabolic Steroids

Urhausen A, Hölpes R, Kindermann W (Univ of the Saarland, Saarbrücken, West Germany)
Eur J Appl Physiol 58:633–640, 1989   7–10

The strength-promoting effect of anabolic steroids remains controversial, but it is assumed that when used in conjunction with a high-protein diet and high-intensity training, these drugs lead to muscle growth. The echocardiographic effects of anabolic drug use combined with intensive strength training over many years were examined in 21 top-ranking male bodybuilders at regional and higher levels; 14 men had taken anabolic steroids regularly for several years, and 5 were taking drugs at the time of the study.

Maximal performances were higher in the steroid users, but ergometric performance was comparable in the users and nonusers. Heart size relative to body size was consistently normal, as was blood pressure. The diastolic left ventricular diameter was lower in the steroid users, whereas the ratio of left ventricular wall thickness to diameter and the left ventricular muscle mass-volume ratio were greater. Systolic function was similar in the 2 groups, but diastolic function measures indicated certain differences (Fig 7–7).

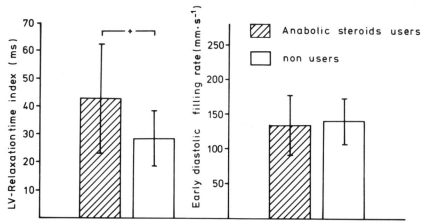

Fig 7–7.—Echocardiographic parameters of diastolic left ventricular (LV) function of 14 anabolic steroid users and 7 nonusers (means ± SD; *asterisk* indicates *P* < .05). (Courtesy of Urhausen A, Hölpes R, Kindermann W: *Eur J Appl Physiol* 58:633–640, 1989.)

Regular anabolic steroid use combined with intense bodybuilding activity can lead to increased left ventricular wall thickness and can impair diastolic function to some extent.

▶ Medical scientists have finally admitted that regular use of massive doses of anabolic steroids can increase muscle bulk, and it is thus logical to anticipate that there would be some effect on cardiac as well as skeletal muscle. Animal experiments have shown both hypertrophy and deleterious functional changes in the myocardium (1,2), and a similar response in humans might be suspected from the predominance of ventricular hypertrophy in weight lifters. The present study sought to tease out the effect of training on the myocardium by separating athletes into 2 groups on the basis of their reported steroid use. The results suggest not only an effect of steroids on ventricular wall thickness, but also an associated slowing of ventricular relaxation. In animals there have been reports that steroids can cause aberrant and chaotically spaced myofibrils, intracellular edema, and mitochondrial swelling (3). It is not yet clear whether any or all of these effects are reversed once drug usage ceases.—R.J. Shephard, M.D., Ph.D.

References

1. Berhendt H, Boffin H: *Cell Tissue Res* 181:423, 1977.
2. Blasius R, et al: *Klin Wochenschr* 35:308, 1957.
3. Appell HJ, et al: *Int J Sports Med* 4:268, 1983.

Anabolic Steroids and Semen Parameters in Bodybuilders
Knuth UA, Maniera H, Nieschlag E (Max Planck Research Inst, Münster, West Germany)
Fertil Steril 52:1041–1047, December 1989   7–11

For ethical reasons, no prospectively controlled clinical trial to assess the long-term effects of anabolic steroids could ever use these drugs at doses commonly self-administered by bodybuilders and other athletes. Thus the long-term effects after anabolic steroid use can be examined only in retrospective case-control studies. A retrospective cross-sectional study was conducted to assess the influence of anabolic steroids on seminal and reproductive endocrine parameters in 41 male bodybuilders (mean age, 26.7 years) who admitted to steroid consumption. Each was asked to complete a detailed questionnaire on past and present drug use, including anabolic steroids, dietary habits, and training performance. All underwent a detailed medical examination, blood testing for endocrine parameters, and semen analysis. Controls were 41 unselected volunteers who were not using steroids or other drugs.

Three subgroups were formed for the purpose of data analysis: 11 men reported 2 months or less of anabolic steroid use and were still taking anabolic steroids at the time of this study; 19 men reported 3–12 months of anabolic steroid consumption up to the time of the study; and

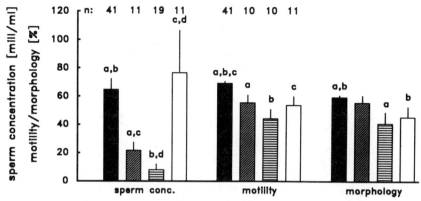

Fig 7–8.—Sperm concentration (mean ± SEM), percentage of motile sperm, and proportion of normally formed sperm in controls *(black bars)* in bodybuilders with short duration of anabolic steroid consumption (group I, *hatched bars*), in bodybuilders with extended anabolic steroid consumption (group II, *horizontally lined bars*), and in athletes after longer than 4 months of drug-free interval (group III, *open bars*). *Identical letters above 2 bars* indicate those pairs of values that are statistically different by analysis of variance and the Student-Newman-Keul test. For analysis of motility and morphology, azoospermic ejaculates were treated as missing values. (Courtesy of Knuth UA, Maniera H, Nieschlag E: *Fertil Steril* 52:1041–1047, December 1989.)

11 men had abandoned anabolic drugs more than 4 months before semen analysis. The amounts of anabolic steroids taken by the bodybuilders per month were considerably greater than the therapeutically recommended doses, reaching extreme ranges of up to 40-fold doses. As a general pattern, different anabolic steroids were taken simultaneously for 3–4 months, interrupted by 3- to 4-month drug-free periods. Despite these enormous doses no side effects were reported, and only 1 of the men had evidence of gynecomastia on physical examination.

In the control group only 2 men had severe oligozoospermia and 2 had moderate oligozoospermia. In contrast, 24 bodybuilders had abnormal sperm counts (Fig 7–8). Depending on the duration of steroid use and the period since last drug intake before testing, the percentages of motile and normally formed spermatozoa were significantly reduced compared with findings in controls. Bodybuilders who had stopped steroid use more than 4 months before testing had normal sperm counts.

Administration of high to very high doses of anabolic steroids may not always stop spermatogenesis. Even after prolonged consumption of extremely high doses of steroids, sperm production may return to normal after drug use is discontinued.

▶ The present report highlights the weakness of studies suggesting that anabolic steroids have no effect on performance. If left to their own devices, some athletes will consume up to 40 times the pharmaceutical dose of anabolic drugs for long periods. Suppression of spermatogenesis is certainly not the only reason for arguing against such use of steroids by athletes, but it would be wrong to conclude from the present paper that there are no long-term effects on sperm counts; 1 of 11 individuals still had pathologically low counts 12 months after stopping steroids, and despite 4 months or more of abstinence, a number of the others had reached no more than the lower limit of normality proposed by the World Health Organization, rather than the average to be anticipated in young, healthy, and well-nourished young men.—R.J. Shephard, M.D., Ph.D.

Effects of Blood Transfusions on Some Hematological Variables in Endurance Athletes
Berglund B, Birgegård G, Wide L, Pihlstedt P (Karolinska Hosp, Stockholm)
Med Sci Sports Exerc 21:637–642, December 1989   7–12

Autologous reinfusion of blood is used in athletes to increase maximal oxygen uptake; however, no method for detecting reinfusion has yet been developed. Transfusion-induced changes in hematologic variables were investigated in 8 men and 4 women. All were formerly competitive endurance athletes now engaged in intense leisure-time endurance training. The athletes ate the same type of mixed diet and continued training regimens throughout the study. One unit of blood was withdrawn on 3 occasions separated by 1–2 weeks. Red blood cells were separated, frozen, and later thawed, washed, and reinfused 3–4 months later. Iron was taken orally from the first phlebotomy until 1 month after the third. Blood samples were analyzed before reinfusion, and 5 hours, 1 day, 2 days, 1 week, 2 weeks, and 4 weeks after reinfusion. No physical training was permitted in the 12 hours before blood sampling.

The hemoglobin concentration in men increased from 146.7 g · L^{-1}

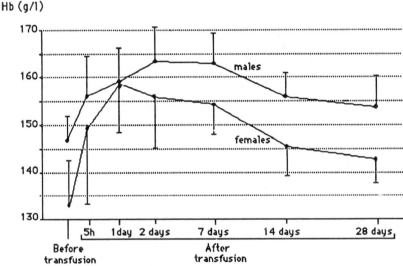

Hb (g/l)

Fig 7–9.—Time course of hemoglobin (Hb) (mean ± SD) in males and females before and during 4 weeks after reinfusion of 1,350 mL of autologous blood. (Courtesy of Berglund B, Birgegård G, Wide L, et al: *Med Sci Sports Exerc* 21:637–642, December 1989.)

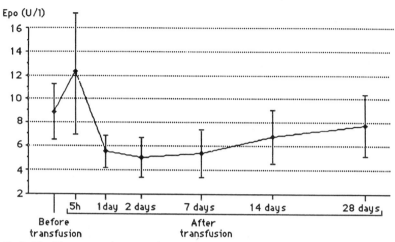

Fig 7–10.—Time course of serum erythropoietin (s-[Epo]) (mean ± SD) before and during 4 weeks after reinfusion of 1,350 mL of autologous blood. (Courtesy of Berglund B, Birgegård G, Wide L, et al: *Med Sci Sports Exerc* 21:637–642, December 1989.)

immediately before reinfusion to a maximum of 163.5 g · L^{-1} 2 days after reinfusion; in women it increased from 131.7 g · L^{-1} to 155.9 g · L^{-1}. Thereafter, in men, the hemoglobin concentration gradually decreased to 153.9 g · L^{-1} and in women to 142.4 g · L^{-1} within 4 weeks after reinfusion (Fig 7–9). Serum iron levels increased significantly 5 hours after infusion but did not increase significantly thereafter. Serum bilirubin levels did not increase, and serum ferritin levels increased gradually for 2 weeks after infusion. Serum erythropoietin levels increased significantly in the afternoon on the day of infusion but decreased to less than preinfusion concentrations 1 day after reinfusion. These values remained significantly decreased until 4 weeks after reinfusion (Fig 7–10). Blood lactate levels decreased significantly within 5 hours after reinfusion and remained significantly lower the first and second days afterward.

An algorithm based on an increase in the serum hemoglobin concentrations and a decrease in serum erythropoietin concentrations might indicate that the patient had been transfused with autologous freezer-stored red blood cells. However, because the transfusion-induced decrease in the serum erythropoietin concentration is relatively small, it is probably impossible to determine unequivocally with this method that an individual athlete has had such a transfusion.

▶ Can we catch blood boosters? Not yet. The algorithm here is imprecise and nonspecific: One week after transfusion, the hemoglobin level was up by 5% or more and the serum erythropoietin level down by 30% or more in 8 of 12 athletes. Not good enough. Worse yet, the recent spate of mysterious deaths in Dutch cyclists raises the fear that some athletes are boosting their blood, perhaps to dangerous levels of viscosity, via injections of erythropoietin.—E.R. Eichner, M.D.

8 Medical Conditions

Physical Fitness and All-Cause Mortality: A Prospective Study of Healthy Men and Women
Blair SN, Kohl HW III, Paffenbarger RS Jr, Clark DG, Cooper KH, Gibbons LW
(Inst for Aerobics Research, Dallas)
JAMA 262:2395–2401, Nov 3, 1989

8–1

The relationship between physical fitness and physical activity and disease is controversial. It is not known whether physical activity sufficient to increase physical fitness is necessary for health benefits. All-cause and cause-specific mortality by physical fitness categories was reviewed for men and women followed for an average of more than 8 years. The 10,224 men and 3,120 women in the study were given a preventive medical examination. A maximal treadmill test measured physical fitness.

Two hundred men and 43 women died. When all-cause mortality was adjusted for age, rates declined with increased physical fitness. In the least fit men the death rate was 64.0 per 10,000 person-years and in the most fit men it was 18.6 per 10,000 person-years. For women the corresponding values were 39.5 per 10,000 person-years and 8.5 per 10,000 person-years, respectively. After statistical adjustments for age, smoking habits, cholesterol levels, systolic blood pressure, parental history of coronary heart disease, fasting blood glucose levels, and follow-up intervals, the trends still remained constant. Mortality from coronary heart disease and cancer of combined sites was also lower in higher fitness categories in both men and women.

Low physical fitness is an important risk factor for all-cause mortality in both men and women. Higher levels of physical fitness appear to defer all-cause mortality primarily because of reduced rates of cancer and cardiovascular disease. The high prevalence of low physical fitness and sedentary habits may be an important public health problem.

▶ Of course, the important question is, what is necessary to achieve the desired level of physical fitness? According to the authors, "A brisk walk of 30 to 60 minutes each day will be sufficient . . . ." In an accompanying editorial, Koplan et al. (1) suggests participating in activities that are pleasurable for the patient and performed on a regular basis at least 3 times a week for 20 minutes.—J.S. Torg, M.D.

Reference

1. Koplan JP, et al: *JAMA* 262:2437, 1989.

An Outbreak of Furunculosis Among High School Athletes

Sosin DM, Gunn RA, Ford WL, Skaggs JW (Centers for Disease Control, Atlanta; Kentucky Dept for Health Services, Frankfort)
Am J Sports Med 17:828–832, November–December 1989   8–2

Furuncles often occur in teenagers, but there have been few reports documented in literature. An outbreak of furuncles was discussed with 118 male football and basketball players; 6 players participated in both sports. There were no furuncles available for laboratory investigation.

Of the athletes, 31 had at least 1 furuncle associated with their sport during the 1986–1987 season. In 81% of the cases the initial lesion developed on the arms or legs. All 31 athletes were seen by either the team trainer or a physician; 71% of initial furuncles were treated with antibiotics. Three athletes were hospitalized and received intravenous antibiotic therapy for recurrent furunculosis unresponsive to oral antibiotics. One athlete had a disseminated *Staphylococcus aureus* infection and a lung abscess. The initial lesion occurred the week before football practice began. After that, the number of new cases rose steadily, and the monthly attack rate increased in football players until the season was over at the end of October (Fig 8–1).

Nearly all athletes sustained abrasions, (e.g., grass and floor burns). Athletes who incurred abrasions more than twice weekly were more than 3 times as likely to have furuncles than those who had few abrasions. In the 43% of players who had close friends with furuncles, the risk of fu-

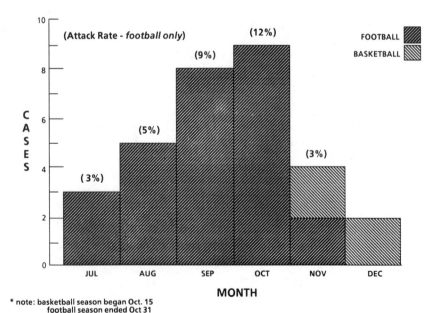

Fig 8–1.—Distribution of cases by month of first furuncle. (Courtesy of Sosin DM, Gunn RA, Ford WL, et al: *Am J Sports Med* 17:828–832, November–December 1989.)

runculosis was more than twice that of other athletes. The risk of furunculosis was also greater for athletes who wore wrist bands or elbow pads.

Skin injury apparently plays a role in the development of furunculosis, but skin injury alone would not be sufficient to cause infection unless *S. aureus* also was present. The highest risk of *S. aureus* exposure in this series appeared to be from contact with other athletes having furuncles. Because 90% of outbreak cases were among varsity athletes, exposure was greater for members of the group than for outsiders.

Fomites appeared to play a minimal role in the outbreak, and use of locker-room facilities did not appear to increase the risk of furunculosis. Early control efforts were directed to the locker room, however. The risk associated with wearing wrist bands or elbow pads may have been related to the greater likelihood for injury in these athletes, rather than from direct contamination. Control measures should be directed toward reducing skin injury and exposure to infectious organisms. Proper showering and washing with soap should be stressed. In this series the systemic administration of antibiotics did not reduce the transmission of infectious organisms.

▶ This systematic study offers tips to prevent or control a team outbreak of furunculosis. Illness requires exposure to *S. aureus,* of course, and perhaps also a skin abrasion. If a buddy has furunculosis, the risk is doubled. Fomites play little role, and systemic antibiotics may not work. Effective control measures include wearing protective gear, taking good care of the skin, curbing exposures to furuncles, and showering properly.— E.R. Eichner, M.D.

Unanticipated Admission to the Hospital Following Ambulatory Surgery
Gold BS, Kitz DS, Lecky JH, Neuhaus JM (Univ of Pennsylvania, Philadelphia; Univ of California, San Francisco)
JAMA 262:3008–3010, Dec 1, 1989   8–3

An increasing amount of surgery is performed in the ambulatory setting, and unexpected hospital admission has become an important measure of outcome. To identify clinical and demographic risk factors for hospital admission after ambulatory surgery, a case-control study was conducted. Of 9,616 adults having ambulatory surgery at a university-affiliated hospital in 1984–1986, 98 patients were admitted 100 times; 1 patient with coagulopathy was admitted after 3 different laparoscopies.

Procedures lasting for more than an hour were associated with a nearly four-fold increase in the risk of admission. Postoperative vomiting and residence more than 1 hour's drive away were other risk factors for admission. Age was not closely associated with admission after ambulatory surgery. American Society of Anesthesiologists' physical status was not a significant factor when adjusted for age. Patients having such medical problems as asthma, hypertension, or diabetes were not more likely than others to be admitted after surgery. On multivariate analysis, independent risk factors for admission included general anesthesia, emesis, abdominal surgery, a lengthy procedure, and age. These findings may help to select patients for ambulatory surgery.

▶ In brief, this study appears to establish that "... the likelihood of unanticipated admission is related more to the type of anesthesia and surgical procedure rather than to the patient's clinical characteristics."—J.S. Torg, M.D.

Quantitative Comparison of Thallium-201 Scintigraphy After Exercise and Dipyridamole in Coronary Artery Disease
Varma SK, Watson DD, Beller GA (Univ of Virginia)
Am J Cardiol 64:871–877, Oct 15, 1989   8–4

Intravenous infusion of dipyridamole as an alternative to exercise for myocardial perfusion imaging with thallium-201 has been suggested. The results in 21 patients who agreed to undergo both procedures were compared. All had been referred for diagnostic evaluation of chest pain. The patients underwent a symptom-limited exercise test using the Bruce protocol followed by thallium-201 scintigraphy. Approximately 2.5 weeks later, they received intravenous infusions of dipyridamole and were imaged by the same procedure. Thallium-201 activity was measured in 9 myocardial segments in initial and delayed anterior and 45-degree left anterior oblique views. There were 184 pairs of segments in the distribution of 63 coronary supply regions available for direct comparison.

There were no significant differences between findings after dipyridamole infusion and exercise with regard to the number of segments with normal thallium-201 uptake or in the number of numerically significant defects. A slightly greater proportion of redistribution defects was found after dipyridamole than after exercise. When segment pairs were classified as either abnormal or normal, there was 87% agreement between the 2 methods (Fig 8–2). Agreement was 92% with regard to coronary supply regions. Cardiac catheterization in 15 patients verified that there was

EXERCISE

NORMAL   ABNORMAL

DIPYRIDAMOLE		NORMAL	ABNORMAL
NORMAL		129	8
ABNORMAL		16	36

AGREEMENT IN 165/189 = 87.5%

Fig 8–2.—A segment-by-segment comparison of thallium-201 uptake after exercise and intravenous dipyridamole. Eighty-seven percent of scan segments showed concordant normal or abnormal uptake. (Courtesy of Varma SK, Watson DD, Beller GA: *Am J Cardiol* 64:871–877, Oct 15, 1989.)

no significant difference in the number of stenoses and normal vessels defined by exercise and dipyridamole protocols.

Dipyridamole-thallium-201 scintigraphy can be substituted for exercise scintigraphy without compromising the sensitivity or specificity for coronary artery disease detection.

▶ In some clinical situations it can be difficult for a patient to undertake vigorous treadmill exercise, and the movement of the body during the activity also makes it difficult to evaluate cardiac function accurately. There has thus been much interest in recent suggestions that dipyridamole infusion is as effective as exercise in provoking coronary vasodilatation and thereby revealing stenosed segments of the coronary arterial tree. The present report is an advance on earlier papers in that sensitivity and specificity of the 2 approaches (exercise vs. dipyridamole) were tested in the same individuals.— R.J. Shephard, M.D., Ph.D.

Comparative Effects of Theophylline and Isosorbide Dinitrate on Exercise Capacity in Stable Angina Pectoris, and Their Mechanisms of Action
Crea F, Pupita G, Galassi AR, El-Tamimi H, Kaski JC, Davies GJ, Maseri A
(Royal Postgrad Med School, Hammersmith Hosp, London)
Am J Cardiol 64:1098–1102, Nov 15, 1989   8–5

Nitrates and theophylline are effective in the treatment of myocardial ischemia; it has been hypothesized that both drugs exert their beneficial action by coronary dilation. The hypothesis has been confirmed for nitrates, but the nature of the anti-ischemic action of theophylline remains uncertain. The effects of theophylline and nitrates on exercise capacity and on the diameter of the large epicardial coronary arteries were compared in 20 patients aged 49–68 years (mean age, 61 years) with stable angina pectoris.

Ten patients were randomized to receive either intravenously administered theophylline ethylenediamine or sublingually administered isosorbide dinitrate on 2 consecutive days, with an exercise test performed within 2 minutes of drug administration. Effects of the 2 drugs were assessed in the remaining 10 patients by means of coronary arteriography.

The time to 1-mm ST segment depression and the heart rate and heart rate-blood pressure product at 1-mm ST segment depression were similar for the patients receiving theophylline or isosorbide dinitrate. Also similar were the time to onset of chest pain, maximum heart rate-blood pressure product, and duration of exercise; these parameters were all greater than those obtained during baseline exercise testing. Arteriography revealed that theophylline, unlike isosorbide dinitrate, did not increase the diameters of the proximal and distal segments of the left anterior descending coronary artery.

Although the effects of theophylline in these patients were similar to those of isosorbide dinitrate, the mechanism of the 2 drugs appears to be substantially different, for theophylline did not dilate epicardial coronary arteries. Theophylline may act by redistributing blood flow from nonischemic to ischemic myocardium, a mechanism that, if confirmed, could open the way for a new class of antianginal drugs.

▶ Nitrates were traditionally regarded as coronary vasodilators, and then for a period their beneficial effect was attributed to a reduction of systemic blood pressure and thus cardiac work-rate. Now the pendulum has swung back, and coronary vasodilatation is seen as making a significant contribution to their effectiveness (1).

Neither of these mechanisms seems to be involved in the therapeutic benefit from theophylline. There is no evidence of coronary vasodilatation (indeed, the tendency is to vasoconstriction), and although venous compliance is increased (2), the inotropic action of theophylline leads to an increase in the cardiac work-rate (3). Crea and colleagues make the ingenious suggestion that the drug is helpful because it is a coronary vasoconstrictor! It is delivered in larger amounts to the superficial coronary vessels, countering metabolic vasodilatation in these regions, and thus allows a diversion of blood flow to the more vulnerable subendocardial tissue.—R.J. Shephard, M.D., Ph.D.

References

1. Brown BG, et al: *Circulation* 64:1089, 1981.
2. Watson WE: *Clin Sci* 22:65, 1962.
3. Rutherford JD, et al: *Circulation* 63:378, 1981.

Impaired Blood Pressure Response to Exercise in Patients With Coronary Artery Disease: Possible Contribution of Attenuated Reflex Vasoconstriction in Non-Exercising Muscles
Okamatsu S, Takeshita A, Nakamura M (Kyushu Univ, Fukuoka, Japan)
Br Heart J 61:149–154, February 1989   8–6

Some patients with severe coronary artery disease (CAD) have an impaired blood pressure (BP) response to ergometric exercise. The impaired response may be caused by acute ischemia-induced pump failure, or by changes in vascular resistance during exercise. To further investigate this issue, 18 patients aged 39–72 years with confirmed CAD were first tested on a treadmill by the Bruce protocol. Eight patients had decreased BP and 10 patients had increased BP in response to exercise testing. Each patient underwent diagnostic cardiac catheterization. After a 20-minute recovery period patients performed leg exercises in the supine position on a bicycle ergometer at a workload of 20 W for 6 minutes.

There were no significant differences between the 2 groups with respect to baseline BP, pulmonary artery wedge pressure, cardiac index, forearm vascular resistance, or oxygen consumption measurements. Patients who had an impaired BP during treadmill testing had similar increases in BP during the supine leg exercises. Increases in cardiac index,

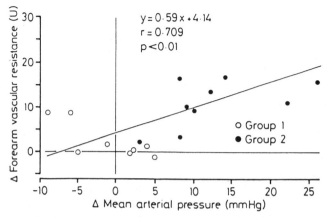

Fig 8–3.—Relationship between increase in mean blood pressure *(x)* and increase in forearm vascular resistance during ergometer exercise *(y)*. There was a positive correlation between them. (Courtesy of Okamatsu S, Takeshita A, Nakamura M: *Br Heart J* 61:149–154, February 1989.)

pulmonary artery wedge pressure, and oxygen consumption during leg exercise were similar in both groups of patients. However, patients with impaired BP responses during exercise had greater increases in forearm vascular resistance than did those who had a decrease in BP. The mean BP changes during leg exercise in patients with impaired BP responses correlated with the mean changes in forearm vascular resistance (Fig. 8–3).

An impaired BP response to ergometer exercise is not caused by the failure to increase cardiac output. Rather, it appears that the impaired BP response during exercise in patients with CAD is a result of attenuation of reflex vasoconstriction in nonexercising muscles.

▶ One of the most worrisome results of a simple progressive exercise test in patients with CAD is failure of the BP to increase or even to decrease. Such an observation is usually taken as a sign of severe CAD with inability of the cardiac output to increase sufficiently because of reduced myocardial contractility (1). We should remind ourselves that the BP response to exercise is the net effect of 2 influences—cardiac output and peripheral vascular resistance—and changes in either or both influence the BP response.

The importance of this article is that both central cardiac function and peripheral vascular tone were measured in 2 groups of cardiac patients: group 1, in whom no increase in BP on exercise occurred, and group 2, in whom the normal increase did occur. Interestingly, both groups appeared to have comparably severe CAD. Cardiac output, left ventricular ejection fraction, and left ventricular end-diastolic pressure were similar in the 2 groups. Thus failure to increase BP appropriately on exercise in group 1 was a peripheral failure—an inability to alter vascular resistance appropriately. However, there was no postural hypotension, as is often seen in patients with autonomic neuropathy, e.g., diabetes or the Shy-Drager syndrome.—J.R. Sutton, M.D.

Reference

1. Thomson PD, Kelemen MH: *Circulation* 52:28, 1975.

Exercise-Induced Myocardial Ischemia in a Cold Environment: Effect of Antianginal Medications
Juneau M, Johnstone M, Dempsey E, Waters DD (Montreal Heart Inst; Univ of Montreal)
Circulation 79:1015–1020, May 1989   8–7

Patients with angina often report worsening symptoms in cold weather, and studies have shown that angina occurs earlier during exercise testing in a cold environment. Ischemic thresholds in patients with stable-effort angina were compared at cold and normal temperatures, as were the rate-pressure products at onset of ischemia at both temperatures. Subjects underwent exercise testing without treatment and after treatment with propranolol and diltiazem.

Twenty-two men and 2 women with stable angina were randomly assigned to undergo exercise testing on a treadmill 90 minutes after administration of either placebo, propranolol, or diltiazem. Each subject was tested after all 3 treatments at room temperatures of −8° C and 20° C. Medical histories indicated that 8 patients were cold sensitive before the study.

With the placebo, exercise end points for the group as a whole did not differ significantly between cold and normal temperatures; however, in the cold-sensitive subjects 1 mm ST depression developed 30% sooner. The rate-pressure product was lower at onset of ischemia at −8° C than at 20° C. At both temperatures propranolol and diltiazem both prolonged time to onset of 1 mm ST depression. The magnitude of improvement at the colder temperature was equal to that at normal temperature, and there were no significant differences between the improvement with propranolol and with diltiazem. However, only diltiazem prolonged the total exercise time.

During exercise, cold does not worsen the ischemic threshold in most patients with stable angina. However, the ischemic threshold does decrease in cold-sensitive patients. Both propranolol and diltiazem are as effective in reducing exercise-induced ischemia in colder temperatures as in normal temperatures.

▶ This is an eminently practical study with simple take home messages:
1. Most patients in the present series with stable angina were not cold sensitive,
2. In those who were cold sensitive the mechanism was probably the result of an increase in coronary artery tone, not because the cold increased the myocardial work (although myocardial work is not easily quantified in the clinical situation).
3. Propranolol or diltiazem are both effective treatments for exercise in the cold, although diltiazem has the added advantage of prolonging exercise time.—J.R. Sutton, M.D.

Physical Training and Relaxation Therapy in Cardiac Rehabilitation Assessed Through a Composite Criterion for Training Outcome
van Dixhoorn J, Duivenvoorden HJ, Staal HA, Pool J (St Joannes de Deo Hosp, Haarlen, The Netherlands; Erasmus Univ, Rotterdam)
Am Heart J 118:545–552, September 1989   8–8

Aerobic exercise training is common in cardiac rehabilitation; however, some patients do not improve their exercise tolerance, and some even have reduced tolerance. A composite criterion was developed to differentiate patients who succeed at exercise training from those who fail, and also whether relaxation therapy has any effect on training outcome.

A total of 156 patients recovering from myocardial infarction were randomly assigned to receive exercise training plus relaxation and breathing therapy (group A) or exercise training only (group B). Exercise training consisted of once-daily 30-minute exercise sessions on a cycle ergometer for 5 weeks. Relaxation therapy centered around a respiratory technique and used several procedures for active and passive relaxation. Relaxation training was given once a week for 1 hour for 5 weeks. To obtain a single measure for overall training outcome, cardiac dysfunction, maximum work rate, maximum heart rate, and systolic blood pressure response were considered sequentially. The 17 patients who dropped out of the program were also classified according to their reasons for not completing training.

Patients receiving treatment A had a more pronounced training bradycardia and a significant improvement in ST abnormalities. Using the composite criterion, 55% of patients in group A and 46% of those in group B had training successes (table). Patients in group A had more successful outcomes and fewer failures than those in group B. The odds for failure were .25 for treatment A and .51 for treatment B. There were failures in 20% of the patients in group A and 33% of those in group B. No changes were noted in 25% of patients in group A and 21% of those in group B.

If relaxation training is added to an exercise regimen, the risk of treat-

Overall Outcome of Training Based on Composite Criterion
for Training Benefit (TB)

	Treatment A	*Treatment B*
TB = + (Success of training)	42(55%)	37(46%)
TB = 0 (No change)	19(25%)	16(21%)
TB = − (Failure of training)	15(20%)	27(33%)
Total	76(100%)	80(100%)

Note: Linear χ^2: 2.85; $df = 1$; $P = .09$, 2-tailed.
(Courtesy of van Dixhoorn J, Duivenvoorden HJ, Staal HA, et al: *Am Heart J* 118:545–552, September 1989.)

ment failure can be reduced. However, not all patients recovering from myocardial infarction will benefit from exercise training regardless of the regimen.

▶ We demonstrated previously that in the first year after myocardial infarction, hypnosis and relaxation training can yield almost as great benefits as regular exercise (1), but that in the second year those who progress to more vigorous training fare better than those who receive hypnotherapy alone. The present report asked whether a combination of exercise plus relaxation therapy would improve the response relative to exercise alone. The study was somewhat biased against a successful outcome, because patients with psychosocial problems were excluded and treatment was followed for only 5 weeks. The authors apparently wanted to find a positive outcome, and concluded that relaxation therapy did reduce the number of patients who failed to respond to treatment. However, if one looks at the "small print" of their statistical analysis, one finds that the critical odds ratio has a probability of only 0.09; in other words, their conclusion is not statistically established.— R.J. Shephard, M.D., Ph.D.

Reference

1. Kavanagh T, et al: *Arch Phys Med Rehabil* 51:578, 1970.

Effects of High Resistance Training in Coronary Artery Disease
Crozier Ghilarducci LE, Holly RG, Amsterdam EA (Univ of California, Davis)
Am J Cardiol 64:866–870, Oct 15, 1989   8–9

Cardiac patients are usually discouraged from participating in resistive exercise. However, such exercise may be both safe and beneficial. The safety and efficacy of an isotonic strength-training program at intensities of more than 60% of maximal capacity were assessed.

Nine stable aerobically trained male cardiac patients underwent a daily 30-minute strength-training program 3 days per week for 10 weeks. They performed the following lifting exercises at 80% of maximum voluntary contraction: quadriceps extension, bench press, hamstring curl, standing biceps curl, and military press. Also, they performed 80% of maximum sit-ups in 1 minute. Body composition was determined before and after the training regimen. Subjects underwent heart monitoring and ECG during all activities.

The men had an 11% increase in quadriceps girth after training; this was the only change in body composition. However, maximum voluntary contractions increased by 12% for miliary press, 17% for bench press, 19% for standing biceps curl, 46% for hamstring curl, and 53% for quadriceps extension after training (Fig 8–4). The number of sit-ups performed in 1 minute increased by 33%. Subjects had no signs or symptoms of ischemia, abnormal heart rate, or blood pressure responses.

Resistance training at 80% of maximum voluntary contraction seems

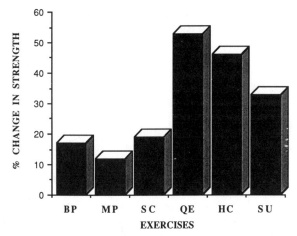

Fig 8−4.—Percent change in strength after a 10-week high-resistance training program in 9 stable, aerobically trained cardiac patients. Strength was assessed by either maximal voluntary contraction lifts for bench press (BP), military press (MP), standing biceps curl (SC), quadriceps extension (QE), and hamstring curl (HC), or by the number of sit-ups (SU) performed in 1 minute. All changes were significant to $P < .001$ except for SU ($P < .005$). (Courtesy of Crozier Ghilarducci LE, Holly RG, Amsterdam EA: *Am J Cardiol* 64:866−870, Oct 15, 1989.)

to be both safe and beneficial in stable aerobically trained cardiac patients. Further research is necessary to determine whether these results would apply to other populations of cardiac patients.

▶ For a long time, cardiologists were frightened by the observations of Lind and McNicol (1), who found an ominous rise in both systolic and diastolic pressures when subjects performed isometric exercise. However, it has more recently been appreciated that their report was based on efforts held to subjective exhaustion, and the rise of pressure can be much smaller with brief muscle overload, particularly if an adequate recovery interval is allowed between individual repetitions. Several recent reports have shown that both cardiac patients and patients as old as 80 years of age can perform circuit training quite safely, without evidence of myocardial ischemia (chest pain, premature ventricular contractions, or ST segmental depression).

Loss of lean tissue is characteristic of the older, coronary-prone individual, and a program to restore muscle mass, as described here, increases the individual's maximal voluntary force. Because the rise in blood pressure during unplanned exercise is proportional to the fraction of maximal voluntary force that is exerted, the end-result of such training is that a given load can be sustained more safely. Particularly for the patient who is returning to heavy work, there is much to commend circuit training as one component of an overall cardiac rehabilitation program.—R.J. Shephard, M.D., Ph.D.

Reference

1. Lind AR, McNicol GW: *Can Med Assoc J* 96:706, 1967.

Effects of Exercise on Left Ventricular Volume and Output Changes in Severe Mitral Regurgitation: A Radionuclide Angiographic Study

Lavie CJ, Lam JB, Gibbons RJ (Mayo Clinic and Found, Rochester, Minn)
Chest 96:1086–1091, November 1989   8–10

Patients with severe mitral or aortic regurgitation often have symptoms of dyspnea during exercise. Because there are few data on the effects of exercise on left ventricular volume and output changes in patients with severe mitral regurgitation, 7 men and 4 women with severe chronic mitral regurgitation underwent radionuclide angiography at rest and after exercise on a supine cycle ergometer. Patients were continuously monitored by ECG during exercise. Patients exercised until they reached 1 of the following end points: moderate angina, marked dyspnea or fatigue, marked dysrhythmias, or ST segment depression of 2 mm or more.

All patients had normal sinus rhythm and a resting left ventricular ejection fraction of more than 0.55; 1 patient had a regurgitant fraction of less than 50%. Most patients could achieve a reasonable exercise workload, but 3 achieved peak workloads of less than 100 W. The end-systolic volume index, end-diastolic index, ejection fraction, and left ventricle regurgitant fraction did not change significantly during exercise; however, the forward cardiac index increased by 86%. There was no significant change in the forward stroke volume index, but there was an 87% increase in the heart rate. The regurgitant stroke volume index decreased by 12% with exercise, but regurgitant flow increased to a mean of 8.2 L/min/m^2, a gain of 64% (Fig 8–5).

To increase forward flow during supine dynamic exercise, patients with severe mitral regurgitation must depend on an increase in heart rate as there is no change in the forward stroke volume index. Blunting of the heart rate response through calcium or β-blockers, or sinus node dysfunction, could severely incapacitate these patients. The marked increase in regurgitant flow during exercise probably contributes to dyspnea.

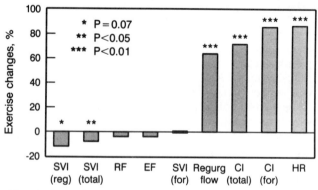

Fig 8–5.—Exercise changes by percentages in patients with severe mitral regurgitation. *SVI*, stroke volume index; *RF*, regurgitant fraction; *EF*, ejection fraction; *CI*, cardiac index; *HR*, heart rate. (Courtesy of Lavie CJ, Lam JB, Gibbons RJ: *Chest* 96:1086–1091, November 1989.)

▶ The orifice of an incompetent valve is relatively fixed, so that the fraction of regurgitant flow depends largely on the pressure gradient across the valve. Vigorous exercise, by raising output impedance and thus systemic pressures, increases the regurgitant flow—in the present series to an average of 8.2 L/min/m², or almost twice the forward flow. It is hardly surprising that such patients have difficulty in exercising, or that the added load on the myocardium sometimes gives rise to angina. Nevertheless, much of the regurgitation occurs during diastole, so that the fraction of regurgitant flow is marginally decreased as the exercise-induced tachycardia brings about a relative shortening of the diastolic phase of the cardiac cycle.

The end-diastolic volume in the patient with mitral regurgitation is much above the normal value even at rest, and there is thus little possibility of increasing the blood flow during exercise by augmentation of stroke volume. In fact, both the end-diastolic volume and the stroke index actually decrease during exercise, so that the doubling of forward flow that is achieved depends entirely on an increase in the heart rates.—R.J. Shephard, M.D., Ph.D.

Sudden Death in Young People Due to Hypertrophic Cardiomyopathy
Gourdie AL, Robertson CE, Busuttil A (Royal Infirmary of Edinburgh; Univ Med School, Edinburgh)
Arch Emerg Med 6:220–224, September 1989   8–11

Hypertrophic cardiomyopathy may cause sudden death in young persons. Five such episodes were encountered.

Woman, 19, with a previously unremarkable medical history, collapsed in the street. The ambulance crew found her in cardiac arrest, and she was given basic life support during transport. Upon arrival at the emergency room she was in ventricular fibrillation. After defibrillation she had a stable sinus rhythm and good cardiac output. A 12-lead ECG showed characteristics of left ventricular hypertrophy and "splintering" of the QRS complex. Her pulse was jerky, and she had an audible systolic murmur maximally at the lower left sternal edge. Echocardiography confirmed a diagnosis of hypertrophic obstructive cardiomyopathy. Despite maintenance of adequate perfusion and a stable rhythm, the patient nevertheless did not regain consciousness and died 3 days later. Postmortem results showed classic features of hypertrophic obstructive cardiomyopathy.

In this study, 4 of 5 persons with hypertrophic obstructive cardiomyopathy who died suddenly had either competed in sports or died during physical activity. There is a need for awareness of this condition in young persons. Those who experience unexplained episodes of syncope, collapse, or chest pain should have appropriate clinical, ECG, and echocardiographic evaluation. Individuals with hypertrophic obstructive cardiomyopathy should avoid strenuous or competitive physical activity, and they should have close cardiologic follow-up. Screening of other family members is also appropriate.

▶ Not a new observation, but a very important one. Since the original descriptions by Brock (1) and by Goodwin et al. (2), we have been made aware of the importance and frequency of hypertrophic obstructive cardiomyopathy as a cause of sudden death in athletes. Maron and colleagues (3) have revealed that the cause of death is most commonly a ventricular arrhythmia or sudden hemodynamic failure caused by an acute increase in outflow tract obstruction. β-Adrenergic antagonists, which form the cornerstone of medical therapy, may help to reduce the gradient across the obstruction, although a variety of surgical procedures from septal myotomy-myectomy to cardiac transplantation have been advocated.—J.R. Sutton, M.D.

References

1. Brock R: *Guys Hosp Gazette* 106: 221, 1957.
2. Goodwin JF, et al: *Br Heart J* 22:403, 1960.
3. Maron BJ, et al: *N Engl J Med* 316:844, 1987.

Heart Rate and Metabolic Response to Competitive Squash in Veteran Players: Identification of Risk Factors for Sudden Cardiac Death
Brady HR, Kinirons M, Lynch T, Ohman EM, Tormey W, O'Malley KM, Horgan JH (Beaumont Hosp, Dublin; Royal College of Surgeons of Ireland, Dublin)
Eur Heart J 10:1029–1035, November 1989   8–12

Squash is associated with a considerable risk of sudden cardiac death. Death is almost always instantaneous and usually occurs during play; however, 23% of these players collapse early after exercise. Autopsy sug-

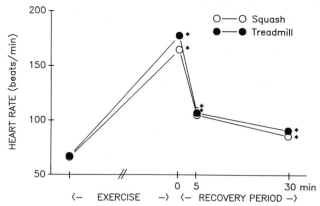

Fig 8–6.—Heart rate during competitive squash and treadmill cardiac stress testing in 10 veteran squash players. All values are mean ± SEM. *Signifies statistical difference compared with preexercise rate (*P* < .05), as determined by analysis of variance. Error bars are within the symbols where not visible. (Courtesy of Brady HR, Kinirons M, Lynch T, et al: *Eur Heart J* 10:1029–1035, November 1989.)

gests that many deaths may be caused by ventricular arrhythmias. Heart rate and metabolism were studied in 10 veteran squash players (mean age, 49 years) during competition and during treadmill exercise to determine whether similar metabolic changes occur in both circumstances.

All 10 athletes played squash at least twice weekly and regularly participated in tournaments. None had known heart disease. The heart rate was measured and phlebotomy was performed immediately before the game, immediately afterward, and at 5 minutes and 30 minutes afterward. Treadmill exercise was performed with a modified Bruce protocol with similar monitoring.

Heart rate and levels of plasma lactate, plasma catecholamines, serum-free fatty acids, and blood glucose were significantly elevated immediately after squash and during the early postexercise period. During recovery, hypokalemia and ventricular arrhythmias were common. The heart rate and metabolic response were similar in pattern and magnitude between squash and treadmill exercise to exhaustion. All subjects had sig-

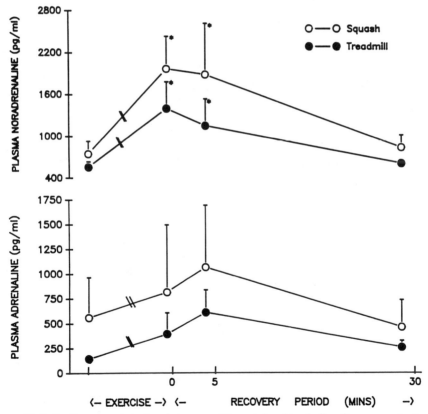

Fig 8–7.—Plasma catecholamines during competitive squash and treadmill cardiac stress testing in 10 veteran squash players. *Signifies statistical difference ($P < .05$) compared with preexercise values, as determined by analysis of variance. All values are mean ± SEM. (Courtesy of Brady HR, Kinirons M, Lynch T, et al: *Eur Heart J* 10:1029–1035, November 1989.)

nificant tachycardia immediately after the game; squash and treadmill exercise caused almost identical changes in heart rate during exercise and recovery (Fig 8–6). Squash also caused a dramatic increase in circulating levels of norepinephrine, epinephrine, lactate, and free fatty acids (Fig 8–7).

The physiologic changes that occur during squash may be appropriate adaptations to exercise in healthy persons, but these changes have been implicated in the pathogenesis of fatal ventricular arrhythmias in persons with ischemic heart disease. Squash may be an inappropriate form of exercise for older men with coronary heart disease.

▶ Squash, which originated at Harrow School in England about 1850, is an old game for young men, or for old men with young hearts. For more, see the analysis of 60 deaths associated with squash in the 1987 YEAR BOOK OF SPORTS MEDICINE, p 14.—E.R. Eichner, M.D.

Isolated Episode of Exercise-Related Ventricular Fibrillation in a Healthy Athlete
Buja G, Meneghello MP, Bellotto F (Univ of Padua, Italy)
Int J Cardiol 24:121–123, July 1989   8–13

The major causes of exercise-related ventricular fibrillation in young athletes are hypertrophic cardiomyopathy and congenital coronary arterial disease. Modifications of neural activity may also be a cause. Exercise-related ventricular fibrillation, a rare event, occurred in a healthy young athlete.

Man, 19, experienced sudden cardiocirculatory arrest during a football match that was caused by a documented ventricular fibrillation. He had been well trained and was asymptomatic previously. Results of blood tests, chest radiography, echocardiography, and exercise stress testing were normal, and there was no evidence of drug abuse. Repeated 24-hour Holter monitoring sometimes demonstrated sporadic and uniform premature ventricular beats. Results were also normal on complete catheterization of the right and left heart chambers, coronary angiography, and right endomyocardial biopsy. An electrophysiologic examination, which included a complete atrial and ventricular stimulation protocol, did not show conduction disturbances, cardiac preexcitation, or atrial or ventricular arrhythmias. Psychological stress testing failed to induce ventricular arrhythmias. Acebutolol, 400 mg/day, taken orally, was prescribed and the patient was discharged. He was perfectly well and continued to play noncontact sports 28 months later.

▶ This extensive and illustrative work-up excluded the most common causes of ventricular fibrillation in the athlete. Other possibilities here include myocarditis, which can be patchy; microscopic conduction tract lesions; or coronary artery spasm, which can be triggered by cocaine, among other drugs (1). This athlete, taking β blockers, returned to noncontact sports. The Hank Gathers tragedy has renewed interest in the proper diagnosis and management of major arrhythmias in athletes (2). Two fine articles provide timely and practical clinical information on the diverse causes of exercise-related sudden deaths in athletes (3,4).—E.R. Eichner, M.D.

References

1. Cantwell JD, Rose FD: *Phys Sportsmed* 14:77, 1986.
2. Munnings F: *Phys Sportsmed* 19:97, 1990.
3. Van Camp SP: *Phys Sportsmed* 16:97, 1988.
4. Thomas RJ, Cantwell JD: *Phys Sportsmed* 18:75, 1990.

Exercise Response in Young Women With Mitral Valve Prolapse
Drory Y, Fisman EZ, Pines A, Kellermann JJ (Chaim Sheba Med Ctr, Tel Hashomer, Israel)
Chest 96:1076–1080, November 1989   8–14

Mitral valve prolapse (MVP), which occurs in about 5% of the general population, is most common among young women. The significance of this condition is not clear. Although serious complications have been reported, MVP is benign in most patients. To study a possible link between MVP and autonomic nervous system dysfunction, exercise responses in young women were evaluated.

The series included 198 women aged 16–29 years with documented MVP on echocardiography. Slightly more than half (53.5%) of the patients were asymptomatic; 46.5% reported palpitations, dizziness, chest pain, and/or fatigue. A control group consisted of 105 healthy young women without MVP. All underwent exercise testing and echocardiography.

Patients with MVP had a significantly lower near-maximal physical working capacity (PWC_{170}) than healthy persons. The presence of symptoms or systolic click did not significantly alter PWC_{170} among patients with MVP. At rest and at moderate exercise, the mean heart rate was significantly higher in patients with MVP than in healthy controls; but at higher workloads the differences between the groups were not statistically significant. Of the women with MVP, 8 had abnormal systolic

---

Nonspecific ST and T Wave Changes in Patients With
MVP and Healthy Persons

	MVP (n = 198) No. of Subjects (%)	Healthy (n = 105) No. of Subjects (%)	P
Rest	29 (14.6)	3 (2.9)	<0.001
Exercise/Recovery	91 (46.9)	24 (22.9)	<0.001

(Courtesy of Drory Y, Fisman EZ, Pines A, et al: *Chest* 96:1076–1080, November 1989.)

blood pressure (SBP) exercise response; the rate of this abnormality was similar for symptomatic and asymptomatic patients with MVP. Both arrhythmias and nonspecific ST and T wave changes were significantly more common in patients with MVP (table). They also had a significantly longer mean corrected QT interval.

Apparently, many patients with MVP have increased adrenergic tone or hypersensitivity to catecholamine stimulation. The abnormal systolic blood pressure response to exercise in some patients may indicate autonomic nervous system imbalance. The fact that a hyperkinetic circulatory state in MVP is not related to symptoms or auscultatory findings may suggest that MVP is a normal physiologic variant in some individuals.

▶ One of the real dangers of modern technology is that we find variants of anticipated physiologic behavior and start to wonder whether these have pathologic significance. Mitral valve prolapse has become a topic of widespread discussion only since echocardiography became commonplace. It is frequently observed in athletes, and if it is insufficient in magnitude to cause regurgitant flow, it probably has no clinical significance. Although the authors found a higher mean blood pressure in those subjects with prolapse, the difference from controls was not impressive. The heart rate in the prolapse group was also a little faster during exercise, so that the double-product is appreciably greater for such individuals; this may explain in part why there is sometimes an association between prolapse and abnormalities of cardiac rhythm.— R.J. Shephard, M.D., Ph.D.

Reproducibility of Exercise-Induced Ventricular Arrhythmia in Patients Undergoing Evaluation for Malignant Ventricular Arrhythmia
Saini V, Graboys TB, Towne V, Lown B (Harvard School of Public Health; Brigham and Women's Hosp, Boston)
Am J Cardiol 63:697–701, March 15, 1989   8–15

Exercise testing is a suitable method for exposing ventricular arrhythmia (VA) and guiding the selection and dosing of antiarrhythmic drugs, but using exercise testing for this purpose is not yet generally accepted. The major reservation focuses on reproducibility of arrhythmia provocation.

The reproducibility of arrhythmia provocation under usual conditions of hospital management of VA was defined in 23 men and 5 women aged 18–76 years referred for evaluation of potentially life-threatening VA. All patients underwent 2 successive exercise studies on a motorized treadmill according to a standard Bruce protocol. A continuous hard copy record of cardiac rhythm was obtained throughout the exercise test, including a 5-minute control period and a 10-minute recovery period. Exercise was maximal and symptom-limited, and continued until the patient wished to stop. However, the attending physician would stop the test for accelerating or lengthening salvoes of ventricular tachycardia increasing angina, a precipitous drop in systolic blood pressure, or signs of poor peripheral perfusion. High-risk patients had an indwelling intravenous catheter in place during testing.

In 27 of the 28 patients, some increase in VA during exercise or recovery was observed, yielding a greater than 80% incidence of exercise-induced VA. The average exercise duration was 7 minutes 50 seconds in the first test and 7 minutes 43 seconds in the second. The reproducibility of a test with a positive outcome was 76%. Similarly, test-retest agreement was more than 74%.

In a population with serious VA, exercise-induced arrhythmia is sufficiently reproducible to serve as an adjunct method in the evaluation and management.

▶ Cardiac arrhythmias on exercise are of considerable clinical significance. Most are simple, and non-life-threatening, but certain malignant ventricular arrhythmias are potentially fatal. Although some will be provoked by exercise, the literature is relatively unconvincing as to the reproducibility of a laboratory-based exercise test for diagnosis (1,2). The interesting aspect of this paper is that the authors found, in 27 of 28 patients being evaluated for ventricular arrhythmias, that a standard Bruce treadmill test increased the arrhythmias. This then enabled the authors to state that treadmill testing in such patients is not only useful for diagnosis but is also useful as a tool to evaluate the effects of antiarrhythmic medications.

One additional point of importance was the observation that in patients with malignant ventricular premature beats the complex forms were not reproducible when their density was low.—J.R. Sutton, M.D.

References

1. Ekbloom B, et al: *Am J Cardiol* 43:35, 1979.
2. Sheps DS, et al: *Circulation* 6:892, 1977.

Is Severe Bradycardia in Veteran Athletes an Indication for a Permanent Pacemaker?

Northcote RJ, Rankin AC, Scullion R, Logan W (Univ Dept of Med Cardiology; Victoria Infirmary, Glasgow; Victoria Hosp, Blackpool, England)
Br Med J 298:231–232, Jan 28, 1989   8–16

Older athletes may be susceptible to severe bradycardia, a condition caused by their years of endurance training and the natural decrease in heart rate that occurs with increasing age. To maintain cardiac rhythm, 2 veteran athletes were given permanent pacemakers.

Case 1.—Man, 66, who was a regular runner for 50 years, ran between 40 and 129 km a week. He had resting bradycardia but no other clinical signs of cardiovascular abnormality. Sinus bradycardia, first-degree heart block, normal ventricular axis, and voltage criteria for left ventricular hypertrophy were detected on resting 12-lead ECG. His mean heart rate in a 24-hour period was 49 beats per minute (Fig 8–8); complete heart block occurred nocturnally. After implantation

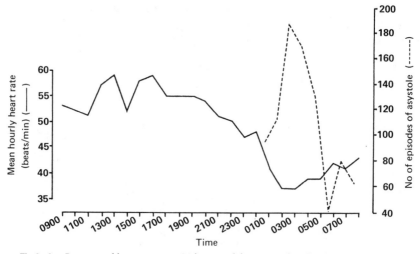

Fig 8–8.—Response of heart rate over 24 hours and frequency of cardiac asystole (longer than 2 seconds). Note maintenance of circadian rhythm. (Courtesy of Northcote RJ, Rankin AC, Scullion R, et al: Br Med J 298:231–232, Jan 28, 1989.)

of a dual-chamber permanent pacemaker, findings on coronary angiography normalized and the patient reported increased energy.

Case 2.—Man, 52, who was a former boxer, experienced periods of lightheadedness and loss of consciousness. His symptoms stopped after he received a permanent pacemaker.

Because neither patient had underlying cardiac disease, the severe bradycardia was probably a result of many years of physical training. This condition carries a risk of syncope, systemic embolism, or sudden death. Reduction of physical training might resolve it, but these patients wanted to continue their athletic activities. Both had improved performance after receiving a pacemaker.

▶ Two interesting case reports of patients who required insertion of a permanent pacemaker. The clinical indications for this—syncope or prolonged and repeated episodes of ventricular standstill—are fairly obvious. However, the causal relationship between life-long endurance training and the onset of ventricular standstill is far less obvious and as yet unproven.—J.R. Sutton, M.D.

Asystole With Syncope Secondary to Hyperventilation in Three Young Athletes
Buja G, Folino AF, Bittante M, Canciani B, Martini B, Miorelli M, Tognin D, Corrado D, Nava A (Univ of Padua, Italy)
PACE 12:406–412, March 1989   8–17

Three male athletes experienced syncope during, or in 1 instance after, an episode of hyperventilation. These were well-trained athletes who

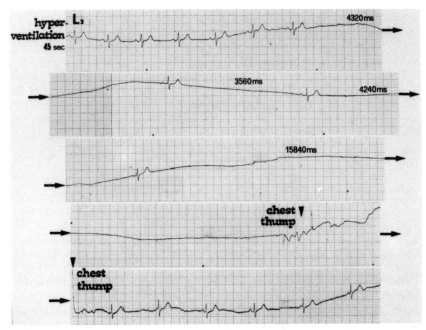

Fig 8–9.—Continuous ECG strip in L2 recorded immediately after cessation (45 seconds) of hyperventilation maneuver. A sinus rhythm of 60–65 beats per minute (bpm) is followed by prolonged sinus arrests (4,320, 3,560, 4,240, 15,840 msec) interrupted by 3 isolated sinus beats. After 2 chest thumps a stable junctional rhythm of 50 bpm appeared dissociated by a sinus rhythm at a slightly lower rate. Paper speed: 25 mm/sec. (Courtesy of Buja G, Folino AF, Bittante M, et al: *PACE* 12:406–412, March 1989.)

were being screened for competitive sports activity. The ECG showed prolonged sinus arrest that was promptly terminated by a chest thump.

Man, 18, well and properly trained, had a sudden fall in heart rate after hyperventilating for 45 seconds, followed by a sequence of prolonged sinus arrests — each interrupted by isolated sinus beats (Fig 8–9). He complained of syncope before several chest thumps restored a stable junctional rhythm. Normal electrolytes and acid-base balance were documented in a blood test 20 minutes later. No bradyarrhythmia occurred when hyperventilation was repeated the next day. Holter monitoring showed an average heart rate of 45 during sleep with a minimum of 38 beats per minute. Conduction appeared to be normal. The athlete remained well 30 months later.

One of the athletes, a mountain climber, was advised to undergo placement of a permanent pacemaker. Prolonged asystole secondary to hyperventilation appears to be rare in athletes without overt heart disease. One possible cause of this condition is a sudden fall in sympathetic activity associated with temporary vagal predominance after hyperventilation. Parasympathetic reflexes induced by cerebral ischemia from vasoconstriction or by emotional stress might be involved.

▶ Prolonged sinus arrest is common in patients with spinal cord transection in the early posttraumatic period. For several weeks after the injury such patients are particularly vulnerable to any procedure such as suctioning that stimulates the vagus. The accompanying hypoxia may serve to augment the vagal stimulus. Some of these patients will have a temporary pacemaker inserted and, rarely, a permanent pacemaker (1).

This report of profound bradycardia in well-trained athletes is included in the YEAR BOOK not because the observations are novel but, rather, because of the severity of the prolonged sinus arrest (Fig 8–9). An increase in vagal tone is a well-known phenomenon in trained athletes, who also will have a lowered intrinsic heart rate (2). However, rarely, if ever, is a permanent pacemaker inserted, and rarely is a permanent pacemaker indicated in an athlete who does not have overt heart disease.—J.R. Sutton, M.D.

References

1. Garner SH, et al: *Arch Phys Med Rehabil* 66:763, 1985.
2. Sutton JR, et al: *Lancet* 2:1398, 1967.

Effect of Isometric Exercise on Cardiac Performance and Mitral Regurgitation in Patients With Severe Congestive Heart Failure
Keren G, Katz S, Gage J, Strom J, Sonnenblick EH, LeJemtel TH (Albert Einstein College of Medicine, Bronx)
Am Heart J 118:973–979, November 1989   8–18

In patients with severe congestive heart failure, systemic arterial pressure increases during isometric exercise as do both systemic vascular resistance and left ventricular filling pressure; however, cardiac output does not increase. Functional mitral regurgitation could contribute to a reduction in cardiac output.

Seventeen patients with longstanding congestive heart failure were studied by invasive right-sided cardiac catheterization and Doppler echocardiography during isometric exercise. Total stroke volume and ejection fraction were calculated from end-diastolic and end-systolic volumes.

Isometric exercise at 30% of maximum produced a decrease in stroke volume index and a significant increase in heart rate from 81 to 92 beats per minute. Systemic vascular resistance also increased. A significant rise in pulmonary wedge pressure was associated with a significant increase in mitral regurgitant volume. Although left ventricular end-diastolic and end systolic volumes did not change significantly, the total stroke volume tended to increase. The increase in mitral regurgitant volume correlated with the decrease in cardiac output (table).

Isometric exercise causes a rise in systemic arterial pressure that is associated with a decrease in cardiac output. Decreased cardiac performance is attributable to an increase in mitral regurgitation. At the same time, forward cardiac output is decreased. Mitral regurgitation can be reduced significantly at rest and during exercise by therapeutic interventions to reduce cardiac afterload.

Echo-Doppler Measurements and Derived Parameters at Rest and During Isometric Exercise

	Rest	Isometric exercise	p Value
End-diastolic volume (ml)	248 ± 51	252 ± 49	NS
End-systolic volume (ml)	185 ± 48	182 ± 52	NS
Total stroke volume (ml)	62 ± 13	67 ± 13	NS
Aortic stroke volume (ml)	48 ± 13	40 ± 12	<0.002
Mitral regurgitant volume (ml)	14 ± 11	27 ± 15	<0.001
Regurgitant fraction (%)	22 ± 15	37 ± 17	<0.001
Mitral regurgitant area (cm²)	0.15 ± 0.12	0.31 ± 0.23	<0.001
Peak systolic pressure/end-systolic volume (mm Hg/ml)	0.69 ± 0.24	0.85 ± 0.32	<0.001

(Courtesy of Keren G, Katz S, Gage J, et al: *Am Heart J* 118:973–979, November 1989.)

▶ As more patients with congestive failure are encouraged to exercise, it is becoming recognized that the rise in afterload associated with isometric activity in particular and the combination of exercise and cardiac failure in general can exacerbate an existing mitral regurgitation, or cause functional regurgitation in patients who have competent mitral valves at rest. Administration of arterial vasodilators has previously been advocated in congestive failure because these patients usually have high peripheral resistance (1, 2); in addition to improving muscle perfusion, such drugs may help to avert the problems associated with mitral regurgitation.—R.J. Shephard, M.D., Ph.D.

References

1. Greenberg BH, et al: *Circulation* 65:181, 1982.
2. Stevenson LW, et al: *Circulation* 78:II, 1988.

Use of the Exercise Test to Predict Prognosis After Coronary Artery Bypass Grafting

Dubach P, Froelicher V, Klein J, Detrano R (Long Beach VA Med Ctr, Calif)
Am J Cardiol 63:530–533, March 1, 1989   8–19

More than 200,000 patients undergo coronary artery bapass grafting (CABG) annually in the United States. Predicting the prognosis in patients who become symptomatic after CABG is therefore an important issue. However, evaluation often is difficult. Symptoms frequently are atypical, and the resting ECG often is abnormal. Several studies have attempted to predict the clinical outcome in patients who become symptomatic after CABG, but none has included treadmill testing.

The use of exercise testing after CABG for predicting cardiac events was evaluated during a 3-year period in 2,044 patients. Previously, 296 of these had undergone CABG. Follow-up data on the latter group were obtained for an average of 2 years after exercise testing. The minimal follow-up was 235 days. Exercise responses considered included MET level, maximal heart rate, maximal systolic blood pressure, chest pain pattern, and ST segment response.

During the 2-year follow-up, 15 patients died, 11 had a nonfatal myocardial infarction, 6 underwent repeat CABG, and 3 had percutaneous transluminal coronary angioplasty (PTCA). The MET level and maximal heart rate were significantly higher in the total patient population compared with patients who died or had experienced a nonfatal myocardial infarction. Patients who had undergone repeat CABG or PTCA had significantly lower maximal systolic blood pressures and significantly greater amounts of ST depression when compared with the total population. Of 80 patients who exceeded 9 METs, only 1 had a myocardial infarction, and none died. In contrast, 10 of 52 patients unable to achieve 5 METS had died or had had a myocardial infarction.

Although MET level and maximal heart rate were significantly related to prognosis and no patient who exceeded 8 METs died, the predictive power of these exercise test responses was low, and ST segment depression was not predictive at all. The exercise ECG is therefore not useful for predicting cardiac events in patients who become symptomatic after undergoing CABG.

▶ Exercise testing continues to enjoy wide popularity in cardiology and for good reason. There is no better way of provoking symptoms of chest pain or dyspnea that are absent or infrequent at rest. An objective assessment of a patient's work capacity, or need of oxygen uptake, can be made and the heart rate and blood pressure responses to the increasing demands of exercise can be observed simply and noninvasively. The ECG is also useful as a diagnostic tool, and provided one is aware of the prevalence of coronary artery disease in the patients under study, one will be realistic about the positive and negative predicted values of the tests.

Now we come to a different patient population—those who have undergone CABG. This study from Froelicher's group urges us to be cautious in estimating prognosis from exercise ECG changes. Although the limitations of retrospective studies must be considered, the simple physiologic observations of power output and maximum heart rate were related to prognosis but not to the exercise ECG. Perhaps additional information provided by an ejection fraction plus other angiographic data quantifying graft patency will remain better prognostic criteria than the exercise ECG (1–3).—J.R. Sutton, M.D.

References

1. Tyras DH, et al: *Ann Thorac Surg* 37:47, 1984.
2. Tyras DH, *Am J Cardiol* 44:1290, 1979.
3. De Feyter PJ, et al: *Am J Cardiol* 55:362, 1985.

Exercise Rehabilitation After Heterotopic Cardiac Transplantation
Kavanagh T, Yacoub MH, Mertens DJ, Campbell RB, Sawyer P (Toronto Rehabilitation Ctr; Harefield Hosp, Middlesex, England)
J Cardiopulmonary Rehabil 9:303–310, August 1989   8–20

In the heterotopic cardiac transplantation procedure, the surgeon implants the donor heart parallel to the recipient heart, placing anastomoses between the donor and the recipient vena cava, left atria, aorta, and pulmonary arteries. The arteries to both sinoatrial nodes are preserved, as are the nerves to the recipient but not the donor heart. The existence of both a denervated and an innervated heart in the heterotopic cardiac transplant recipient offers an opportunity to study the simultaneous effect of an endurance training program on both structures.

Ten men who had heterotopic cardiac transplantations because of end-stage ischemic heart disease were studied to determine their initial capacity for dynamic exercise and their responses to exercise rehabilitation. All patients were ≥30 months post transplant and currently well. Fourteen patients with orthotopic transplantations were used for comparison. All subjects underwent an 18-month walk/jog training program after initial assessment on a cycle ergometer. Training progressed from walking 1.6 km 5 times per week to walking/jogging 6.5 km per session for a total distance of 32.5 km per week. Training lasted from 30 minutes to 1 hour.

Heterotopic cardiac transplant patients (heterotopes) had poorer compliance with the training regimen because of minor medical problems, but lean body mass increased in both groups after training. The resting heart rate in the heterotopes' donor hearts did not change significantly, but the recipient resting heart rates fell by 14 beats per minute. On the cycle ergometer both groups had increases in peak power output, peak oxygen consumption, and absolute ventilatory threshold. Patients with heterotopic transplantations experienced recipient-heart training bradycardia and less exercise-induced ventricular ectopy than at initial testing. Donor submaximal heart rates were unchanged. Patients with orthotopic transplantations also tended toward training bradycardia. There was no correlation between any changes and the time between surgery and entry into the program.

Training effects corresponding to the walk/jog distances and intensities achieved were evident in both heterotopes and orthotopes. Heterotopes had training bradycardia in the recipient heart that was associated with less ventricular ectopy. Exercise training after heterotopic heart transplantation is recommended to improve physical capacity and maximize the benefits of reparative surgery to the recipient heart.

▶ One of the pioneers of exercise therapy in postmyocardial infarction patients, Terry Kavanagh, has now successfully trained a number of patients after cardiac transplantation and several of them completed the Boston marathon. In the present study he has collaborated with a group from the Harefield Hospital in England, one of the few groups who continue to do heterotopic cardiac transplantation; in this procedure both the recipient and donor hearts occupy the same chest cavity. A unique physiologic aspect of this surgical procedure is that there is both a neurogenically intact and a neurogenically isolated heart present in the same chest cavity. The authors took the opportunity to explore what effects training has on the 2 hearts of the heterotopic transplant patients and compared the responses with those of orthotopic cardiac transplant patients and age-matched controls.

In an 18-month period, the 2 groups of patients trained and improved their fitness. The resting heart rate decreased and maximum exercise heart rates increased. Even in the recipient hearts of those heterotopic transplant patients the resting heart rates were high (an indication of a failing heart), but the elevated resting heart rates of the donor heart in both the heterotopic and orthotopic transplants is indicative of the neurogenic isolation of the pacemaker tissue. Of interest is that the resting heart rate in the orthotopes was some 9 beats lower before training and 11 beats lower afterward, compared to the donor hearts of those heterotopes. This seems strange initially, but it may be attributed in part to the age of the donors for the 2 groups. The orthotopic hearts were from donors an average 6 years younger than the donors to the heterotopic group, and Jose (1) has previously demonstrated an age-related reduction in the intrinsic heart rate. In such isolated hearts it is not surprising that the maximum heart rates achieved were lower in the donor hearts of both groups when compared with the normal population. However, the maximum heart rate in the recipient heart of the heterotopic group was also reduced when compared with normal, both before and after training. Although training did produce a mean increase in maximum heart rate from 136 beats per minute to 143 beats per minute, it was still considerably lower than that in age-matched controls (171 beats per minute). One wonders if there is still some degree of chronotropic impairment of the pacemaker in these patients, or if after training the limitation to performance is now noncardiac.—J.R. Sutton, M.D.

Reference

1. Jose AD: *Am J Cardiol* 18:476, 1966.

Effects of Physical Training on Peripheral Vascular Disease: A Controlled Study
Mannarino E, Pasqualini L, Menna M, Maragoni G, Orlandi U (Univ of Perugia, Italy)
Angiology 40:5–10, January 1989   8–21

Physical activity can improve the walking capacity of patients who experience intermittent claudication. Whether physical exercise causes a real increase in local blood flow and/or in local oxygen delivery in patients with peripheral vascular disease (PVD), or intermittent claudication (stage II PVD), was investigated in 16 patients who received either placebo therapy or participated in a physical training program for 6 months. Physical training consisted of a daily walk outdoors for 1 hour, or gymnastics program consisting of exercise for total motor coordination, postural exercises, and specific lower limb exercises. Patients given placebo therapy took 3 tablets daily. Patients were evaluated by treadmill test,

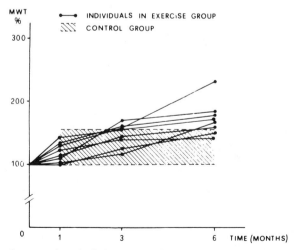

Fig 8–10.—Changes in the individual maximal walking times *(MWT)*. The values are given in percentage of the basal walking time. (Courtesy of Mannarino E, Pasqualini L, Menna M, et al: *Angiology* 40:5–10, January 1989.)

Doppler velocimetry for ankle/arm pressure ratio before and after exercise, and plethysmography for rest flow and peak flow. Local oxygen delivery was measured using basal transcutaneous oxygen pressure and transcutaneous oxygen pressure half-recovery time to basal values after induced ischemia.

Patients who exercised had increased maximum walking capacity and increased pain-free walking capacity compared with those undergoing placebo therapy (Fig 8–10). There were no significant differences between the groups with regard to the other parameters studied.

Physical training reduces claudication in patients with stage II PVD; however, the increase in overall walking and pain-free walking capacity could not be attributed to an increase in collateral circulation or to greater local oxygen delivery or absorption. Nevertheless, exercise was beneficial and is recommended for treatment of all patients with stage II PVD, either alone or in combination with pharmaceutical therapy.

▶ The concept that exercise training benefits the patient with intermittent claudication goes back at least to Larsen and Lassen (1). The present results confirm these findings; actively treated patients increased their pain-free walking time by 87%, whereas there was no change in the control group. However, the training-induced gains of performance could not be linked to any increase in overall limb perfusion. There are at least 3 possible explanations of these observations: (1) regular walking may have increased the patient's pain threshold; (2) there may have been local improvement in perfusion of the painful muscle (3), possibly linked to strengthening of the active muscles; or (3) there may have been an increase in tissue enzyme activity. Plainly, earlier reports of the development of a collateral circulation (4) need to be examined with some scepticism.—R.J. Shephard, M.D., Ph.D.

References

1. Larsen OA, Lassen NA: *Lancet* 2:1093, 1966.
2. Clifford PC, et al: *Br Med J* 280:1503, 1980.
3. Waibel PP, Wolff G: *Surgery* 60:912, 1966.
4. Sanne M, Siversson R: *Acta Physiol Scand* 73:259, 1968.

Effects of Oral Morphine on Breathlessness and Exercise Tolerance in Patients With Chronic Obstructive Pulmonary Disease
Light RW, Muro JR, Sato RI, Stansbury DW, Fischer CE, Brown SE (VA Med Ctr, Long Beach, Calif; Univ of California, Irvine)
Am Rev Respir Dis 139:126–133, January 1989   8–22

Administration of opiates increases the exercise tolerance of patients with chronic obstructive pulmonary disease, but the mechanism responsible has not been identified. The effects of oral opiate administration on exercise tolerance, dyspnea, and arterial blood gas levels were assessed in 13 eucapnic men aged 58–70 years with stable chronic obstructive pul-

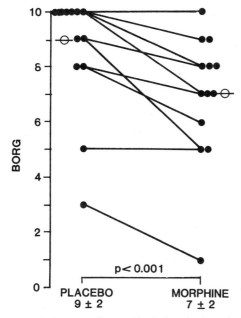

Fig 8–11.—Borg scores at highest equivalent workload after placebo and after morphine on the main study day. (Courtesy of Light RW, Muro JR, Sato RI, et al: *Am Rev Respir Dis* 139:126–133, January 1989.)

monary disease. The men performed duplicate incremental cycle ergometer tests to exhaustion after ingesting a placebo or a morphine solution. An arterial line was inserted for arterial blood determination on the day of active medication.

Analyses after subjects ingested morphine revealed that the mean maximal workload increased by 18.6% from 78.5 W to 93.1 W, and the mean duration of exercise increased from 6.5 minutes to 7.5 minutes. The mean oxygen uptake increased by 19.3%, and the mean carbon dioxide output increased by 13%. Despite the higher ventilation at maximum workload after morphine ingestion, the mean Borg score was not significantly higher (Fig 8–11).

The improved exercise tolerance appears to be related to a higher arterial carbon dioxide pressure and a reduced perception of breathlessness for a given level of ventilation.

▶ One of the major obstacles to rehabilitation of the patient with chronic obstructive pulmonary disease is unpleasantly severe breathlessness on exertion. Any factor that reduces ventilation, and thus the respiratory work rate, will make the patient more comfortable. One option is to breathe oxygen during the early phases of training (1–3). However, in many patients the respiratory problem arises from accumulation of carbon dioxide as much as from a lack of oxygen, and a high arterial oxygen pressure may therefore hinder rather than help performance by fostering a build-up of carbon dioxide in the tissues (including the respiratory centers). An alternative approach is to reduce the central drive to ventilation by administering depressant drugs; these allow arterial carbon dioxide levels to increase for a given work rate and also reduce the sensation of breathlessness associated with a given external ventilation. The main objection to such therapy is the use of an addictive drug in a patient who is likely to live for a substantial time. There is also a strong possibility that such addiction will be associated with a reduced impact of the morphine on respiratory sensations (4). A third therapeutic option (which I prefer) is to strengthen the working muscles. This reduces breathlessness by facilitating their perfusion and thus reducing the build-up of lactate during exercise (5).—R.J. Shephard, M.D., Ph.D.

References

1. Bradley BL, et al: *Am Rev Respir Dis* 118:239, 1978.
2. Scano G, et al: *Eur J Respir Dis* 63:23, 1982.
3. Yas MN, et al: *Am Rev Respir Dis* 103:401, 1971.
4. Santiago TV, et al: *J Appl Physiol* 47:112, 1979.
5. Mertens D, et al: *Respiration* 35:96, 1978.

Airway Responses to Hypertonic Saline, Exercise and Histamine Challenges in Bronchial Asthma

Belcher NG, Lee TH, Rees PJ (Guy's Hosp, London)
Eur Respir J 2:44–48, January 1989   8–23

Patients with asthma have enhanced bronchoconstrictor responses to various stimuli. Respiratory fluid loss during exercise may trigger exercise-induced asthma (EIA) by inducing transient hyperosmolarity of the respiratory epithelium. If this is so, there should be a close relationship between responses to inhaled hyperosmolar aerosols and exercise.

Airway responses were compared to hypertonic, exercise, and histamine challenges in 10 asthmatic patients. Also, the reproducibility of the hypertonic challenge was compared to the reproducibility of exercise challenges in another group of 11 asthmatic patients.

Responses to hypertonic saline did not differ significantly whether the same volume of aerosol was given in 10 *l* aliquots or in a single dose, a finding suggesting that the challenge is cumulative. The response to hypertonic saline correlated significantly both with exercise and with histamine response (Fig 8–12). However, the correlation between exercise and histamine was not statistically significant. The variability of the response to challenge with hypertonic saline did not differ significantly from the variability of the response to exercise.

Exercise-induced asthma apparently is more closely related to the bronchial response to hypertonic saline aerosol than it is to the response to a nonspecific histamine challenge. A closer relationship between EIA and the bronchial response to histamine might have been detected if the patients had had lower histamine reactivity, however. The reproducibility

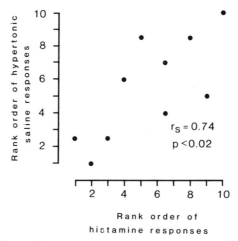

Fig 8–12.—Correlation of the rank orders between the airway responsiveness to histamine, expressed as the concentration producing a 20% decrease in the forced expiratory volume in 1 second (FEV_1) (PC_{20}) and the dose of hypertonic saline producing a 20% decrease in FEV_1 (PD_{20}). Each point is an individual patient. (Courtesy of Belcher NG, Lee TH, Rees PJ: *Eur Respir J* 2:44–48, January 1989.)

of challenge with hypertonic saline was similar to the reproducibility of exercise challenge in the same patients.

▶ The fact that exercise-induced bronchospasm is particularly likely to develop when the air is cold and dry has for a long time suggested that drying of the respiratory mucosa is an important step in provoking this disorder (1, 2). The present paper supports this view and suggests that a face mask that allows prewarming and humidification of inspired air should do much to protect against spasm.—R.J. Shephard, M.D., Ph.D.

References

1. Anderson SD: *J Allergy Clin Immunol* 73:660, 1984.
2. Smith CM, et al: *J Allergy Clin Immunol* 79:85, 1987.

Exercise-Induced Angioedema and Asthma
Leung AKC, Hegde HR (Alberta Children's Hosp, Calgary)
Am J Sports Med 17:442–443, May–June 1989   8–24

Exertion can be complicated by urticaria, angioedema, asthmatic attacks, laryngospasm, cardiac arrhythmias, and vascular collapse. One boy was seen in whom angioedema and asthmatic attacks developed on more than 6 occasions after physical exertion.

Boy, 15 years, had sudden onset of painless facial and periorbital swelling and breathing difficulty after playing basketball for 30 minutes. He had no itchiness or rash, and there was no urticaria. Similar episodes had occurred 6 times within the preceding 6 months, usually after 20–30 minutes of exercise in the gymnasium. He had not been taking medication. On previous occasions physical examination had confirmed angioedema and wheezing. Neither hot baths nor nervousness brought on periorbital edema or asthmatic attacks, and there was no family history of angioneurotic edema. Results of laboratory tests were within normal limits. His bronchospasm was relieved promptly after being given 0.3 mL of 1:1,000 epinephrine subcutaneously and salbutamol by inhalation. He then received 25 mg of diphenhydramine every 4 hours. His periorbital and facial edema resolved within 2 days. Cimetidine prophylaxis, 300 mg twice daily, reduced the frequency and severity of these attacks.

Angioedema, a nonitchy swelling in the deep dermis or subcutaneous tissue, has a predilection for the face and oral soft tissues. The nonpruritic nature of the lesion is unexplained by the paucity of sensory nerve endings in affected areas. Cimetidine is a useful prophylactic agent in this condition.

▶ Another rare allergic reaction to exercise: angioedema and asthma, without urticaria or anaphylaxis. See recent editions of the YEAR BOOK OF SPORTS MEDICINE for articles on exercise-induced anaphylaxis and exercise-related cholinergic urticaria (1986, p 105, and pp 161–164; 1988, pp 168–169). Measures that may help to control these attacks include not eating for several hours before exercising, antihistamine therapy, and, as suggested here, cimetidine.—E.R. Eichner, M.D.

Cardiorespiratory Responses to Aerobic Training by Patients With Postpoliomyelitis Sequelae
Jones DR, Speier J, Canine K, Owen R, Stull GA (Sister Kenny Inst, Minneapolis; State Univ of New York, Buffalo)
JAMA 261:3255–3258, June 9, 1989   8–25

Estimates are that approximately 400,000 survivors of poliomyelitis are at risk for postpoliomyelitis sequelae. Controversy exists over the use of exercise as a treatment modality should postpolio sequelae develop. Whereas some reports have discouraged vigorous physical activity because of the belief that overuse of muscles will result in increased muscle weakness, others have concluded that a modified aerobic exercise program has a positive effect on both muscle weakness and fatigue.

The effects of a 16-week modified aerobic exercise program on cardiorespiratory fitness levels were evaluated in 37 patients aged 30–60 years with postpolio sequelae. The disease had been contracted between 1952 and 1959. Twenty-one patients were randomly assigned to a control group and 16 to an exercise group. Four of the 16 patients in the exercise group had significant preexisting muscular atrophy and weakness in 1 leg; 1 of these patients required bracing for exercise. After undergoing a preliminary stress test, patients trained on a cycle ergometer at 70% of maximal heart rate. Metabolic measurements were obtained at the beginning and end of training.

The mean duration of the exercise bouts during the program was 4.21 minutes. Each patient trained for an average of 20.33 minutes per session for 2.89 sessions per week. The mean training heart rate was 128.9 beats per minute, representing 69.2% of the reserve heart rate plus resting heart rate. Six patients withdrew from the study during training, and 6 patients in the exercise group were eliminated for various reasons, including nonattendance. Values in the exercise group were superior to those in the control group with regard to watts, exercise time, maximum expired volume per unit time, and maximum oxygen consumption. All exercise patients found their endurance improved and fatigue with normal daily activities decreased. None of the patients experienced adverse events or loss of leg strength as a result of the exercise regimen.

The aerobic training program used in treating patients with postpolio sequelae is safe and improves cardiorespiratory fitness in a manner comparable with that of age-matched healthy counterparts.

▶ The widespread vaccination program to prevent the dreaded "infantile paralysis" or poliomyelitis has meant that few younger physicians in the developed worlds have seen an epidemic of polio, as occurred the 1950s. This, of course, is not so in developing countries in which such vaccinations are not commonplace. However, it is now 30 or 40 years since the last generalized epidemics occurred in the Western world, and a new and unusual series of symptoms is evident in those polio sufferers who recovered and have been relatively stable for years. These symptoms include (1) fatigue-exhaustion and decreased effort tolerance, (2) new joint and muscle pain, (3) progressive weakness in both affected and (?) unaffected muscles, and (4) respiratory difficulties that may result in sleep apnea, even to the point of requiring supported ventilation.

In the present series 37 such patients were enrolled in an activity program (16 exercise, 21 control), which was found to improve their endurance and lessen their fatigue, and was accompanied by the same physiologic improvements as are found in the healthy adult population. Another important finding was the failure to observe any untoward effects of exercise.

This latter observation is of particular significance in the reported group of patients with polio from the Sister Kenny Institute. Ironically, one of the current fears about the postpolio syndrome is that exercise may make matters worse! This, of course, was the original fear with acute polio and was the basis of the "immobilization therapy," which was shown subsequently to do more harm than good.

We have much to thank Sister Kenny for. A prophet in her time, she grew up in the small Australian bush town of Warialda and was convinced that the therapeutic practices of the day were doing more harm than good to patients with acute polio. Unfortunately, very few of the medical community listened. However, she revolutionized treatment programs and instituted movement and activity. She deserves an exalted place in the annals of medicine and especially sports medicine. How fitting it is that the institute that perpetuates her memory in honor of her contributions to the treatment of acute poliomyelitis continues to help those same patients more than 30 years later when this new and unusual debility, the postpolio syndrome, has developed.—J.R. Sutton, M.D.

Exercise Training in Individuals With Diabetic Retinopathy and Blindness
Bernbaum M, Albert SG, Cohen JD (St Louis Univ)
Arch Phys Med Rehabil 70:605–611, August 1989   8–26

Exercise is important in the management of patients with diabetes, and it is also helpful in improving coordination and self-confidence in individuals with visual impairment. Previous studies have not addressed exercise training in patients with both diabetes and visual impairment, however. These individuals often have cardiovascular autonomic dysfunction and may also be at risk of becoming hypoglycemic, so guidelines for exercise would be helpful.

Twenty-one visually impaired patients with either insulin-dependent or non-insulin-dependent diabetes mellitus were studied. They underwent graded exercise testing on a cycle ergometer and standardized noninvasive testing to evaluate cardiovascular autonomic function. The exercise program consisted of low-intensity exercise performed 3 times per week. The exercise training target heart rate was 60% of maximum predicted heart rate. Exercise programs were designed individually according to preference and physical status. Most subjects chose to use stationary cycles or walked in the gymnasium with the aid of a guidewire. They used chairs for support and orientation during warm-up and stretching exercises.

Twenty-eight patients had inadequate heart rate responses to respiratory variation, 23 patients had abnormal heart rate responses to postural maneuvers, and 9 patients had postural hypotension. Patients with symptomatic postural hypotension could exercise on a stationary cycle; however, they had hypotensive episodes on walking or prolonged standing. After each exercise session the blood glucose level consistently decreased by a mean of 76 mg/dL even though exercise was performed at low intensity. No relationship between the degree of autonomic neuropathy and the level of decrease in blood glucose was found. However, there was a significant correlation between the decrease in blood glucose and the amount of insulin used in the routine morning dose.

The principal determinant for exercise-induced hypoglycemia was the amount of subcutaneous regular insulin taken. It is important to anticipate hypoglycemia and monitor blood glucose before and after exercise. With appropriate hemodynamic and glucose monitoring, it is safe for patients with both diabetic retinopathy and autonomic neuropathy to exercise.

▶ There is often involvement of the autonomic nerves in advanced diabetes, and because of poor vascular regulation exercise can lead to hypotensive collapse, particularly if it is performed in a warm environment (1–3). Less frequently, there may also be hypertension during exercise (4). It is nevertheless important to distinguish a true diabetic pathology from poor vasoregulation caused by lack of fitness; this problem may possibly explain why the usual test of autonomic dysfunction [respiratory variation (3)] was unable to distinguish the likelihood of an adverse exercise response.

Exercise on a cycle ergometer provides a setting for improving the physical condition but in which fewer demands are placed on the venous reservoirs. In terms of quality of life, however, the ultimate goal must be to get the blind diabetic patient back to a state in which they can walk about confidently and without risk of vasomotor collapse. It is particularly important to recognize that the dose of insulin may have been calculated for a patient having a very sedentary life-style, and a substantial downward revision of the dosage is commonly needed once training is begun.— R.J. Shephard, M.D., Ph.D.

References

1. Hilsted J, et al: *Diabetologia* 22:318, 1982.
2. Kahn JK, et al: *Diabetes Care* 9:389, 1986.
3. Margonato A, et al: *Am Heart J* 112:554, 1986.
4. Karlefors T: *Acta Med Scand Suppl* 449:3, 1966.

A New Case With Hereditary Xanthinuria: Response to Exercise
Landaas S, Borch K, Aagaard E (Ullevaal Univ Hosp, Oslo; Norwegian College of Physical Education and Sport, Oslo)
Clin Chim Acta 181:119–124, May 15, 1989   8–27

Xanthinuria is a rare metabolic imbalance caused by a deficiency of the enzyme xanthine oxidase. Because some patients have muscular symptoms and histologic changes in muscle fibers, patients with xanthinuria should avoid physical exercise. Investigations were made in a healthy 37-year-old man suspected of having hereditary xanthinuria. On routine physical examination he had a very low plasma level of urate but no urinary tract symptoms and no stone formation. The man was physically fit and accustomed to running. Four healthy men served as controls.

The subject and controls underwent a treadmill running test at maximal aerobic power. Heart rate, PO_2, and PCO_2 were monitored. Lactate was measured from a blood sample drawn from the fingertip. The subject also participated in a 5-km running competition. Blood samples were collected before and after the run and in the next morning. Urine samples were analyzed as well as blood.

The study subject had a persistent increase in xanthine and a slight elevation of hypoxanthine. After treadmill running and long-distance running, his hypoxanthine concentration increased to approximately the same level as in healthy controls; however, ellimination from plasma was considerably slower (Fig 8–13).

The subject tolerated exercise extremely well, and there was no evi-

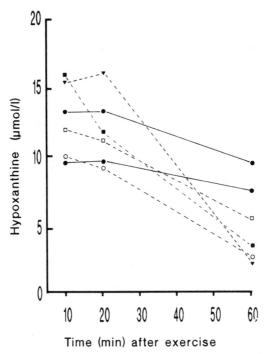

Fig 8–13.—Plasma concentrations of hypoxanthine after treadmill running, in the patient (examined twice, *solid lines*) and in 4 healthy controls *(dashed lines)*. (Courtesy of Landaas S, Borch K, Aagaard E: *Clin Chim Acta* 181:119–124, May 15, 1989.)

dence of muscular damage. Others have reported myopathy and microscopic changes in the myofibrils in patients with hereditary xanthinuria, however. A standardized exercise test followed by determinations of plasma concentrations of hypoxanthine and xanthine should determine whether a patient with xanthinuria should restrict physical activity.

▶ Hereditary xanthinuria is an interesting medical curiosity. The diagnosis is usually based on a low plasma level of urate. To date, about 50 cases have been described, the usual clinical manifestation being urinary xanthine stones. The xanthine is derived from the guanidine nucleotides. Even in normal subjects, exercise causes some breakdown of adenosine triphosphate to adenosine and thus to hypoxanthine. As there is little xanthine oxidase in muscle, the hypoxanthine accumulates during exercise. In patients with this anomaly, mechanisms for the hepatic breakdown of hypoxanthine to xanthine and uric acid are impaired, so that high blood levels of hypoxanthine are sustained after exercise. Although the present patient seemed to tolerate exercise quite well, others have observed muscle damage associated with the local deposition of crystalline material, supposedly xanthine or hypoxanthine (1–3). Exercise should thus be held below a level that causes major elevations of the plasma hypoxanthine concentration in such individuals.—R.J. Shephard, M.D., Ph.D.

References

1. Engelman K, et al: *Am J Med* 37:839, 1964.
2. Chalmers RA, et al: *Q J Med* 38:493, 1969.
3. Isaacs H, et al: *S Afr Med J* 49:1035, 1975.

Effect of Physical Activity on Lumbar Spine and Femoral Neck Bone Densities

Zylstra S, Hopkins A, Erk M, Hreshchyshyn MM, Anbar M (State Univ of New York, Buffalo)

Int J Sports Med 10:181–186, June 1989   8–28

Osteoporosis is a common disease in elderly persons and particularly in women. Preventing bone loss is important to maintaining mobility in later years. Much has been written about exercise but few studies have considered the effects of physical activity on bone mineral densities of the lumbar spine (LS) and femoral neck (FN).

Dual-photon absorptiometry was used to measure bone mineral densities of the LS in 123 women aged 35–65 years. The same procedure was used to measure bone mineral densities in the FN in 151 women of similar ages. These values were correlated with the number of hours spent in walking daily in conjunction with regular daily activities.

Both the LS and FN values were significantly correlated with walking (Fig 8–14). The LS values increased by .8% and the FN values by 1.9% in average bone density per hour of daily walking. The age-related rate of bone loss in the LS was .7% and the FN, .5%, in the same population. On average, a woman walking 1 additional hour daily would have an FN bone density comparable to that of a woman 4 years younger who did not pursue this activity.

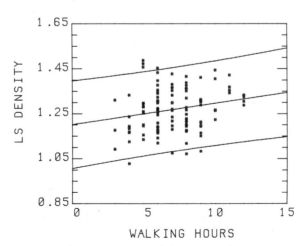

Fig 8–14.—Comparison between lumbar spine bone mineral density (gm/cm²) and walking hours (hr/day). (Courtesy of Zylstra S, Hopkins A, Erk M, et al: *Int J Sports Med* 10:181–186, June 1989.)

Walking can enhance bone mineral densities in both the LS and the FN. One additional hour of walking daily as part of normal daily activities can greatly reduce age-related bone loss and may help to prevent osteoporosis.

▶ At first reading this paper gives the very encouraging impression that one can turn back the osteoporotic clock by 4 years simply by walking for an hour per day. However, the true conclusion is probably a little more complicated. The authors noted all moving about by foot that involved being fully upright and weight-bearing. Some women reported 12 hours of walking per day, with the mean for the sample being 7 hours. This is hardly the volume of walking (as normally conceived) that one would anticipate in Caucasian 50-year-old women living in Buffalo, particularly as the authors suggest that they excluded about 20% of their sample for reporting excessive activity!

Presumably, the report of walking serves, rather, as a loose measure of general weight-bearing activity. The looseness of the measure may mean that one could get a larger advantage than 4 years from an hour of deliberate, vigorous walking, but a more tightly controlled measure of activity patterns is needed to answer this question definitively.—R.J. Shephard, M.D., Ph.D.

The Relationship of Swimming Exercise to Bone Mass in Men and Women

Orwoll ES, Ferar J, Oviatt SK, McClung MR, Huntington K (VA Med Ctr, Portland, Ore; Oregon Health Sciences Univ, Portland)
Arch Intern Med 149:2197–2200, October 1989   8–29

Physical activity helps to maintain skeletal health. For the exercise to be beneficial, weight-bearing must be involved; therefore, swimming has been considered ineffective in the prevention of bone loss. The potential usefulness of swimming in the prevention and treatment of osteopenia was explored in 58 men and 41 women aged 40–85 years who swam regularly, and 78 nonexercising men and 41 nonexercising women of similar ages. The swimmers engaged in no other form of regular exercise, and no person had conditions known to affect mineral or bone metabolism. Dietary protein and calcium intakes were similar in the 2 groups. Radial and vertebral bone mineral density was measured in all persons using single-photon absorptiometry.

Men in the exercising group had been swimming regularly for a mean of 13 years and women for a mean of 11 years. Both radial and vertebral bone densities were significantly greater in male swimmers than in nonswimmers. In women, however, there was apparently no relationship between swimming and bone mineral density. This was true whether women were premenopausal, postmenopausal, or postmenopausal taking estrogen supplements. In men, there was a positive association between bone mineral density and swimming.

Although no such correlation was found in women, swimming may be beneficial in the prevention or treatment of osteopenia in some individuals. The merits of swimming for this purpose should be further investigated.

▶ Debate continues as to whether swimming provides useful protection against osteoporosis. The question is an important one to resolve, because swimming is a valuable form of exercise for the obese and those with degenerative joint conditions.

The present report suggests a substantial effect on both vertebral and radial density in men but not in women. It could be that the men were more vigorous swimmers and indulged in more butterfly work, imposing greater stresses on the vertebral column. The subjects were all competitors in a Masters swim contest and had been swimming for "at least 3 hours per week for at least 3 years"; however, many Masters competitors participate for fun rather than compete seriously, which may well have made a difference between the 2 sexes.

The other possibility is one that affects most studies of swimmers. Did swimming serve as an indicator of a more general vigorous life-style? Individuals were excluded who undertook other types of exercise "regularly" or who used resistance training. However, bone density is influenced by the individual's lifetime activity history, and it is conceivable that several years earlier the swimmers had engaged in other types of sport, switching to swimming when joint problems precluded continuation of their initially selected activity. Further study of this important question is necessary.— R.J. Shephard, M.D., Ph.D.

Efficacy of Physical Conditioning Exercise in Patients With Rheumatoid Arthritis and Osteoarthritis
Minor MA, Hewett JE, Webel RR, Anderson SK, Kay DR (Univ of Missouri, Columbia)
Arthritis Rheum 32:1396–1405, November 1989   8–30

Physical inactivity increases the risk for the development of degenerative and chronic conditions. Because patients with arthritis often have poor physical fitness, the effects of aerobic and nonaerobic exercise were compared in 120 patients with rheumatoid arthritis (RA) or osteoarthritis (OA).

After baseline evaluation, patients were stratified by diagnosis and randomized to aerobic walking, aerobic aquatics, or range of motion (ROM) exercise groups. Groups met for 1 hour, 3 times per week, for 12 weeks. Target exercise heart rates were individually assigned to members of the aerobic exercise groups. Walkers exercised on a level course, progressing from 10 to 30 minutes. Those exercising in the pool jogged in shallow and deep water and performed calisthenics in chest-high water. The ROM nonaerobic group performed gentle active ROM and isometric strengthening and relaxation exercises.

Patients were evaluated for exercise tolerance, flexibility, disease and

Mean Change Scores at 1 Year (Over Baseline Levels) in Exercise Tolerance,
Disease-Related Measures, and Health Status in Patients with RA and OA Randomly
Assigned to 12 Weeks of Aerobic or Nonaerobic Exercise*

	Pool group (n = 37)	Walk group (n = 26)	ROM group (n = 20)	P†
Aerobic capacity (ml/kg/minute)	3.17 ± 4.41‡	4.72 ± 4.9‡	3.59 ± 4.9‡	0.6823
Exercise endurance (minutes)	2.7 ± 2.9‡	3.2 ± 3.4‡	2.6 ± 4.1§	0.9728
Resting blood pressure (mm Hg)				
Systolic	−8.1 ± 17‡	−8.0 ± 15§	−9.6 ± 22	0.7071
Diastolic	−6.3 ± 10‡	−8.6 ± 10‡	−7.2 ± 13§	0.8998
Exercise heart rate (bpm)	3.5 ± 15	1.6 ± 15	−2.7 ± 19	0.3426
Heart rate recovery (change in 5 minutes)	2.9 ± 14§	3.9 ± 8.0§	6.1 ± 12	0.5521
Clinically active joints (number)				
Total	−3.4 ± 6.7‡	−3.4 ± 8.5§	−4.4 ± 8.6§	0.3873
Lower extremity	−1.5 ± 3.4‡	−1.1 ± 4.5	−1.5 ± 3.8	0.6067
Morning stiffness (hours)	−0.5 ± 1.1‡	−0.2 ± 0.8	−0.1 ± 0.6	0.0851
50-foot walking time (seconds)	−1.5 ± 1.7‡	−1.3 ± 1.4‡	−0.8 ± 3.3	0.8132
Grip strength (mm Hg)	25 ± 33‡	36 ± 38‡	23 ± 35§	0.5810
Trunk flexibility (cm)	5.5 ± 6.9‡	2.1 ± 5.3	7.2 ± 6.9‡	0.0530
AIMS scores (0–10)				
Pain	−0.7 ± 1.8§	−0.6 ± 1.9	−1.1 ± 1.9§	0.2898
Physical activity	−1.4 ± 2.6‡	−1.1 ± 2.0§	−0.7 ± 2.5	0.6472
Anxiety	−0.6 ± 1.4§	0.01 ± 1.5	0 ± 1.3	0.4181
Depression	−0.3 ± 1.0	−0.1 ± 0.8	−0.2 ± 1.2	0.7325

*Values are the mean ± SD. Patients in the pool group were taught aquatic exercise, those in the walk group were taught walking exercise, and those in the ROM group were taught ROM exercise (nonaerobic control group). *AIMS*, Arthritis Impact Measurement Scales.
†Change scores for the aerobic exercise groups combined vs. change scores for the nonaerobic control group, by Wilcoxon rank sum test.
‡$P ≤ .01$ for within-group change, by Wilcoxon signed rank test.
§$P ≤ .05$ for within-group change, by Wilcoxon signed rank test.
(Courtesy of Minor MA, Hewett JE, Webel RR, et al: *Arthritis Rheum* 32:1396–1405, November 1989.)

health status, activity level, self-concept, and use of medications at baseline, at the end of the 12-week program, and at 3 months and 9 months later.

At 12 weeks both aerobic groups showed significant improvement over the ROM group in aerobic power, 15-m (50-ft) walking time, anxiety, depression, and physical activity. The aerobic aquatic group significantly improved in the number of clinically active joints, duration of morning stiffness, and grip strength, whereas the aerobic walking group improved significantly only in grip strength. There were no significant differences in change scores for joint counts, duration of morning stiffness, or grip strength between exercise groups. All groups had improved trunk, shoulder, and ankle flexibility. At 9-month follow-up, both aerobic groups had significant decreases over baseline in resting blood pressure, physical activity dysfunction, 15-m walking time, and total number of clinically active joints (table). The aerobic groups also had significantly increased aerobic power, exercise endurance, heart rate recovery, flexibility, and grip strength. The ROM group had significant increases in mean aerobic power, exercise endurance, grip strength, and flexibility, and significant decreases in the total number of clinically active joints. At 9 months 57% of the patients exercised for at least 60 minutes per week.

Both enjoyable and effective exercise programs can be developed for persons with arthritis. Many patients continued to engage in an exercise regimen 9 months after the formal study was completed.

▶ The present report shows clearly that patients with rheumatoid arthritis and osteoarthritis can engage usefully in walking and in aquatics programs. However, 2 findings may limit the conclusions that can be drawn. Although a substantial number of subjects were allocated randomly to each of the 3 treatments, the 2 exercised groups had a decreased number of clinically active joints. Did a modest stimulation of immune function help the underlying rheumatoid arthritis, or is this an expression of the tremendous week-to-week variation in disability with rheumatic problems? The second issue is involvement of the control group in exercise programs. This has been a problem in a number of recent cardiac rehabilitation trials. The benefits of exercise are now so widely known that it has become almost impossible to dissuade patients assigned to a control group from exercising. In the present experiment, half of the controls were undertaking an hour or more of conditioning per week after the experiment had been running for a year. It is good news that exercise has become socially so acceptable, but it is now almost impossible to carry out a well-designed experiment to test the benefits of exercise.—R.J. Shephard, M.D., Ph.D.

Effect of Exercise and Physical Fitness on Large Intestinal Function

Bingham SA, Cummings JH (Univ of Cambridge; Dunn Clinical Nutrition Ctr, Cambridge, England)
Gastroenterology 97:1389–1399, December 1989   8–31

Because individuals with high-activity occupations have a lower relative risk of large bowel cancer, physical activity has been thought to affect colonic function. The relationship between exercise and colonic function was investigated by measuring fecal weight, frequency, and transit time in 14 volunteers, all healthy but normally sedentary men and women aged 22–34 years. Measurements were obtained during a control period of minimal activity and during 3 training schedules that included jogging for 30–60 minutes per day 5 days a week. Diet was kept constant during the experiment. Data from the 3 protocols were combined and the differences between high- and low-activity periods noted (table).

The volunteers achieved the maximum amount of exercise recommended for developing and maintaining fitness in healthy adults. No significant differences were found in average fecal weights during periods of high- (126 g wet weight) and low- (127 g wet weight) physical activity. Nor did an increase in physical activity cause an overall increase in frequency of bowel habit, average intestinal transit time, fecal solids, pH,

Effect of Exercise on Colonic Function

	Control	Weeks 6–7	Change*
Protocol 3 (n = 6)			
No. of specimens per 24 h	1.3 ± 0.3	1.3 ± 0.3	0.002 ± 0.1
Fecal weight (wet) (g/day)†	161 ± 19	162 ± 46	1.3 ± 39.5
Fecal weight (dry) (g/day)†	37.2 ± 4.4	38.8 ± 9.7	1.6 ± 6.6
Transit time (h)	42.8 ± 9.1	44.0 ± 4.1	1.2 ± 7.0

	Control (last 14 days)	High exercise (last 14 days)	Change‡
All subjects (n = 14)			
No. of specimens per 24 h	1.0 ± 0.4	1.0 ± 0.3	0.004 ± 0.1
Fecal weight (wet) (g/day) †	124 ± 39	129 ± 49	4 ± 33
Fecal weight (dry) (g/day)†|	29.8 ± 7.8	31.4 ± 10.9	0.7 ± 6.7
Transit time (h)	54.9 ± 20.1	54.4 ± 23.5	0.4 ± 14.3

*Weeks 6–7 vs. control. No significant differences.
†Marker corrected.
‡High exercise vs. control. No significant differences.
(Courtesy of Bingham SA, Cummings JH: *Gastroenterology* 97:1389–1399, December 1989.)

ammonia concentration, or fecal nitrogen. The 7- to 9-week exercise periods did, however, result in considerable changes in cardiovascular function. A significant increase was noted in high-density lipoprotein cholesterol.

Thus exercise and a constant diet improve physical fitness but do not consistently affect large bowel habit. Dietary changes, in contrast, can markedly affect fecal weight and transit time.

▶ There have now been at least 7 reports looking at the incidence of colonic tumors among workers in physically active occupations; 5 of the 7 have found significantly lower tumor rates in active workers, and a sixth study tended in the same direction. The benefit was modest, but it seemed to be consistent across ethnic groups and social classes; it was also seen after standardizing for age and area of residence (1).

The reason for the protection remains unclear, although some authors have suggested a connection with the "runner's trots" (2), the tendency for competitive running to produce bowel movements and/or diarrhea. The postulated mechanism for the "trots" is intestinal ischemia, caused by a diversion of blood flow from the gut to the working muscles. Other expressions of this same response can include abdominal cramps and intestinal blood loss. Although such changes are likely in long-distance competitive runners, they are unlikely to be seen in the usual type of aerobic fitness program discussed by Bingham and Cummings, and it is thus not surprising that their more modest activity prescription had little impact on intestinal transit times.

Even in the long-distance runners and heavy workers it is by no means certain that a faster intestinal transit is responsible for the protection against colonic cancer. Other candidate mechanisms include a change of diet (particularly replacement of protein by refined carbohydrate, with alterations of bacterial flora) and the overall adoption of a more healthy life-style.—R.J. Shephard, M.D., Ph.D.

References

1. Shephard RJ: *Int J Sports Med.* In press, 1990.
2. Fogoros RN: *JAMA* 243:1743, 1980.

Bladder Carcinoma Presenting as Exercise-Induced Hematuria
Mueller EJ, Thompson IM (Walson Army Community Hosp, Fort Dix, NJ; Brooke Army Med Ctr, Fort Sam Houston, Tex)
Postgrad Med 84:173–176, December 1988   8–32

As the number of runners has increased in the past several years, so has the number of patients seen for evaluation of hematuria. Several urologic diseases can mimic hematuria secondary to exercise and may be overlooked if a urologic examination is not done. Four men aged 22–68 years with exercise-induced hematuria were found to have papillary transitional cell carcinoma of the bladder.

The first was aged 31 years and had a 13-year history of intermittent, total, painless hematuria. He had gross hematuria after strenuous exercise in high school and after joining the military. Cystoscopy showed a papillary lesion above the right ureteral orifice. The second patient, aged 68 years, had gross, total, painless hematuria after a 2-mile run on 1 day and a 2-mile walk on the second. He had been a jogger for more than 10 years without any previous hematuria. Cystoscopy in this patient revealed 3 papillary lesions 1–1.5 cm in size on the left lateral bladder wall.

The third patient was aged 22 years and had 4 episodes of gross, total, painless hematuria in the 3 months preceding examination. Three of these episodes followed morning training runs. Cystoscopy demonstrated a 1-cm papillary lesion on the right lateral wall of the bladder. The fourth, age 41 years, had participated in a vigorous aerobics class 3 days before being seen at the urology clinic. His urine was dark brown after the class; urinalysis showed red blood cells that were too numerous to count. In this patient cystoscopy showed a 1–1.5 cm papillary lesion on the bladder dome.

Genitourinary tract diseases that cause gross and microscopic hematuria include obstruction of the ureteropelvic junction, hydronephrosis, stones, tumors, and prostatic disease. Any patient with gross or microscopic hematuria after exercise should be referred to a urologist. A delay in referral may result in significant morbidity. Intravenous urography and cystoscopy are recommended.

▶ Athletes are prone to diverse causes of hematuria, and proper diagnosis hinges on careful history, physical examination, and urinalysis, as well as the judicious use of screening tests, intravenous pyelography, and cystoscopy (1). Hematuria in runners can be benign, e.g., pseudonephritis (see the 1988 YEAR BOOK OF SPORTS MEDICINE, pp 126–128), or painful and gross, apparently as a result of bladder trauma; the latter can trouble male distance runners especially. Painless gross hematuria, however, as reported here, can be ominous, and calls for a careful work-up. Another case of gross hematuria caused by bladder cancer in a young athlete, a 29-year-old recreational runner, was reported to the 1990 annual meeting of the American College of Sports Medicine (2). Perhaps running or other vigorous aerobic exercise can act as an "exercise stress test" to unmask bladder cancer long before it would otherwise be diagnosed and when it is easily cured.— E.R. Eichner, M.D.

References

1. Eichner ER: *Phys Sportsmed.* In press, 1990.
2. Elliott DL, Goldberg L: *Med Sci Sports Exerc* 22:797, 1990 (abstr).

Effects of Aerobic Interval Training on Cancer Patients' Functional Capacity
MacVicar MG, Winningham ML, Nickel JL (Ohio State Univ)
Nurs Res 38:348–351, November–December 1989   8–33

Functional capacity is defined as the highest metabolic rate an individual can achieve on exertion. It is estimated that one-third or more of the decline in functional capacity experienced by cancer patients, regardless of disease stage, is attributable to hypokinetic conditions caused by prolonged physical inactivity. Exercise during treatment for cancer has been recommended to maintain functional capacity, but data on exercise response are not available. The effect of a 10-week exercise intervention protocol on functional capacity was assessed in women with stage II breast cancer.

Of 45 women who were undergoing standard postsurgical chemotherapy, 18 were randomly assigned to aerobic interval exercise training, 11 were assigned to placebo exercise training, and 16 served as controls. Aerobic exercise training consisted of alternating higher and lower exercise intensity involving the use of large muscle groups, preceded by a set of flexibility and stretching exercises, performed 3 times a week for 10 weeks. Placebo exercise training consisted of flexibility and stretching exercises only, performed 3 times a week for 10 weeks. All participants underwent standard pre- and posttraining evaluation.

The women enrolled in aerobic interval training had a mean 40% improvement on functional capacity between pre- and posttesting. Mean workload and test time were also improved. No significant changes were observed in the placebo and the control groups on any of the parameters measured. Because an increase in functional capacity could improve the potential ability for self-care and daily living activities in patients with cancer, it is recommended that intervention aerobic training be implemented during therapy for cancer.

▶ Some patients who are receiving chemotherapy for advanced cancer become so weak that they cannot even open the refrigerator door to get some food. The authors are correct to suggest an important potential for exercise to improve the quality of life after a diagnosis of cancer. In addition to ameliorating the loss of conditioning associated with bed rest, exercise may help to counteract the loss of appetite and encourage retention of protein in the face of large energy demands from the tumor cells. It can also have a very positive effect on mood. Finally, there is growing evidence that moderate amounts of exercise can stimulate natural killer cell activity, thereby increasing the efficacy of treatment.

The one note of caution concerns the location of the tumor. It is important that an increase of blood flow not be directed to the region in which the tumor is located, as this could cause further dissemination of cancer cells through the circulation and might also precipitate local hemorrhage. But if a patient enjoys exercise, and the prognosis is for an early demise, it would be wrong for the physician to deny such activity except in unusual circumstances.—R.J. Shephard, M.D., Ph.D.

9 Athletic Training

Introduction

In many of the past YEAR BOOKS I have introduced this chapter with an article on the need for athletic trainers in high schools. This year is an exception, however, and I will make a plea to athletic trainers that is quite different. We as athletic trainers must protect ourselves, our student trainers, and our athletes from AIDS. I would like to quote from the article review in Abstract 9–1: "Athletic trainers need to be aware of the recommendations for the prevention of the transmission of HIV. Universities with student athletic trainers need to establish written guidelines to ensure that AIDS information is disseminated to all such student athletes."

Athletic trainers must face the facts. The nature of our work can expose us to HIV. We are called upon daily to fix a bleeding cut or treat an open wound. Be smart and safe: Wear gloves when you treat these athletes, and use a 10% bleach solution to clean the training room. Some of the athletes we treat may be in the so-called high-risk group.

Francis J. George, ATC, PT

Should Athletic Trainers Be Concerned About HIV? Guidelines for Athletic Trainers
Welch MJ, Sitler MR, Horodyski MB (US Military Academy, West Point, NY; Temple Univ)
Athletic Training 24:27–28, Spring 1989   9–1

An estimated 1 to 1.5 million Americans are infected with HIV, and half may progress to AIDS in the next 9 years. Virtually all of those who are infected can transmit infection to others. Once infected with HIV, a person remains a carrier for life. The chief high-risk groups are homosexuals, intravenous drug users, and sex partners of these groups, but health care workers are also at risk of acquiring HIV.

A survey of athletic trainers at 20 universities or colleges in the northeastern United States showed that 14 had implemented changes in the way they care for bleeding wounds in athletes. However, only 5 schools had made wearing gloves mandatory and only 2 schools had formalized this practice in writing. Most schools reported that AIDS was addressed in the athletic training curriculum. Only 2 schools used 10% bleach solution, which kills HIV, to clean up the training room.

Gloves are recommended whenever a health care worker is exposed to mucous membranes, nonintact skin, or materials contaminated by blood or body fluids. Precautions to prevent injury from a needle or scalpel are necessary. Training room tables and other surfaces should be cleaned with a 10% bleach solution.

Quality Assessment of Athletic Trainers
Foster DT, Yesalis CE, Ferguson KJ, Albright JP (Univ of Iowa; Pennsylvania State Univ, University Park)
Am J Sports Med 17:258–262, March–April 1989   9–2

Because athletic trainers have an acknowledged role in the overall health care of sports participants, the competence of 30 certified athletic trainers (ATCs) who were part of the health care team at the 1985 Junior Olympic Games was assessed. During the games, 121 significant injuries were managed, and the ATCs collected standard injury information; the same information was gathered separately by physicians. Telephone interviews with the injured participants were conducted 9 months after the games. Physicians completed assessment questionnaires.

The injured athletes usually did not inform parents of their injuries or medical care during the games. Both athletes and physicians were in overwhelming agreement that the ATCs with whom they had contact were capable. According to the athletes' reports, approximately 70% recovered from their symptoms and the limitations imposed by the injuries within a month after the games. About 17% had some type of injury recurrence to the same body part, but 97% had fully recovered from their injuries at 9-month follow-up.

▶ For many years the medical community has been concerned about the quality of care its members deliver. Athletic trainers, representing an integral part of the health care team testing athletes, should be included in these assessments. Since 1970 the athletic training profession has improved its standards a great deal through education and certification of its members.

This paper examined the performance of athletic trainers at the 1985 Junior Olympic Games. Specifically, the authors attempted to determine whether certified athletic trainers were qualified to assess and treat minor athletic injuries and make a determination of the athlete's ability to return to participation. The responses of the supervising physicians and the athletes who were treated indicated that their quality assessment of these athletic trainers was very favorable.—F.J. George, ATC, PT

The Background Required of Athletic Trainers to Evaluate Knee, Shoulder, and Ankle Injuries: Survey of Orthopaedists
Rauls BL, Frazier CL, Thorpe WP (Southeast Missouri State Univ, Cape Girardeau)
Athletic Training 24:36–38, Spring 1989   9–3

Evaluation of an injured joint by someone who lacks adequate preparation and experience can result in further damage to the joint, either by its improper manipulation during examination or faulty interpretation of the findings. A random sample of 113 orthopedic surgeons, a third of those asked, participated in a survey of the level of education and experience needed to evaluate injuries to a specific joint. All of the respondents had worked with an athletic trainer, usually at the college or high school level. About half of the respondents were associated with trainers at sports medicine clinics, and about a third worked with trainers for professional teams.

Nearly half of the respondents believed that all athletic trainers should know how to palpate for tenderness. Most preferred to have at least an experienced trainer do range-of-motion testing. A definite majority indicated that a trainer should be certified before doing joint stability tests. More education and experience was considered necessary for evaluating the knee than for evaluating the shoulder.

These physicians believe that specific levels of education and experience are needed for most aspects of injury evaluation by athletic trainers.

▶ The authors have raised a number of significant questions that should be addressed by the athletic training profession. Should student athletic trainers be allowed to do joint testing? How much experience or supervision should they have before administering these tests? Which tests are safe and which are dangerous and should be avoided?

Many of those physicians surveyed indicated that, in the final analysis, the interpretation of test results and management of the injury are the responsibilities of certified athletic trainers and the supervising physician.—F.J. George, ATC, PT

The Use of Instruction and the Behavioral Approach to Facilitate Injury Rehabilitation
DePalma MT, DePalma B (Cornell Univ, Ithaca, NY)
Athletic Training 24:217–219, Fall 1989   9–4

Athletic trainers should be able to assist in the rehabilitation of athletes. The behavioral approach, or the use of short-term realistic goals, can be adapted for use in injury rehabilitation. The behavioral approach distinguishes between long-term goals and short-term subgoals. Athletes often set long-term goals for themselves, such as when they will return to competition. Short-term subgoals based on what can be done to achieve the long-term goals should be presented to the athlete. Subgoals should be extremely specific, with detailed instructions for daily work, and should also be realistic, challenging, and attainable; this will result in reinforcement and support. Having subgoals also restores the opportunity for hard work, immediate feedback, satisfaction, and reward as each subgoal is reached. Both athlete and trainer must be flexible, because subgoals might need restructuring if they prove too difficult.

It is especially helpful if the injured athlete can talk with an athlete who has recovered from a similar injury using a similar program. This builds confidence that the program is useful and successful. The athlete should contribute input to the program design, helping to outline an individualized timetable for achievement of subgoals. If rehabilitation is scheduled at the usual practice time, alienation from the team is reduced. The trainer should provide positive feedback to the athlete as subgoals are achieved.

▶ The authors have presented a number of excellent ideas to improve an athlete's attitude and ensure his or her cooperation and compliance during the rehabilitation program. Establishing achievable subgoals is a must. They stress how important it is to be very specific with these subgoals and to make the athlete feel that they are a vital part of the rehabilitation process.—F.J. George, ATC, PT

Role of the Athletic Trainer in the Use of Inhaled Bronchodilators
Clifton EJ, Clifton GD (Eastern Kentucky Univ, Richmond; Univ of Kentucky, Lexington)
Athletic Training 24:325–328, Winter 1989   9–5

Many asthmatic individuals now participate in sports events thanks to advances in the pharmacologic treatment of asthma and exercise-induced asthma. Because β_2-agonists administered by inhalation are the drugs of choice for acute episodes of chronic asthma, for intermittent symptoms, and for protection from exercise-induced asthma, trainers should be familiar with their properties and correct use.

The β_2-agonists stimulate β_2-receptors in the airway smooth muscles, leading to bronchodilation. Common adverse effects include tachycardia, skeletal muscle tremor, and nervousness; rare adverse effects include cardiac arrhythmia, myocardial ischemia, and infarction. Toxicity is related to the method of administration, with adverse side effects negligible after inhalation of normal doses of these agents.

Metered-dose inhalers are preferred for administration of these bronchodilators, because the drug is delivered directly to the site of action, minimizing systemic concentrations. Metered-dose inhalers can easily be

---

Steps for Correct Use of Metered Dose Inhalers

1. Shake the canister thoroughly.
2. Breath out slowly and steadily.
3. Place the mouthpiece between lips; make sure teeth and tongue are out of the way.
4. Just after beginning a slow, deep breath, activate the canister.
5. At the end of the complete inspiration, hold breath for approximately 10 seconds.
6. If a second inhalation is called for, wait at least 2 minutes.

(Courtesy of Clifton EJ, Clifton GD: *Athletic Training* 24:325–328, Winter 1989.)

---

overused, incorrectly used, or used with improper timing, however. For exercise-induced asthma, prophylactic use 15 minutes before exercise prevents symptoms for 2–4 hours. Trainers should be able to instruct athletes in the proper use of these devices (table).

The National Collegiate Athletic Association allows the use of bitolterol, metaproterenol (orciprenoline), albuterol (salbutamol), and terbutaline by all routes. The United States Olympic Committee permits aerosol forms of albuterol, terbutaline, and rimiterol. Both associations allow the use of theophylline and cromolyn sodium, and the National Collegiate Athletic Association also permits aerosol beclomethasone and atropine. Neither agency permits the use of the over-the-counter β_2-agonist bronchodilator epinephrine.

▶ Athletic trainers must be able to instruct their athletes in the proper use of inhaled bronchodilators. Too many athletes use these bronchodilators incorrectly. The authors recommend that they be used 15 minutes before exercise begins (see the instructions in the table for the correct use of these inhalers).

Please be aware that both the NCAA and USOC have banned the use of over-the-counter (nonprescription) inhaled bronchodilators that contain epinephrine.—F.J. George, ATC, PT

The Athletic Trainer's Role in Saving Avulsed Teeth
Krasner P (Temple Univ)
Athletic Training 24:139–142, Summer 1989   9–6

Tooth avulsion, which is frequent in the United States, can cause pain and necessitate great expense. Up to 16% of injuries involving the mouth lead to avulsion of a tooth despite all precautions. Nearly any avulsed

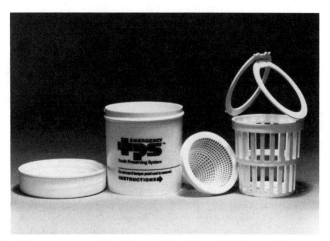

Fig 9–1.—Component parts of the Emergency Tooth Preserving System. (Courtesy of Krasner P: *Athletic Training* 24:139–142, Summer 1989.)

tooth can be replanted and retained permanently, but it is essential to maintain the viability of the attached periodontal ligament.

There may be problems in replacing the tooth in the socket immediately. If so, the best storage media are pH-balanced cell culture fluids, (e.g., Hanks' solution and Eagle's medium). The worst are dry media, (e.g., gauze and sterile saline). Saliva is adequate for a brief period. The Emergency Tooth Preservation System (Fig 9–1) is a convenient means of transporting avulsed teeth.

The athletic trainer should inform all school personnel that avulsed teeth should be saved. Tooth-preserving devices should be on hand at strategic locations. If possible, the tooth is rinsed with saline or a pH-balanced preservative solution and replanted immediately, having the patient bite on gauze. A tooth that is not replanted immediately should be kept in a secure, biocompatible environment; fresh whole milk may substitute for a designated preserving system. The tooth should not be scraped or cleaned in any way.

▶ The author has made some excellent suggestions for preserving avulsed teeth. The Emergency Tooth Preserving System is inexpensive and can easily fit into a trainer's kit. Athletic trainers should be familiar with its use. Whole, cold milk can be used as a storage medium for short periods of time. This article also gives me a chance to reinforce the importance of wearing a mouthpiece in all contact sports and in any other sport in which a high incidence of tooth or facial injuries occurs.—F.J. George, ATC, PT

Airway Obstruction: Recognition and Immediate Management
Rund DA (Ohio State Univ)
Physician Sports Med 17:173–174, October 1989   9–7

Airway obstruction requires immediate treatment, as irreversible brain damage occurs within 4–6 minutes. The rescuer must be able to identify the obstruction and open the airway while protecting the cervical spine.

When the airway is completely blocked, air flow cannot be heard or felt at the victim's nose or mouth. Certain sounds are characteristic of partial airway obstruction. Snoring may occur when the tongue obstructs the hypopharynx. When stridor (crowing) is heard, edema, a tumor, or a foreign body may be blocking the larynx. A gurgling sound indicates that a liquid such as vomitus or blood is present in the airway.

A victim with complete airway obstruction progresses from violent agitation to exhaustion, loss of consciousness, and cardiac arrest. Agitation, restlessness, and confusion may signify partial obstruction. Once these signs are recognized, the rescuer must open the airway, provide ventilation, and administer supplemental oxygen. Care must be taken to prevent movement of the cervical spine in trauma patients.

Airway opening maneuvers include the mandibular lift, the chin lift, and the triple-airway maneuver (Fig 9–2). Patients with good muscle relaxation may be treated with the mandibular lift. The jaw is brought for-

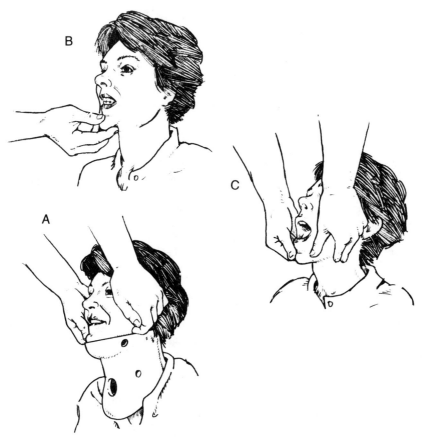

Fig 9–2.—Airway opening maneuvers demonstrated on model. **A,** mandibular lift: place fingers behind vertical rami of the mandible, and thrust the jaw forward. **B,** chin lift: grasp chin and pull the mandible forward. **C,** triple-airway maneuver: while standing at the patient's head, grasp ascending rami with fingers 2 through 5. Open the mouth with thumbs and tilt head backward. (Illustration courtesy of Terry Boles, Cottage Grove, Minn. From Rund DA: *Physician Sports Med* 17:173–174, October 1989.)

ward and the tongue lifted away from the hypopharynx. For the chin lift, the rescuer grasps the chin and pulls the mandible forward. In certain situations the tongue itself must be grasped and pulled forward. When neck injury is suspected, the triple-airway maneuver may be necessary. The patient's head is tilted backward, the mouth opened, and the mandible displaced forward.

After opening the airway, the rescuer should attempt to ventilate the patient. Manual clearing of the mouth or hypopharynx may be required. The patient is placed on his or her side in order to force the mouth open. If the patient still cannot be ventilated, deeper sweeps into the throat may be needed to remove obstructing debris.

▶ Athletic trainers must be proficient in cardiopulmonary resuscitation (CPR) techniques and should review these techniques periodically. A CPR refresher course, given by a certified instructor, should be mandatory yearly.—F.J. George, ATC, PT

A Musculoskeletal Approach to the Preparticipation Physical Examination: Preventing Injury and Improving Performance

Kibler WB, Chandler TJ, Uhl T, Maddux RE (Lexington Clinic Sports Medicine Ctr, Ky)

Am J Sports Med 17:525–531, July–August 1989   9–8

When information specific to the musculoskeletal system is acquired in a preparticipation examination, injury may be prevented and performance improved. Specific tests for flexibility, strength, and endurance were used to evaluate 2,107 athletes who participated in a range of sports activities from the junior high school to the college level. The station method was used, and athletes were examined preferably within a month of the start of preseason drills. Tests of strength or endurance (e.g., sit-ups, push-ups, grip testing, and knee or shoulder Cybex testing) were supplemented by estimates of total-body flexibility.

Male athletes were significantly stronger than female athletes, but female athletes were significantly more flexible. Upper-body athletes were less flexible in dominant side internal rotation and more flexible in dominant side external rotation. Lower-body athletes, especially females, had tighter leg muscles.

By combining data from the preseason physical examination concerning athletes in a range of sports with injury records, sport-specific profiles (table) can be developed. These in turn will be helpful in designing a training program to improve performance and prevent injury in a given sport.

▶ We have done a preseason physical screening examination for our football team for many years. Screening is done after a complete medical examination

Importance of Each Variable to Given Sport or Sport Function

Sport or function	Flexibility	Strength	Speed	Endurance	
				Anaerobic	Aerobic
Football	2	4	4	4	2
Basketball	3	3	4	4	4
Tennis	3	3	4	4	4
Baseball	3	3	3	3	2
pitching	4	3	2	4	2
Runner	3	2	2	2	4
Sprinter	4	3	4	4	2

Note: 4, variable is essential to best performance of sport or sporting function; 3, variable is synergistic to best performance of sport or sporting function; 2, variable is needed at certain level, usually for injury prevention; 1, variable is needed at minimal level.

(Courtesy of Kibler WB, Chandler TJ, Uhl T, et al: Am J Sports Med 17:525–531, July–August 1989.)

that includes vision and auditory testing. We use the station method and measure height and weight as well as quadriceps and hamstring flexibility; Cybex testing of the quadriceps and hamstrings is done, and knee and ankle joint laxity is tested; also, the percent body fat is measured. As athletic trainers, the most valuable portion of this screening in our view has repeatedly been the knee and ankle joint laxity tests. When an athlete sustains an ankle or knee injury with joint laxity, we always refer to the previous test results when determining the extent of injury. In addition to the preceding tests, a podiatric biomechanical analysis is done for our distance runners.—F.J. George, ATC, PT

Accuracy of Spring and Strain Gauge Hand-Held Dynamometers

Bohannon RW, Andrews AW (Univ of Connecticut, Storrs; Univ of North Carolina)
J Orthop Sports Phys Ther 10:323–325, February 1989   9–9

Hand dynamometers, fixed dynamometers, isokinetic dynamometers, and hand-held dynamometers have been used extensively for measuring muscle strength in clinical settings. The accuracy of 2 spring gauge and 2 strain gauge hand-held dynamometers was determined by using certified weights.

Each dynamometer, which had extensive prior use, was vertically loaded with the weights in 5-lb increments from 5 to 55 lb. The actual certified weights were compared with the weights measured by each dynamometer by using analysis of variance. Pearson product moment correlations were calculated between weights measured by each dynamometer.

The 2 spring gauge dynamometers measured comparably, as did the 2 strain gauge devices. However, only the 2 strain gauge devices registered weights not significantly different from the actual weights with which they were loaded. The correlations between the measurements of each device were 0.98 or higher.

Strain gauge dynamometers may be more accurate than spring gauge dynamometers after extensive use. Using these 2 types of gauges interchangeably is not appropriate. The accuracy of hand-held dynamometers should be checked over time because these devices may not maintain their accuracy equally. Spring gauge dynamometers appear to be especially prone to losing accuracy over time.

▶ The authors have concluded that strain gauge dynamometers are more accurate than spring gauge dynamometers. It is also not appropriate to use them interchangeably.—F.J. George, ATC, PT

Reliability of an Isokinetic Test of Muscle Strength and Endurance

Montgomery LC, Douglass LW, Deuster PA (Uniformed Services Univ of the Health Sciences, Bethesda, Md; Univ of Maryland, College Park)
J Orthop Sports Phys Ther 10:315–322, February 1989   9–10

An attempt was made to develop a concise protocol for evaluating muscle strength and endurance by isokinetic dynamometry. Eleven men and 9 women in their late 20s were tested on 3 occasions 2–4 days apart. The velocity spectrum test includes 5 repetitions at velocities of 90–330 degrees per second. The muscle endurance test is performed in 45 seconds at 180 degrees per second.

The velocity spectrum test of the knee extensors and flexors showed no significant intraindividual differences at any velocity. Reliability generally was greater at the slower velocities and greater for knee extension than for flexion. The mean correlation coefficients for peak torque across velocity were 0.88 for extension and 0.79 for flexion. In the endurance test, both total work performed and average power were reliable measures.

The velocity spectrum test should prove useful in intervention studies, e.g., rehabilitation or drug testing. In testing muscle endurance, absolute measures are highly consistent, but relative measures (e.g., percent decline in performance) exhibit greater inherent variation.

▶ The authors used a Biodex to determine the isokinetic values measured in this study. (Please see Abstract 9–21). They developed a testing protocol for evaluating strength and endurance with the Biodex that can be done in 30 minutes and have concluded that it is reliable over repeated test sessions.—F.J. George, ATC, PT

Measurement of Upper Extremity Torque Production and Its Relationship to Throwing Speed in the Competitive Athlete
Bartlett LR, Storey MD, Simons BD (Sports Medicine Clinic, Seattle)
Am J Sports Med 17:89–91, January–February 1989   9–11

The upper body exercise and testing table developed by Cybex allows accurate testing of torque of the upper extremity. Studies correlating upper body torque with throwing velocity, body weight, free arm speed, and mass moved by the upper extremity have principally involved a nonathletic population. To establish whether a correlation exists between peak torque production and throwing speed in professional athletes, 11 professional baseball players underwent testing for upper extremity peak torque production using a Cybex II Isokinetic Dynamometer.

During shoulder and elbow tests, pelvic and chest straps were used to prevent use of trunk muscles. Each player performed 4 repetitions of maximal effort. After an adequate rest period, the opposite extremity was tested for the same motion. The shoulder motions tested were shoulder flexion and extension, shoulder abduction and adduction, shoulder horizontal abduction and adduction, shoulder internal and external rotation with the arm in 90 degrees of abduction, elbow flexion and extension, forearm pronation and supination, and wrist flexion and extension. The peak torque for each motion was recorded. In a separate session, throwing speed was measured by radar gun for each participant.

A significant relationship was found between shoulder adduction and throwing speed. Although it was not statistically significant, shoulder extension was the only other motion strongly associated with throwing speed. The shoulder adductor musculature of the dominant arm was capable of producing significantly more torque than was this musculature in the nondominant arm.

No positive correlation was found between upper extremity torque production in general and throwing speed. However, the specific torque produced by dominant-arm shoulder adductors in baseball players was positively correlated with throwing speed.

▶ In this study the athletes were tested at 90 degrees per second. Other studies have tested athletes at slower and faster speeds and have come to different conclusions. We have traditionally included all major muscle groups of the shoulder in our preseason conditioning drills. The results of this study may influence us to emphasize the shoulder adductors and extensors more than we have been. Related studies were presented in the 1989 YEAR BOOK OF SPORTS MEDICINE, pp 48–57.—F.J. George, ATC, PT

Comparison of Values Generated During Testing of the Knee Using the Cybex II Plus and Biodex Model B-2000 Isokinetic Dynamometers
Thompson MC, Shingleton LG, Kegerreis ST (Univ of Indianapolis)
J Orthop Sports Phys Ther 11:108–115, September 1989   9–12

Historically, Cybex has dominated the isokinetic testing and exercise machine market and Cybex instruments have been used in most isokinetic research. Now several other companies have entered this growing market. Values generated during knee testing with 2 isokinetic dynamometers, the Cybex II Plus and the Biodex Model B-2000, were compared in 28 healthy women and 20 healthy men aged 21–46 years. The same knee of each volunteer was tested at speeds of 60, 180, and 240 degrees per second on both machines. Peak torques, angle of peak torques, peak torque to body weight ratios, and flexion to extension ratios were compared.

Several pairs of values were significantly related. However, results of paired *t* tests revealed many statistically significant and nonuniform differences, indicating that caution is necessary when attempting to extrapolate test data from 1 machine to another. These results suggest that manufacturers' claims that the machines measure the same variables may be questioned.

▶ In comparing the test results done on a Cybex and a Biodex there were significant value differences recorded. This should caution all of us to be sure we know which testing devices are being used and how the data may be compared or not compared.—F.J. George, ATC, PT

Prediction of Torque Acceleration Energy and Power of Thigh Muscles From Peak Torque

Kannus P, Järvinen M (Tampere Univ Central Hosp, Finland)
Med Sci Sports Exerc 21:304–307, June 1989   9–13

Patients with complete anterior cruciate ligament (ACL) rupture face a difficult period of rehabilitation before the thigh muscle returns to normal strength. A number of strength testing protocols have been developed to measure thigh muscle functions.

To determine the relationships between peak torque (PT) and PT acceleration energy (PTAE), and between PT and average power (AP) in multiple, low-speed (0, 60, and 180 degrees per second^{-1}) contractions of the quadriceps and hamstring muscles, studies were done in 38 patients who had chronic, complete ACL deficiency of 1 knee. None had an injury to the opposite knee. An isokinetic dynamometer was used to measure muscle function parameters of the injured and normal knees.

Average hamstring musculature PT, PTAE, and AP findings in the ACL-insufficient knee were somewhat lower than those for the uninjured knee, but the differences were not significant. In the quadriceps, however, peak torques were significantly lower in the injured knee. At all test speeds the Pearson product moment and the Spearman rank correlation coefficients between the PT and PTAE were highly significant for both muscle groups in both knees. The correlation coefficients increased simultaneously with the speed of movement in both knees and both muscle groups.

Both isokinetic and isometric PT measurements give a good indication of the ability of knee extensor and flexor muscles to emit torque throughout the range of motion. The predictability of PTAE and AP from PT is statistically and clinically significant. Because PT analysis is simple and highly reliable, little additional information is to be gained from PTAE or AP tests.

▶ How many different measurements do we need to give us an indication of how a muscle is functioning? The authors have concluded that ". . . the PTAE or AP analysis may offer little additional information about thigh muscle function to that attained by [a] more simple measurement, the PT analysis."—F.J. George, ATC, PT

Effect of Standard and Aircast Tennis Elbow Bands on Integrated Electromyography of Forearm Extensor Musculature Proximal to the Bands

Snyder-Mackler L, Epler M (Boston Univ; Temple Univ)
Am J Sports Med 17:278–281, March–April 1989   9–14

Classic tennis elbow, also called lateral epicondylitis, is a form of tendinitis primarily involving the extensor carpi radialis brevis (ECRB) and extensor digitorum communis (EDC). Treatment generally involves the use of a constrictive band placed several centimeters distal to the origin of these 2 muscles.

The Aircast band, which uses an air-filled bladder as the counterpressure element, was tested in the right upper extremities of 10 healthy individuals from 20 to 43 years of age.

Procedure.—The forearms were stabilized in a Cybex II forearm stabilization V-pad. The wrist was placed in neutral flexion/extension and full pronation. Monopolar electromyographic (EMG) electrodes were inserted into the ECRB and the EDC, and the recording electrode was placed on the surface of the skin within 2 cm of the needle electrodes. Participants were tested at 80% of maximum voluntary isometric contraction without any band, with a standard band, and with an Aircast band.

The EMG activity was significantly lower in both the EDC and the ECRB with the Aircast band than with either no band or the standard band. In both muscles tested the mean standard trial integrated EMG was lower than the control with the standard band, but differences were not significant.

In healthy humans the Aircast tennis elbow band decreased the integrated EMG of both the EDC and ECRB muscles in comparison with applying no band or using the standard band. Because the trial sample was small, the insignificant effect of the standard band should be viewed cautiously.

Effect of the Counterforce Armband on Wrist Extension and Grip Strength and Pain in Subjects With Tennis Elbow
Wadsworth CT, Nielsen DH, Burns LT, Krull JD, Thompson CG (Univ of Iowa; Spokane, Wash; Iowa Musculoskeletal Ctr, Cedar Rapids; Grantwood AEA, Coralville, Iowa)
J Orthop Sports Phys Ther 11:192–197, November 1989   9–15

A lateral counterforce armband is often prescribed for patients with tennis elbow. Theoretically, the armband controls intrinsic muscle forces, directing potential overloads to healthy tissues or to the band itself; it neither alters agonist-antagonist muscle balance nor restricts joint range of motion. It may alter wrist extension strength, but this effect may be different in patients with and without pathology. The armband's effect on both strength and pain was investigated in 14 patients with tennis elbow. All 14 underwent strength tests and had pain analogue scale assessments on both arms, with and without an armband (Fig 9–3).

In both affected and unaffected arms the armband led to increased strength on grip and wrist extensor tests. The affected arm was significantly improved. Wrist extension strength was the more sensitive measure. A nonsignificant reduction in pain was noted with the armband.

The increase in wrist extension and grip strength of the affected arm may be related to dispersal by the armband of stresses generated by mus-

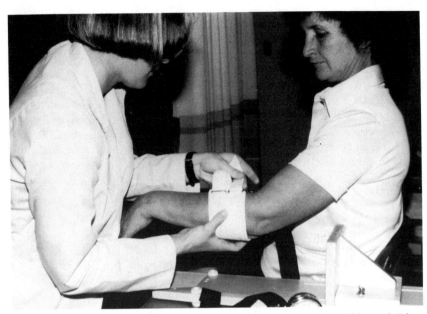

Fig 9–3.—Investigator positions counterforce armband, made of contoured, rigid fabric with Velcro fasteners, 1 in. distal to lateral humeral epicondyle. (Courtesy of Wadsworth CT, Nielsen DH, Burns LT, et al: *J Orthop Sports Phys Ther* 11:192–197, November 1989.)

cle contraction. This might reduce painful inhibition and permit more forceful contraction. In the unaffected arm contraction may be facilitated by the armband, either by superficial sensory stimulation or deep muscle belly pressure.

▶ The authors of the article reviewed in Abstract 9–14 caution that the number of subjects in their study is small. They also were healthy, compared to those described in Abstract 9–15, who had tennis elbow. The Aircast band was effective in reducing EMG activity in the EDC and the ECRB of the healthy subjects. In the group reported in Abstract 9–15, the lateral counterforce armband used significantly improved strength in the affected arm but did not significantly reduce pain. The authors explain that this increase in strength resulted from the dispersal of stresses by the armband.—F.J. George, ATC, PT

Sports-Related Muscle Injuries: Evaluation With MR Imaging
Fleckenstein JL, Weatherall PT, Parkey RW, Payne JA, Peshock RM (Univ of Texas, Dallas)
Radiology 172:793–798, September 1989   9–15

The underlying pathophysiology of muscle pain associated with strenuous exercise has not been precisely identified. Also, the severity and duration of muscle injury are difficult to quantify because of limitations in methodology. Magnetic resonance imaging (MRI) was used to evaluate acute strains and delayed-onset muscle soreness in 3 groups of individuals.

Group 1 consisted of 3 sedentary persons who complained of the acute onset of thigh pain while playing softball. Magnetic resonance imaging was performed within 4 days. The group was followed up at 1 month and again after 9–18 months. The 6 sedentary individuals in group 2 were examined prospectively for delayed-onset muscle soreness. These subjects were imaged before and immediately after calf plantar-flexion exercise. Five were also imaged after a delay of 2–5 days. Two individuals underwent repeat imaging at 24, 36, 48, and 72 hours, and at 13, 23, and 48 days after exercise. These 2 individuals also underwent testing for serum creatine kinase levels and evaluation of pain. Group 3 comprised 10 trained runners imaged after completion of all or part of a marathon run.

Muscles that were painful after exercise showed altered signal intensity, particularly in the periphery of muscles, in all persons with acute strains, 2 individuals with delayed-onset muscle soreness, and 3 marathoners. Another rim pattern showed a brighter and thinner rim appearing in the perifascial and intermuscular spaces near the injured muscle. This rim was found within 5 days of the inciting event in patients with the most severe injuries clinically. Two of the more severe injuries showed streaks of an undefined material in the subcutaneous fat adjacent to the bright rim.

Pain associated with strain or pain occurring several days after exercise was associated with prolongation of muscle T1 and T2. In the prospective evaluation of delayed-onset soreness, abnormalities seen on MRI persisted for up to 3 weeks after cessation of symptoms. The highly trained marathon runners tended to have relatively mild injuries involving the myotendinous junctions.

Painful muscles after exercise show focal signal-intensity abnormalities on MRI. Changes in relaxation times appear to correlate with serum creatine kinase levels, but alterations in signal intensity on MRI may persist for weeks beyond other indications of injury.

▶ This is an excellent preliminary study demonstrating sports-related muscle sequelae on MRI. The MR demonstration of signal abnormalities provides objective confirmation of heretofore unexplainable pains and muscle soreness. Localized individual muscle abnormalities were identified, with the characteristic distribution that is not necessarily related to the primary muscles used during exertion. It was also demonstrated that muscle recovery lags beyond clinical relief of symptoms. Focal hematomas and facial herniations were not seen, eliminating the necessity for surgical intervention, and no evidence of fatty infiltration or fibrosis that would indicate long-term sequelae was noted. Recognition of the MR patterns associated with exercise, and distinguishing them from pathologic lesions, is of critical importance to physicians who are responsible for treating these patients. Studies of larger samples of patients and various exercise regimens should be encouraged.—J.S. Torg, M.D.

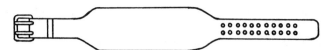

Fig 9–4.—The weight-lifting belt drawn to scale. Fabricated of 0.6-cm thick leather, it is 108 cm long, 15 cm wide in the center, and 6.2 cm wide at the ends. The belt is worn with the buckle centered over the navel. (Courtesy of Harman EA, Rosenstein RM, Frykman PN, et al: *Med Sci Sports Exerc* 21:186–190, April 1989.)

Effects of a Belt on Intra-Abdominal Pressure During Weight Lifting
Harman EA, Rosenstein RM, Frykman PN, Nigro GA (US Army Research Inst of Environmental Medicine, Natick, Mass)
Med Sci Sports Exerc 21:186–190, April 1989   9–17

Lifting belts have been used by weight lifters for many years, but there are few data on whether belts are effective in increasing intra-abdominal pressure (IAP), reducing injury, or improving lifting capacity. The IAP changes during lifting using high-speed computed data. were investigated in 9 weight lifters who dead-lifted a barbell both with and without a lifting belt at 90% of maximum (Fig 9–4). During the lifts, IAP and vertical ground reaction force (GRF) were monitored by computer using a catheter transducer and force platform.

Both IAP and GRF increased steeply before lift-off. After the initial surge, GRF usually plateaued; IAP either plateaued or declined. The IAP rose significantly earlier when belts were worn, and significantly earlier than did GRF. Both with and without the belt, the IAP surge ended significantly earlier than did the GRF surge. Significantly greater variables with the belt included peak IAP, area under IAP in relation to the time-curve from the beginning of the IAP surge to lift-off, peak rate of IAP increase after termination of the initial surge, and average IAP from lift-off to completion of the lift. However, the average rate of IAP increase during the initial surge was significantly lower with the belt.

A lifting belt augments IAP during dead-lifts and probably reduces compressive force on spinal disks, thus improving lifting safety. However, all weight lifting need not be performed with a belt. Training with a belt may inhibit strengthening of the abdominal muscles that contribute to generation of IAP. The IAP-generating muscles may also develop differently if a belt is used in training.

The Effects of a Weight Training Belt on Blood Pressure During Exercise
Hunter GR, McGuirk J, Mitrano N, Pearman P, Thomas B, Arrington R (Univ of Alabama, Birmingham)
J Appl Sport Sci Res 3:13–18, February–March 1989   9–18

To determine what effect wearing a weight-lifting belt (WLB) has on rate and blood pressure during exercise, 5 healthy men and 1 woman were tested for peak oxygen uptake during cycle ergometer exercise, maximum 1-arm bench press, and maximum isometric dead-lift. Submaximal tests were performed on each person twice for each exercise, once while wearing a WLB and once without a belt. Blood pressure was determined by auscultation. Heart rate and WLB pressure on the abdominal wall also were monitored continuously during exercise and during recovery.

The pressure of the WLB on the abdominal wall increased across exercise time in the bench press and dead-lift. After an initial significant increase in abdominal pressure during cycle ergometer exercise, pressure from the WLB stabilized and remained constant. The mean systolic blood pressure was significantly increased during both aerobic and isometric exercises with the WLB. Aerobic exercise was associated with a significant increase in heart rate when the WLB was worn. The rate-pressure product was also significantly higher with all exercises when the WLB was worn. The use of a WLB may put an added strain on the cardiovascular system. Persons with compromised coronary arteries may be at added risk when exercising while wearing a WLB.

▶ Weight-lifting belts—why do lifters wear them? Do they prevent injuries? Do they increase strength? Can more weight be lifted wearing one? Do they affect heart rate or blood pressure? Do they have an effect on intra-abdominal pressure?

The authors of the article reviewed in Abstract 9–17 concluded that weight-lifting belts augment internal abdominal pressure during dead-lifts and probably reduce compressive force on spinal disks. However, they also caution their use during training, as they may inhibit abdominal muscle strengthening. The authors of the article reviewed in Abstract 9–18 concluded that a weight-lifting belt may put an added strain on the cardiovascular system and caution users who have compromised coronary arteries.—F.J. George, ATC, PT

Tibiofemoral Joint Forces During Isokinetic Knee Extension
Nisell R, Ericson MO, Németh G, Ekholm J (Karolinska Inst and Hosp, Stockholm)
Am J Sports Med 17:49–54, January–February 1989   9–19

Isokinetic exercises are often used in muscle-strengthening programs. After anterior cruciate ligament (ACL) surgery it is important that knee rehabilitation not cause excess stress on the ligament, but it is not known which activities are safe and which are dangerous during ligament healing.

Eight healthy men performed isokinetic knee extensions at 30 degrees per second and 180 degrees per second with the resistance pad in both proximal and distal positions. A Cybex II isokinetic dynamometer recorded the maximum moment of force produced by the right knee extensor muscles.

At 180 degrees per second, the maximum moments produced by the quadriceps muscle reached mean peak magnitudes at 65 degrees of knee flexion when the resistance pad was placed distally. When the pad was placed proximally, the peak moment occurred at the same degree of knee flexion, but the peak moment was lower: 181 Nm when the pad was distal versus 163 Nm when the pad was proximal. At knee angles of 65 degrees or more, the difference was statistically significant. At 30 degrees per second, the mean magnitude of the peak moment was significantly higher—284 Nm—than at the faster speed. The peak also occurred somewhat earlier during knee extension at 70 degrees of knee flexion.

The tibiofemoral compressive force was of the same magnitude as the patellar tendon force, with a maximum approaching 9 times body weight. The tibiofemoral shear force changed from a negative to a positive magnitude of about 700 N, indicating that high forces occur in the ACL when the knee is extended more than 60 degrees. Placing the resistance pad in a proximal position on the leg lowered the anteriorly directed shear force considerably.

During rehabilitation after ACL repair or reconstruction, stress on the ligament may be controlled by using the model presented here. When the lowest possible ACL stress is indicated during isokinetic knee extensions, the resistance pad should be placed proximally.

▶ The authors of the 2 previous articles reviewed (Abstracts 9–18 and 9–19) remind us of how careful we must be in the rehabilitation programs of our ACL patients. Quadriceps exercises that require the knee to be extended from 90 degrees of flexion should be avoided. When sufficient hamstring strength has been attained, we teach a co-contraction of the hamstrings and quadriceps muscles, and we use the Johnson Anti-Shear Device to prevent anterior tibial translation during knee extension exercises. We also use relatively high speed isokinetic exercises until the very late stages of knee rehabilitation.

The authors of the article discussed in Abstract 9–19 state that stress on the ACL may be relieved during knee extension if the resistance pad is placed proximally on the tibia.

Related abstracts may be found in the 1987 YEAR BOOK OF SPORTS MEDICINE, Abstracts 6–25, 6–26, and 6–27.—F.J. George, ATC, PT

The Influence of Velocity-Specific Resistance Training on the In Vivo Torque-Velocity Relationship and the Cross-Sectional Area of Quadriceps Femoris

Petersen SR, Bagnall KM, Wenger HA, Reid DC, Castor WR, Quinney HA (Univ of Alberta, Edmonton; Univ of Victoria, Victoria, BC)
J Orthop Sports Phys Ther 10:456–462, May 1989   9–20

Strength training has been widely used to improve athletic performance. Although the effects of velocity-specific training have been studied, the nature, and even the existence, of such velocity-specific adaptations has not been sufficiently clarified. The effects of velocity-specific resistance training were examined in 30 healthy, male varsity athletes who were assigned to high-velocity resistance (HVR) training, low-velocity resistance (LVR) training, or control group. Every other day for 6 weeks the men completed 2 or 3 sets of 20-second maximal exercises at 6 hydraulic resistance stations for the lower extremity. Resistances were adjusted to maintain average angular velocities of about 1.05 and 3.14 rad/sec for the LVR and HVR groups, respectively.

In the LVR group peak knee extension torques were improved at all 7 angular velocities tested between 1.05 and 4.19 rad/sec. The HVR group also improved, but only at angular velocities of 2.62, 3.14, 3.66, and 4.19 rad/sec. In both training groups the cross-sectional area of the quadriceps femoris muscle group was increased. There were no significant changes in strength or cross-sectional area among the men in the control group.

Resistance training at high velocity appears to be no more effective than training at low velocity in increasing high-velocity peak torque. Low-velocity resistance training seemed to have a greater and more consistent effect on the in vivo torque velocity relationship than HVR training.

These findings do not resolve the apparent controversy over velocity-specific training effects or potential transfer of enhanced function from high-speed training to low-speed performance, or vice versa.

▶ In both high-velocity and low-velocity groups the cross-sectional area of the quadriceps muscle was increased. Then things got confusing. This study did not support the theory of velocity-specific training. The authors did support the theory that "High resistance, slow-velocity (LVR) resistance training appears to induce more strength gains over a wide range of angular velocities than does low resistance, high-velocity (HVR) training.—F.J. George, ATC, PT

Effect of an Adjustable Pedal Shaft on ROM and Phasic Muscle Activity of the Knee During Bicycling

Goodwin C, Cornwall MW (Louisiana State Univ)
J Orthop Sports Phys Ther 11:259–262, December 1989   9–21

To determine whether a shortened bicycle pedal shaft in comparison to a standard-length pedal shaft significantly alters the amount of flexion required of the knee during cycling, and whether the phasic activity of the lower leg musculature changes as a result of cycling under 2 different conditions, 6 healthy experienced cyclists were tested using a Fitron stationary bicycle equipped with a pedal shaft with a length of 8.9–17.0 cm; tests were conducted at both extremes.

The range of motion (ROM) during cycling was measured with an electrogoniometer; surface electromyographic activity of the right rectus femoris, biceps femoris, lateral gastrocnemius, and gluteus maximus were sampled with Ag-AgCl surface electrodes. The cyclists pedalled using toe clips. The seat height was adjusted so that the knee was in 15 degrees of flexion with the pedal completely down; the handlebars were adjusted so that the trunk was in 20 degrees of flexion.

Using the standard-length pedal shaft, an average of 87.9 degrees of knee flexion was required for cycling. Using the shortened shaft, only 53.3 degrees of flexion was required, significantly less than with the standard length. The rectus femoris muscle became active later in the cycle using the shortened shaft, whereas the gastrocnemius muscle ceased activity earlier using the shortened shaft. The activity of the other muscles was unaffected by pedal shaft length.

These findings indicate that use of a shortened pedal shaft results in a significant decrease in knee ROM. At the same time, the muscle contraction patterns of 4 leg muscles were not greatly affected. The use of a shortened bicycle pedal shaft should allow patients with moderate restrictions in knee ROM to benefit from the use of a stationary bicycle.

▶ The results of this study indicate that a shortened pedal shaft decreases knee ROM by 41.6%. This would certainly allow many patients with reduced knee ROM to use a stationary bicycle.—F.J. George, ATC, PT

The Effect of the Squat Exercise on Knee Stability
Chandler TJ, Wilson GD, Stone MH (Auburn Univ)
Med Sci Sports Exerc 21:299–303, June 1989   9–22

Weight training has become popular to improve sports performance and fitness. However, there is controversy about the effect of the squat exercise on the functional integrity of the knee.

Twenty-nine men and 10 women who were beginning an 8-week weight-training program were assigned to a half-squat group, 31 men and 7 women were assigned to a full-squat group, and 10 men and 13 women were assigned to a control group. Measurements of knee stability were taken before training, at midpoint, and after training was completed. Nine tests for knee stability were performed using a knee ligament arthrometer. To measure the long-term effects of squatting, the same measurements were made in 27 male power lifters and 28 male weight lifters.

During the 8 weeks performance of neither full nor half squats significantly affected knee stability, compared to stability in controls who did not squat. In the long-term study, power lifters were significantly tighter than controls on the anterior drawer at 90 degrees of knee flexion, and both power lifters and weight lifters were significantly tighter than controls on the quadriceps active drawer at 90 degrees of knee flexion. When data for power lifters and weight lifters were analyzed by years of experience and by level of skill, squat training did not appear to affect knee stability in any of the tested groups.

Knee stability was neither increased nor decreased by 8 weeks of weight training that included either full squats or half squats. Knee stability in athletes who performed the squat over long periods of time was also unaffected. Therefore, the full squat appears to be safe in terms of not causing permanent stretching of the knee ligaments.

▶ This article is good news for those who wish to use squatting exercises in their conditioning regime. As the authors state, there has been a good deal of controversy about the safety of this exercise with regard to knee injuries. I'm sure the controversy will continue, but here is one article that supports the safety of doing the squat. Of course, the exercise must be taught and performed correctly. The heavier the weight used, the more important it is to use proper technique.—F.J. George, ATC, PT

Nautilus Training System Versus Traditional Weight Training System
Kosmahl EM, Mackarey PJ, Buntz SE (Univ of Scranton, Pa; Scranton Rehabilitation Services, Inc; Allied Services for the Handicapped, Scranton)
J Orthop Sports Phys Ther 11:253–258, December 1989   9–23

To investigate whether Nautilus exercise equipment might be a more effective and time-efficient method of strength training than traditional, progressive resistive exercise, the strength gains of the dominant quadriceps femoris muscle achieved with the Nautilus equipment were compared with those achieved with traditional methods. Eighteen college students were divided into 3 groups. Group N used a Nautilus knee extension machine, performing 1 set of 15 repetitions to failure, with a 15 RM (repetition maximum) for a count of 5 contract-1 hold-5 release. Group T used an NK table, performing 3 sets of 10 repetitions for a count of 1 contract-1 release. Group C did not undergo any training. Training was carried out for 6 weeks (with a 1 week rest between the third and fourth weeks), 3 times weekly. All workouts were supervised. A Cybex II Dynamometer was used for pre- and posttest evaluation of bilateral quadriceps femoris strength.

Based on the analysis of variance with F-ratio, no significant differences among the different groups were found in the strength gain of the dominant quadriceps femoris muscle, but significant differences were found between groups T and C for average quadriceps femoris strength. Although not significant, other measures suggested that group T had made greater strength gains.

Further investigations are needed to determine whether the traditional or Nautilus method is superior at increasing quadriceps femoris strength. In the meantime, clinicians must consider many factors, including patient comfort and convenience, when designing a program for a given patient.

Comparison of Muscle Capability and the Resistance Patterns Provided by Nautilus Leg Extension and Leg Curl Machines
Kramer J, Clarkson H (Univ of Western Ontario, London; Univ of Alberta, Edmonton)
Physiother Can 41:256–261, September–October 1989   9–24

Many pieces of commercial equipment might be of value to patients undergoing strength rehabilitation. A widely promoted machine uses an

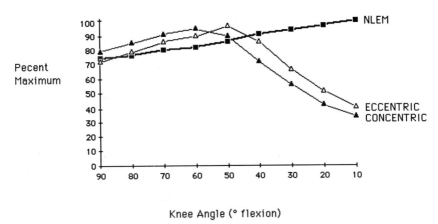

Fig 9–5.—Resistance pattern of the NLEM and human capability patterns. (Courtesy of Kramer J, Clarkson H: *Physiother Can* 41:256–261, September–October 1989.)

irregularly shaped pulley, called a cam, to provide variable resistance. Little scientific information is available on such machines. To provide the clinician with useful data on cam-based equipment, the Nautilus Leg Extension Machine (NLEM) and the Nautilus Leg Curl Machine (NLCM) were evaluated.

The resistance patterns of the 2 machines were compared with knee extensor and flexor capability patterns during both concentric and eccentric muscle actions. The resistance torque patterns of the 2 machines were determined with a Cybex II Isokinetic dynamometer. Testing was completed using an angular velocity of 30 degrees per second to represent slow movements. Human torque patterns were determined using a computer controlled dynamometer. The dominant leg of 20 healthy young

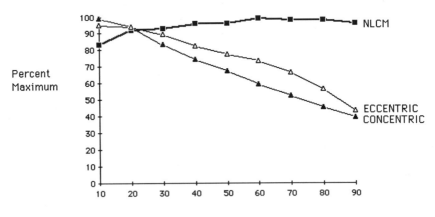

Fig 9–6.—Resistance pattern of the NLCM and human capability patterns. (Courtesy of Kramer J, Clarkson H: *Physiother Can* 41:256–261, September–October 1989.)

male volunteers was tested in body positions similar to those in which the NLEM and NLCM would be used.

The concentric and eccentric capability patterns of the knee extensors and flexors did not correspond to the resistance patterns provided by the 2 Nautilus machines (Figs 9–5 and 9–6). A high correlation was found between the resistance patterns of the machines and the cam perpendicular distances, but only slight correlations between the NLEM and NLCM and muscle capability.

When using moderately heavy weight-plate loads, the manner in which most trainees use the equipment, the cam is the primary determinant of the resistance pattern. Although muscle capability and machine resistance patterns did not match, the decision to use the tested equipment may not be based solely on this measure.

▶ Abstract 9–23 indicates that Nautilus equipment is not superior to a traditional NK table for increasing quadriceps muscle strength. The authors used an unusual training regime of 6 weeks with a 1-week rest between weeks 3 and 4. The authors of the article reviewed in Abstract 9–24 conclude that the concentric and eccentric capability patterns of the knee extensors and flexors did not correspond to the resistance pattern provided by the Nautilus machines.

Nautilus and Universal had virtual control of the muscle machine market for many years. There is now a great deal of competition from other manufacturers and a resurgence of the proponents of free weights. As I stated in an earlier YEAR BOOK, the effort an athlete puts into his or her training regime is much more important than the device that is used.—F.J. George, ATC, PT

High Frequency Electrical Stimulation in Muscle Strengthening: A Review and Discussion
Selkowitz DM (Oakland, Calif)
Am J Sports Med 17:103–111, January–February 1990   9–25

Electrical stimulation (ES) for strengthening is useful clinically in a variety of circumstances. Although experiments on this topic have involved much variability in procedural details, 2 major categories of reported ES strength-training programs have been described: a muscle endurance type regimen, with short intervals between contractions and use of frequencies of 50–200 Hz, and a more typical muscle strength training regimen with longer rest intervals, shorter total stimulation times, and higher frequencies, e.g., 2,500 Hz. The major findings from studies of muscle strength training regimens on the strengthening effects of ES on the quadriceps femoris muscles of healthy persons were reviewed. Most of these studies used ES at frequencies of 2,500 Hz.

Isometric ES training can significantly increase both isometric and isokinetic strength. It is unclear whether differences exist in the effects of ES on men and women. Electrical stimulation training results in increases in isometric strength that correlate positively with mean training contraction intensity and that may depend on mean training contraction duration. However, upper limits to training contraction intensity and duration may exist and may be affected by neuromuscular and muscle fiber fatigue factors. No consistent physiologic changes in muscles have been shown to accompany strength increases attributable to ES training. Motor learning may be involved in the increased isometric strength that results from ES training. Increases in isometric strength are similar whether ES, voluntary contractions, or both are used. No consistent relationship has been found between current amplitude tolerated and torque produced during a contraction.

These conclusions were not drawn from clinical studies. Although ES may be useful for strengthening, it is necessary to consider research methods when conducting or evaluating clinical studies.

▶ There has been a good deal of controversy regarding the effectiveness of ES on strengthening the quadriceps muscle. Much of the controversy has arisen because of vast differences in the studies that were done. In some studies the subjects were healthy, in others they were postoperative or injured. Further, different machines and different modes of treatment were used in these studies.

In the author's summary he states, "There are no significant differences in isometric strength increases between testing groups using ES alone, VC [voluntary contraction] alone, or ES and VC simultaneously."

There are related abstracts in the 1989 YEAR BOOK OF SPORTS MEDICINE, Abstract 8–34, and in the 1988 edition, Abstracts 7–32 to 7–36.—F.J. George, ATC, PT

Hamstring Injuries in Sprinting: The Role of Eccentric Exercise
Stanton P, Purdam C (Belconnen, Australia)
J Orthop Sports Phys Ther 10:343–349, March 1989   9–26

Athletes involved in power-based events have long been frustrated by hamstring injuries despite attempts at prevention through stretching and strengthening. A specific connective tissue insufficiency-induced hamstring injury that occurs in the late swing-early stance phase of sprinting and jumping activities was studied, and an exercise regimen for strengthening the hamstrings and preventing such injury was investigated.

Eccentric muscle action can produce high forces within the series elastic component (SEC) of the hamstrings in the sprinting phase, and these high forces have been related to hamstring injury. Eccentric exercise training regimens can prevent this injury by strengthening the SEC, resulting in a musculotendinous structure that is theoretically able to generate and withstand higher eccentric and concentric forces.

In an eccentric exercise regimen for strengthening the hamstrings patients rapidly extend the knee and decelerate at about 20 degrees to 30 degrees via an eccentric hamstring contraction. This is followed by a quick concentric contraction. Patients begin the exercise with no weights or .5-kg weights. Three sets of 15 repetitions are done every other day. Once patients feel no discomfort during or after the first catches, weight is added to the foot. Patients then return to a slow catch speed before progressing to fast catches. The weight is increased slowly to the point just below which a noticeable drop in catch speed occurs. The exercise must be done carefully, because increasing the speed or weight too fast results in pronounced delayed muscle soreness. The exercise can be done standing, lying prone, or lying over a couch. A recent pilot study suggested that this exercise is a valid way of preventing and rehabilitating hamstring injury.

Such exercise should prove valid for retraining and preventing hamstring injury resulting from connective tissue insufficiency and possibly for enhancing performance in terms of torques produced, joint positions used, and angular velocities achieved. This exercise may then be added to other methods of training and rehabilitation to achieve more complete recovery and to reduce the incidence of reinjury.

The Effect of Stretching Neural Structures on Grade One Hamstring Injuries

Kornberg C, Lew P (Metropolitan Spinal Clinic, Prahran, Australia; Moonee Ponds Physiotherapy Ctr, Moonee Ponds, Australia)
J Orthop Sports Phys Ther 10:481–487, June 1989   9–27

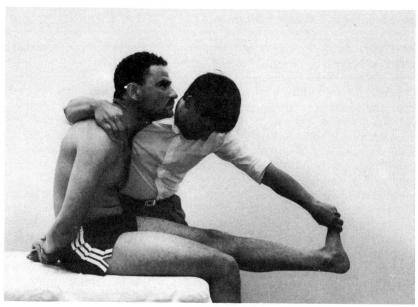

Fig 9–7.—Slump test, cervical extension. (Courtesy of Kornberg C, Lew P: *J Orthop Sports Phys Ther* 10:481–487, June 1989.)

Hamstring strain is one of the most difficult and refractory conditions to treat in sports medicine. The effect of stretching neural structures was studied in 28 professional Australian Rules football players with grade I hamstring injuries who had positive responses to the slump test, a neural tension test (Fig 9–7). Sixteen men were treated traditionally, and 12 had slump stretch added to the traditional regimen.

The slump stretching technique combined with traditional treatment modalities was a more effective treatment than traditional treatment alone for grade I hamstring strains in athletes who had a positive slump test. The slump test can be used as a differentiation test in assessing hamstring strain, thus permitting the best treatment regimen to be used.

▶ The previous 2 abstracts (9–26 and 9–27) present relatively new theories in the treatment and prevention of hamstring injuries. Abstract 9–26 describes a series of "catch" type exercises using eccentric muscle contractions. The theory is that, through the use of eccentric exercises, the musculotendinous unit is able to generate and withstand higher forces.

Abstract 9–27 describes how neural structures are stretched, using what the authors describe as a "slump" technique. The slump test is a spinal test to determine the relationship between the mobility of the pain-sensitive structures in the vertebral canal and or intervertebral foramen. The authors' theory is that abnormal neural tension predisposes to hamstring muscle pathology.—F.J. George, ATC, PT

Therapeutic Effect of High Speed Voluntary Muscle Contractions on Muscle Soreness and Muscle Performance

Hasson S, Barnes W, Hunter M, Williams J (Univ of Texas, Galveston; Texas A & M Univ, College Station; Virginia Polytechnic Inst and State Univ, Blacksburg)
J Orthop Sports Phys Ther 10:499–507, June 1989   9–28

Muscular pain and soreness can result from disease, trauma, or exercise, and soreness resulting from exercise can have a rapid or delayed onset. To determine the effects of a high-velocity therapeutic exercise regimen on muscle soreness and muscular performance, 6 male and 4 female subjects participated in a regimen that consisted of 20 voluntary maximum knee extension-flexion contractions at about 300 degrees per second with a 3-minute recovery, repeated for 6 sets. Data on eccentric stepping exercise were collected just before inducing muscle soreness, immediately after inducing the soreness, at 24 hours, and at 48 hours.

Maximum voluntary contraction by the quadriceps, peak torque by the quadriceps at high resistance, and total work by the quadriceps at low resistance showed a percent decrease from baseline that was significantly lower in the experimental group than in the control group at 48 hours after muscle soreness was induced. The soreness perception index was also significantly lower at 48 hours in the experimental group.

High-speed voluntary muscle contractions are effective in reducing delayed muscle soreness and in facilitating return of normal muscle performance. Further research is needed to examine the effects of high-speed voluntary muscle contractions on the inflammatory process and intra-muscular compartmental fluid pressures after a bout of eccentric muscle contractions.

Does Postexercise Static Stretching Alleviate Delayed Muscle Soreness?
Buroker KC, Schwane JA (Good Shepherd Hosp, Longview, Tex; Univ of Texas, Tyler)
Physician Sportsmed 17:65–83, June 1989   9–29

Delayed muscle soreness (DMS) is common after strenuous or unaccus-tomed exercise. It is widely believed that postexercise stretching can alle-viate DMS, but there are few data confirming this hypothesis.

Seven women and 16 men performed a 30-minute step-test to induce DMS in thigh and calf muscles. Each person was randomly assigned to 1 of 3 groups after the test: group 1 performed no stretching exercises, group 2 stretched only the left knee extensor muscles, and group 3 stretched both the right and left eccentric muscle groups. Stretching exer-cises were performed immediately after exercise, at 2-hour intervals for 24 hours after exercise, and at 4-hour intervals for the next 48 hours.

The step test produced DMS in eccentric muscles but not in concentric muscles. Stretching did not alleviate DMS either immediately after exer-cise or during the 3-day postexercise period. All individuals reported soreness in the left knee extensor muscles after exercise, and all but 2 had soreness in the right plantar flexor muscles. Serum creatine kinase levels, markers of muscle damage, were increased after exercise. The strength of the sore thigh muscle also was reduced. Stretching had no effect on these responses.

Static stretching to relieve DMS after exercise was ineffective in this study; however, these results do not prove that stretching is never effec-tive. Further research is needed to determine whether and under what conditions stretching might relieve DMS in other situations.

Effectiveness of 10% Trolamine Salicylate Cream on Muscular Soreness Induced by a Reproducible Program of Weight Training
Hill DW, Richardson JD (Miami-Dade Community College-North Campus, Mi-ami)
J Orthop Sports Phys Ther 11:19–23, July 1989   9–30

The effect of an over-the-counter topical analgesic cream on soreness resulting from weight training was evaluated in 34 untrained college stu-dents who exercised on 5 consecutive days and rated soreness 4 times daily. The exercise consisted of 3 sets of up to 20 repetitions of arm curls using 80% of 1-repetition maximum. The students applied either 10% trolamine salicylate cream or a placebo cream over sore muscles 4 times daily. Increased plasma levels of creatinine kinase indicated muscle damage.

Students given placebo reported meaningful levels of soreness that occurred sooner and persisted longer than those reported by the treatment group. When soreness occurred, levels were lower in the treatment group.

A 10% trolamine salicylate cream is effective in reducing the muscular soreness associated with unaccustomed exercise. The regular application of this odor-free, nongreasy cream would be well tolerated by patients in physical therapy and could be a beneficial adjunct to their care.

▶ It is theorized that delayed-onset muscle soreness (DMS) is caused by tissue damage within the muscle, which leads to inflammation and increased fluid pressure. Eccentric contractions are considered the culprit for most of this tissue damage. The previous 3 studies deal with methods of preventing or alleviating this soreness.

The conclusion in Abstract 9–28 is that high-speed voluntary muscle contractions (300 degrees per second) are very effective in decreasing DMS and facilitating the return of normal muscle performance. The authors propose that these contractions decrease inflammation and fluid compartment pressure. The authors of the article reviewed in Abstract 9–29 conclude that static stretching does not relieve DMS, nor does it have an effect on creatine kinase levels, which are markers of muscle damage. Abstract 9–3 reports that 10% trolamine salicylate cream is effective in reducing the muscle soreness associated with unaccustomed exercise. But these authors could not deduce whether soreness was reduced directly by the analgesic effects of the trolamine salicylate or indirectly by its anti-inflammatory effects.—F.J. George, ATC, PT

Knee Orthoses for Valgus Protection: Experiments on 11 Designs With Related Analyses of Orthosis Length and Rigidity
Carlson JM, French J (Gillette Children's Hosp, St Paul)
Clin Orthop 247:175–192, October 1989   9–31

Many knee orthoses are now available, and some designs seem sturdy, but others seem frail. To obtain objective data on the relative effectiveness of orthoses used to protect the medial collateral ligament (MCL) during sporting activities, 11 different commercially available knee orthoses and a leg model were tested with static loading.

The leg model was made of stainless steel tubing covered by polyethylene foam. A polyurethane plug was used to separate the simulated tibial and femoral sections. The orthoses tested included Lenox Hill, NUKO, OTI, CTi, Lorus, Polyaction 404, Lerman Multi-Ligamentus, Ecko II, Anderson Knee Stabler, Am Pro, and Three-way Knee Stabilizer. The effectiveness of each orthosis was calculated in terms of the rigidity contributed to the leg-orthosis combination. Both length and rigidity of the orthosis were analyzed.

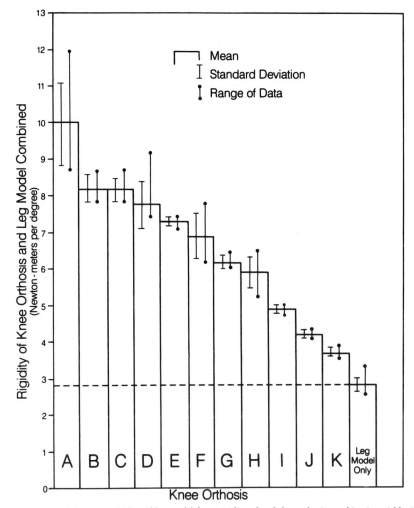

Fig 9–8.—Subtracting rigidity of leg model from rigidity of each leg-orthosis combination yields rigidity provided by orthosis. *Bar graph* compares external rigidity provided by each of 11 knee orthoses at 78 Nm loading. (Courtesy of Carlson JM, French J: *Clin Orthop* 247:175–192, October 1989.)

At a static valgus loading of 78 Nm, the unbraced leg had a rigidity of only 2.8 Nm per degree of valgus, but the leg-orthosis combination that produced the most rigidity, the Lenox Hill, had a rigidity of 10.0 Nm per degree of valgus (Fig 9–8). Even with this orthosis, however, a valgus increase of 8 degrees initiated injury to the MCL. Theoretical design deficiencies correlated with data from laboratory tests.

Both adequate length and rigidity are required for an orthosis to be biomechanically effective. Wide variation in efficacy of the devices was noted, with the Lenox Hill providing the most rigidity.

Controlling Anterior Tibial Displacement Under Static Load: A Comparison of Two Braces

Branch T, Hunter R, Reynolds P (Univ of Minnesota)
Orthopedics 11:1249–1252, September 1989   9–32

Two knee braces were compared to determine whether bracing improves static knee stability, enhances or alters muscle firing amplitude or timing to create dynamic stability, alters gait, and affects oxygen expenditure during running. Nine men and 6 women (average age, 25.9 years) who had used the Lenox Hill brace for an average of 24 months were studied. All 15 had a complete anterior cruciate insufficiency on the involved side. The contralateral leg in all cases was normal. The knee injury had occurred an average of 62 months previously. Six affected knees were left and 9 were right; 6 dominant knees were involved. Both normal and affected knees were tested; then the affected knee was tested with both the Lenox Hill brace and the CTi brace in random order. The unaffected knee served as a control.

In differentiating the affected knee from the control knee, the anterior drawer was more sensitive at 25 degrees than at 90 degrees. During passive and active drawer tests both the Lenox Hill and the CTi braces improved the affected knee significantly at 25 degrees. With 15 lb of passive loading both braces improved the drawer to within normal limits; however, only the CTi brace was able to return the drawer to within the normal range at 20 lb of force. Neither brace could improve the drawer to normal when it was subjected to the higher loads created by the active drawer test.

At 90 degrees the results with 15 lb of passive loading were similar, whether the knee was braced or unbraced, and whether the affected or the unaffected knee was tested. At 20 lb of force only the CTi brace improved the drawer significantly and placed the drawer within the normal range.

The CTi brace was superior to the Lenox Hill brace for controlling the anterior drawer in flexion and at 20 lb of passive load under static testing conditions. However, when higher loading forces were used for the active anterior drawer test, neither brace could control anterior tibial translation.

▶ The 2 articles reviewed in Abstracts 9–31 and 9–32 compared the effectiveness of different models of knee braces. Abstract 9–31 reports a study of 11 different braces that provide protection for the MCL. The authors determined that the Lenox Hill knee brace is the most effective. I have used the Lenox Hill brace for many years and also have found that it provides adequate protection for our MCL-injured athletes.

The second paper, reviewed in Abstract 9–32, evaluated the Lenox Hill and CTi knee braces and assessed how well they control anterior tibial displacement under a static load. The authors determined that neither brace was effective with higher static loads. Both were effective with 15 lb of load, but only the CTi at 20 lb. I have tried both of these braces with ACL-deficient knees and found them to be equally effective or equally ineffective when providing protection for our ACL patients. The Lenox Hill brace has been a more durable brace.—F.J. George, ATC, PT

The Knee Brace Controversy
Montgomery DL, Koziris PL (McGill Univ)
Sports Med 8:260–272, November 1989   9–33

Many athletes wear prophylactic knee braces during contact sports. However, there is a lack of clinical data to support their value. Because many other factors can affect the rate of knee injuries, these factors should be examined before any changes in injury patterns are ascribed to the use of prophylactic knee braces.

More than 20% of all American football injuries are to the knee, and these injuries account for the greatest loss in participation. Up to 22% of such injuries require surgery. Three of 8 studies of knee injuries supported prophylactic knee bracing, 3 found no significant change in injuries with bracing, and 2 found an increased incidence of injuries with bracing.

Two biomechanical studies showed that knee bracing modified function of a lower extremity, causing greater impact forces plus a time delay in achieving maximum impact force. Bracing reduced knee flexion during the swing and support phases in this series, and also reduces knee extension and internal rotation and torque variables.

Some studies have shown that knee braces increase expenditure during play and also impair forward speed and agility; other studies have found no effect on running speed, agility, strength, power, or endurance of the quadriceps and hamstring muscles.

The current level of knowledge regarding knee braces does not provide conclusive proof that prophylactic knee braces reduce the number and severity of knee injuries. The American Academy of Orthopedic Surgeons has stated, "There is no credible, long-term scientifically conducted study that supports using knee braces on otherwise healthy players." The use of rehabilitative and functional knee braces, on the other hand, is approved by the academy as an effective means of treating knee injuries. Further studies with unbiased evaluations are needed to determine the efficacy of prophylactic knee braces.

▶ This paper is an excellent review of the subject matter. The original article is recommended for those interested in the subject.—J.S. Torg, M.D.

Comparison of Rehabilitation Knee Braces: A Biomechanical Investigation
Cawley PW, France EP, Paulos LE (DonJoy Biomechanics Research Lab, Carlsbad, Calif; Intermountain Orthopedic Research Lab, Salt Lake City; Salt Lake Knee and Sports Medicine Clinic)
Am J Sports Med 17:141–146, March–April 1989   9–34

Research into the functional characteristics of various types of knee orthoses has been hampered by medicolegal problems in testing orthoses on human subjects and difficulties with testing on cadaveric specimens. Therefore, a special mechanical surrogate of the left lower limb was constructed and 8 different braces were tested for comparison. The braces tested were Zimmer Flex-10 (ZIM), DonJoy ROM Splint, Medical Technology Bledsoe Brace (MED TECH), Medical Designs Universal Leg Bracing System, DonJoy ROM Splint with Shells, Orthopedic Systems, Inc., Limited Motion Functional Knee Brace, 3-D Orthopedic 2 Way Brace, and the Orthopedic Technology, Inc., Universal Brace. The unbraced limb was tested before and after testing with each brace. Five repetitions of each test procedure were performed. Tests included passive extension, valgus rotation, and anterior posterior tibial translation.

Most braces significantly reduced both translations and rotations compared to the unbraced limb under static test conditions. During passive extension, the hinges of MED TECH and Orthopedic Systems Inc, Limited Motion Functional Knee Braces failed to hold a set extension stop. All but the ZIM and 3-D Orthopedic 2 Way Brace significantly reduced valgus rotation relative to the unbraced limb. The ZIM also failed to reduce anterior translation of the tibia relative to the unbraced limb. Overall, braced vs. braced performance varied and depended on a number of mechanical and design factors.

The principal factors affecting the choice of a rehabilitative brace are number, arrangement, and means of interfacing straps with the brace; design and alignment of hinge bars; the means of interfacing hinge bars with the limb; and hinge design. Most braces significantly reduce both translations and rotations.

▶ It should also be noted that observations revealed that ". . . joint line contact is a principal key in controlling varus/valgus contact is a principal key in controlling varus/valgus rotation in rehabilitative braces." Also, overall brace stiffness, not simply pure mechanical stiffness but that caused by the complex interrelationship of the individual brace parts, is an important component. As concluded by the authors, "Since the loads applied in all test conditions in this study were certainly well below those we would expect in normal physiologic loading conditions, the data presented here may be clinically relevant only in those patients who are either in a nonweightbearing or partial weightbearing status while using the rehabilitative brace."—J.S. Torg, M.D.

The Effect of Prophylactic Knee Bracing on Performance
Sforzo GA, Chen N-M, Gold CA, Frye PA (Ithaca College, NY)
Med Sci Sports Exerc 21:254–257, June 1989   9–35

Bracing and taping are standard treatments for improving joint stability so injured athletes may resume competition. Prophylactic bracing has also become popular. The effects of prophylactic knee braces on athletic performance were examined in 25 male football players and 10 female lacrosse players of college age.

All 35 completed 2 sets of tests to determine peak torque, rise time, anaerobic power, time to fatigue, and concentrations of lactate in blood. Baseline blood samples were obtained before the tests. Eighteen athletes wore a prophylactic dual-hinged knee brace during the first testing session; the others wore the brace during the second test period.

Bracing did not significantly affect the performance of the football players, but it did decrease the overall performance of the lacrosse players. The rise time, time to develop peak torque, was the most significant factor in the multivariate difference found in the female athletes. However, repeated-measures *t*-tests found no isolated variable that was significantly different among the conditions. Familiarity with wearing a brace, the order of testing, or a learning period did not alter performance results.

Wearing a prophylactic knee brace does not improve performance during athletic activity. In some asymptomatic athletes performance may be diminished. Athletes and coaches should reexamine the use of prophylactic knee braces. Other factors such as cost and the potential for inducement of muscle cramps add to the negative possibilities.

▶ The introduction to Chapter 6 of the 1987 YEAR BOOK OF SPORTS MEDICINE addressed the use of prophylactic knee braces for football. In the same edition there were 5 different abstracts on this subject (3–4 and 6–1 to 6–4). In the 1988 YEAR BOOK OF SPORTS MEDICINE there were also 5 abstracts (7–10 to 7–14). In the 1989 YEAR BOOK there was only 1 abstract (3–12).

Believe me, as athletic trainers we wanted to buy a knee brace that would prevent these injuries. We spent a great deal of money, time, and effort to make our players wear them. There has been no conclusive evidence that any prophylactic knee brace tried to date has been effective. I wish they were successful. We would be happy to pay for one if it were available. We hope that in the future such a brace will be designed, manufactured, and become available. We no longer make it mandatory for our athletes to wear braces. If they want them, we provide them.—F.J. George, ATC, PT

Differential Diagnosis: Exertional Compartment Syndromes, Stress Fractures, and Shin Splints
Genuario SE (Univ of Cincinnati)
Athletic Training 24:31–34, Spring 1989   9–36

Overuse injuries result from repeated trauma to tissues with insufficient time for healing. A compartment syndrome results when tissue fluid pressure rises in a closed fascial space and compromises circulation to the nerves and muscles. The acute form is seen when muscle volume increases after fracture or severe soft tissue injury.

Trainers are much more likely to encounter an exertional compartment syndrome, in which exercise raises intercompartmental pressure to the point that small vessels are compromised. With chronic exertional compartment syndrome there is pain, muscle weakness, and paresthesias. Bilateral involvement is frequent.

In stress fractures changes on films are noted within 2–3 weeks after onset of pain as new callus begins to form. The patient often reports an increase in training 2–5 weeks before pain develops. If training continues, pain worsens and is not relieved by rest. Examination may show localized tenderness and soft tissue swelling.

The anterior shin splint syndrome most often involves an inflamed anterior tibial muscle. Pain and tenderness commonly occur along the lateral border of the tibia at the medial crest, and pain worsens on active dorsiflexion and passive plantar flexion. Posterior shin splint syndrome involves the posterior tibialis longus, flexor digitorum longus, and flexor hallucis longus muscles. Pain often is localized to the insertion of the posterior tibialis at the tibia and is increased on active inversion of the ankle.

Medial tibial stress syndrome refers to pain in the distal tibia, possibly associated with the tibialis posterior muscle. Bone scans can distinguish the syndrome from stress fracture by showing involvement of the posterior tibial cortex and longitudinal activity of one third or more of the length of the bone. Pain is present on weight-bearing and is relieved by rest.

▶ When teaching student trainers the differential diagnosis of an acute compartment syndrome, we stress the importance of recognizing the symptoms and the dire consequences if they go undetected. We use the 5 Ps as our guide in recognizing this injury: pain, pallor, paresthesia, pulselessness, and paralysis. If a compartment syndrome is suspected, immediate referral is made to the team physician.—F.J. George, ATC, PT

10 Injuries

Epidemiology and Prevention

Bicycle Helmet Use by Children: Evaluation of a Community-Wide Helmet Campaign
DiGuiseppi CG, Rivara FP, Koepsell TD, Polissar L (George Washington Univ; Univ of Washington)
JAMA 262:2256–2261, Oct 27, 1989   10–1

Less than 5% of school-aged children wear helmets while riding a bicycle. Yet bicycling injuries to children account for 300,000 emergency department visits and 500–600 deaths per year in the United States. To determine whether a community-wide education campaign focused solely on bicycle helmet use would increase the use of helmets by school-age children, trained observers counted helmet use among 9,827 school-aged children riding bicycles at sites located in high-income, middle-income, and low-income census tracts in Seattle and Portland.

An interventional campaign was implemented in Seattle but not in Portland, which served as a nonintervention control city for the study. Direct observations of helmet use by children were carried out during 2-week intervals before and 4, 12, and 16 months after the start of the campaign. The campaign included distribution of posters and stickers at various bicycling events and offered incentives for wearing a helmet. More than 100,000 discount coupons for $25.00 toward the purchase of a helmet were distributed. Children from low-income families were given free helmets.

There were 4,940 children observed in Seattle and 4,887 in Portland. In Seattle, helmet use increased from 5.5% before the educational campaign to 15.7% afterward. In Portland, helmet use increased from 1% to 2.9%. The increase in helmet use in Seattle was found at sites in all 3 socioeconomic levels, whereas very little increase in helmet use over time was seen in low- and middle-income areas in Portland.

Statistical analysis revealed strong associations between helmet use and white race; riding geared bicycles; riding in playgrounds or parks, and on bicycle paths; riding with adults; and riding with other children, compared with black or other race, riding nongeared bicycles, riding on city streets, and riding alone. Adjustment of the data for these variables increased the proportions of helmet wearers in Seattle from 4.6% to 14% and in Portland from 1% to 3.6%. A focused community-wide bicycle helmet campaign can increase helmet use among school-age children.

▶ This study, supported in part by a grant from the Centers for Disease Control, concludes that a community-wide bicycle helmet campaign can increase helmet use among children. The statement that this type of program may reduce "the substantial morbidity and mortality of children who are involved in bicycle crashes" is conjectural and certainly not supported by the data.—J.S. Torg, M.D.

A Case-Control Study of the Effectiveness of Bicycle Safety Helmets
Thompson RS, Rivara FP, Thompson DC (Group Health Cooperative of Puget Sound; Univ of Washington)
N Engl J Med 320:1361–1367, May 25, 1989   10–2

The most common cause of morbidity and mortality in bicycle accidents is head injury. Although wearing a bicycle helmet has been advocated as a way to reduce head injuries, evidence of the effectiveness of this approach is inadequate. A case-control study was conducted to evaluate the effectiveness of wearing a bicycle helmet in reducing the risk of head and brain injury. Case patients included 235 bicyclists who sought emergency room treatment in 1 of 5 hospitals for head injury after a bicycling accident in a 1-year period. One control group consisted of 433 patients seeking emergency room treatment for bicycling injuries other than head injuries and another control group consisted of 558 members of a health maintenance organization involved in bicycling accidents during the year. Data were collected from emergency rooms and hospital records. Population-based controls responded to postcards and completed detailed questionnaires.

At the time of injury, 7% of the cases were wearing helmets, as were 24% of emergency room controls and 23% of population-based controls. Serious head injuries occurred in 99 bicyclists of whom only 4% were wearing helmets. Regression analyses controlling for age, sex, education, income, cycling experience, and severity of the accident demonstrated that wearing a helmet reduced the risk of head injury by 85% and the risk of brain injury by 88%.

Wearing a helmet while bicycling is a highly effective means of reducing the risk of both head and brain injury. Because most serious head injuries from bicycling accidents occur in children, the wearing of helmets is particularly important in this segment of the population.

▶ Many serious head injuries in children could be avoided if they would wear a helmet when riding a bike. I have heard a number of different reasons why children don't wear helmets, ranging from expense to cosmetic aspects to availability. I sincerely believe that the biggest problem is peer pressure and how children are perceived by their friends if they wear a helmet.

There is an article in the May/June 1990 *NEA Today* health section about bike helmets. In that article Dr. William Boyle states that there are 400 to 500 bicycle accident deaths yearly in children under age 15, and that many are preventable. He also states that if a child is allowed to help buy a helmet he or she is often more willing to wear it. He recommends buying only a helmet that bears an ANSI- or Snell-approved sticker.—F.J. George, ATC, PT

Cerebral Concussion Rates in Various Brands of Football Helmets
Zemper ED (Univ of Oregon, Eugene)
Athletic Training 24:133–137, Summer 1989   10–3

Cerebral concussions are relatively common in football players. The risks associated with the use of various types of helmets were examined by reviewing data concerning 15,610 college football players over 4 seasons. There were more than 1,200,000 athlete exposures to injury in a game or practice.

There were no significant differences in the incidence of concussion associated with the type of helmet worn in the first 3 seasons evaluated. In the fourth, however, certain differences were noted. Two brands of helmets were associated with concussion rates substantially above or below expected values. It is not clear whether these data reflect a statistical aberration or whether different brands of helmets actually do differ in protective capacity. It is not possible at present to recommend changing brands of helmets.

▶ We all want to have our athletes in the safest helmet available. To date, there has not been an independent study clearly indicating that one brand of football helmet is safer than another. If the results of the 1987 NCAA study are repeated, there may be evidence to indicate that there is a safer helmet available.—F.J. George, ATC, PT

Training Activities, Competitive Histories, and Injury Profiles of Elite Boardsailing Athletes
Allen GD, Locke S (Darling Downs Inst of Advanced Education, Toowoomba, Queensland; Sunnybank Med Clinic, Brisbane, Queensland, Australia)
Aust J Sci Med Sport 21:12–14, June 1989   10–4

Boardsailing has grown rapidly in popularity. The training and competitive histories, as well as medical problems, were reviewed in questionnaires completed by 41 selected Australian and international boardsailing athletes. The 36 males and 5 females included members of the Australian Olympic team and others of national or international ranking. The athletes ranged in age from 15 to 44 years. Questions were related to personal, training, and competitive histories, injury patterns, and length of competitive involvement.

Internationally ranked sailors had greater competitive experience, and they spent more time per week in sailing and dry-land training than athletes of lesser standing. Abrasions, lacerations, and muscle strains were the most common injuries. Gender did not affect the relative frequency of injuries. Injuries were most often caused by rocks, centerboards, mast tracks, footstraps, and fins. Some athletes also contracted secondary infections from coral cuts. The most common chronic injury was low back pain, with most athletes reporting this problem. Overuse, equipment problems, and trauma led to these injuries.

Boardsailing appears to be a relatively safe sport with few serious injuries associated; however, specific and appropriate training programs are reommended. The frequency of low back pain justifies further study.

▶ The conclusion that boardsailing appears to be a relatively safe sport with few serious injuries is somewhat contradicted by Ullis and Anno (1) and Habal (2) who have reported intervertebral disk herniations, significant fractures, cerebral concussions, pneumothorax, cervical spine fractures, cruciate ligament injury, and a drowning death.—J.S. Torg, M.D.

References

1. Ullis KC, Anno K: *Phys Sports Med* 12:86, 1984.
2. Habal MB: *J Fla Med Assoc* 73:609, 1986.

Warm-Up and Muscular Injury Prevention: An Update
Safran MR, Seaber AV, Garrett WE Jr (Duke Univ)
Sports Med 8:239–249, 1989   10–5

Many muscular injuries are preventable. One of the factors implicated in muscle injury is an inadequate warm-up. Others are incorrect or no stretching, weakness, strength imbalance, overall fatigue, and undernourished muscle. Warm-up relaxes the athlete by promoting calm and aiding concentration. Circulation and respiration are increased, and oxygen is more accessible to the cells. Myocardial ischemia at the onset of vigorous exercise is less likely. More force may be needed to tear "warmed-up" muscle tissue.

Increased flexibility after stretching may lower the risk of musculotendinous injury, minimize soreness, and possibly improve athletic performance. Ballistic stretching may extend a muscle to near its physiologic limit and produce reflex contraction. Repeated stretching at a constant length lowers tension at that length in experimental studies.

Strong athletes are said to perform better and to sustain fewer injuries. Part of the explanation is the overall effect of conditioning. A stronger muscle might absorb more energy than a weak one before failing. In this way, the likelihood of strain would be reduced by the need for greater energy to rupture the muscle.

▶ This is an excellent review of the subject matter. The interested reader is referred to the original article.—J.S. Torg, M.D.

The Ontario Cohort Study of Running-Related Injuries
Walter SD, Hart LE, McIntosh JM, Sutton JR (McMaster Univ)
Arch Intern Med 149:2561–2564, November 1989   10–6

Although running is a popular fitness activity, few studies have examined the incidence and causes of running injuries. The frequency and types of injuries experienced by runners were characterized and identification of risk factors was attempted in 1,680 runners who participated in 2 community road race events that included both a longer and a shorter race. All participants completed a baseline questionnaire, and as many as possible underwent a brief physical evaluation. The questionnaire covered training, running environment, use of stretching, warm-up and cooldown exercises, other physical activities, occupational activity level, characteristics of shoes, height and weight, race participation, smoking status, and injuries during the previous year. Participants were followed by telephone interview at 4, 8, and 12 months after enrollment.

Forty-eight percent of runners experienced at least 1 injury; of these, 54% were new injuries, whereas the remainder were recurrences of previous injuries. Competitive runners apparently had a substantially elevated risk for new injuries compared with fitness runners. Excess risk also was associated with running more than 40 miles per week, increasing daily mileage on running days, length of the longest run during the week, number of running days per week, and running year round. The relative risks for these variables were similar in men and women. Runners who never warmed up had less risk than those who did, and runners who sometimes stretched appeared to be at higher risk than those who usually or never did. An injury during the previous year was highly predictive of sustaining a new injury. Tall men appeared to be at greater risk but not tall women. Factors such as pace, running surface, hill running, or intense training had little effect on the incidence of injury. Injury rates were similar in all age-sex groups and were unrelated to years of running experience.

Running is associated with a high incidence of injuries; however, many injuries might be prevented by a reduced training load. Running in moderation does not entail undue risk, but athletes who wish to train at high levels are at risk for more frequent injuries.

Predicting Lower-Extremity Injuries Among Habitual Runners
Macera CA, Pate RR, Powell KE, Jackson KL, Kendrick JS, Craven TE (Univ of South Carolina, Columbia; Ctrs for Disease Control, Atlanta)
Arch Intern Med 149:2565–2568, November 1989   10–7

Running is thought to be beneficial to the cardiovascular system but potentially deleterious to the musculoskeletal system. Although the rate of lower-extremity injuries in habitual runners seems to be substantial, neither risk factors nor incidence rates have been clearly defined.

A lengthy questionnaire was sent to all persons on a mailing list for road races in South Carolina. The questionnaire was used to elicit information on running practices, history of illnesses and injuries, and demographic characteristics. In all, 583 runners returned the questionnaire and agreed to participate in follow-up. They were sent a log and a monthly newsletter for the next 12 months. The log was used to detail daily running habits, participation in other physical activities, and injuries incurred.

During the 12-month follow-up, 52% of men and 49% of women reported at least 1 injury. Through multiple logistic regression, investigators identified that running 64 km or more per week was the most important predictor of injury in men. Other risk factors were having incurred an injury in the preceding year and having been a runner for less than 3 years. For women the only statistically significant predictor of lower extremity injury was the practice of running more than two thirds of the time on concrete.

There is a high incidence of lower extremity injury in habitual runners, those new to running, and those with previous injuries. Reducing the weekly running distance is suggested as a suitable preventive measure.

▶ The definition of "injury" was similar for both studies (Abstracts 10–6 and 10–7). Specifically, it is defined as a problem severe enough to cause a reduction in weekly distance, a visit to a health professional, or the use of medication. Using this definition of injury, Walter et al. (Abstract 10–6) reported an overall 1-year accumulative incidence of 48% for all injuries, whereas Macera et al. (Abstract 10–7) reported that 49% of the women who responded reported at least 1 running-related injury to the lower extremities during the preceding 12-month period. Lacking from their data are an expression of permanence and whether there was any subsequent disability. The difficulty that these papers present in interpretation is their failure to designate injuries in terms of objective findings as opposed to subjective complaints of the participants.—J.S. Torg, M.D.

Musculoskeletal Injuries Associated With Physical Activity in Older Adults
Matheson GO, Macintyre JG, Taunton JE, Clement DB, Lloyd-Smith R (Univ of British Columbia)
Med Sci Sports Exerc 21:379–385, August 1989   10–8

Lifelong physical activity is recognized as a requisite for good health, but injury is often a barrier to sports participation in older age groups. In the past decade there has been a significant increase in the incidence of overuse injuries. To compare the clinical presentation of overuse injuries in older and younger athletes, data were obtained on 685 patients at least age 50 years who had been referred to an outpatient sports medicine clinic over a 5-year period; 722 younger patients served as controls.

Charts of all patients were reviewed for demographic information, sports activity at the time of injury, historical data, clinical evaluation, specific diagnosis, and the use of confirmatory diagnostic studies. Subjective evaluation of muscle weakness was also obtained from the records.

Both groups cited running as the most common physical activity at the time of injury. In the older group racquet sports and walking were the next most common. In 15% of the older group it was not possible to identify a causal relationship between a single sport and onset of injury. In both populations there was a high proportion of injuries to the knee, lower leg, and foot. Foot injuries were more common in older patients and knee injuries were more common in the younger group.

Tendinitis occurred with similar frequency in both groups, but older patients had more metatarsalgia, Morton's neuroma, plantar fasciitis, and meniscal injury; younger patients were more prone to stress fracture-periostitis and patellofemoral pain syndrome. Osteoarthritis and degenerative disk disease were more common in the older group, as expected. The incidence of osteoarthritis increased significantly with advancing age, and the frequency of muscle weakness was greater in patients with osteoarthritis; however, muscle weakness was not greater with advancing age alone.

Approximately 85% of injuries in older athletes were overuse injuries known to respond to conservative treatment. Less than 5% of older patients required surgery. It appears that injury should be no more of a deterrent to exercising in the elderly than it is at any age.

▶ The authors point out that ". . . since this study is a retrospective survey, a comparison of these two populations cannot be used to predict the injury rate or prevalence for the entire population or to correlate specific sports with specific injuries." They also point out that, "Although it remains to be determined whether the component of functional loss associated with inactivity can be separated from the functional loss due to disease or aging, increased physical activity has been shown to be associated with reductions in age-related morbidity, improvements in functional capacity, and preservation of independence."—J.S. Torg, M.D.

Age, Physical Activity, Physical Fitness, Body Composition, and Incidence of Orthopedic Problems
Macera CA, Jackson KL, Hagenmaier GW, Kronenfeld JJ, Kohl HW, Blair SN
(Univ of South Carolina; Inst for Aerobics Research, Dallas)
Res Q Exerc Sport 60:225–233, September 1989   10–9

The effects of age, physical activity, physical fitness, and body mass index (BMI) were studied on the incidence of orthopedic problems in a large population of men and women followed for up to 8 years. Active persons would be at increased risk for these problems, but the other factors studied might have a modifying effect.

Using a proportional hazards approach to evaluate the effects of the variables, studies were made in 5,582 men and women. Orthopedic problems were physician diagnosed but were self-reported in response to a questionnaire mailed to persons who had come to a preventive medicine center for advice. Physical fitness was determined by treadmill testing, and physical activity was ranked on a scale of 1 to 5. The BMI was calculated by dividing the subject's weight by height.

Overall, 16% of men and 14% of women reported a problem in the foot, knee, back, or hip at least once during follow-up. The expected risk of orthopedic problems per person-year was .045 for men and .046 for women. Physical fitness, BMI, and physical activity were associated with orthopedic problems. The main predictor for women was physical activity. Age was not a factor for either gender. Change in physical activity and a decrease in BMI were associated with orthopedic problems in women, but neither these factors nor change in physical fitness were significant for men.

The yearly risk for orthopedic problems was similar for both sexes; an increase in activity paralleled an increase in orthopedic problems. However, baseline physical fitness was related to orthopedic problems in men but not in women. The fact that age was not a factor suggests that moderate physical activity in generally healthy persons can be recommended for those of any age.

Prevention and Treatment of Overuse Tendon Injuries
Hess GP, Cappiello WL, Poole RM, Hunter SC (Hughston Orthopaedic Clinic; Rehabilitation Services of Columbus, Ga)
Sports Med 8:371–384, 1989   10–10

Up to half of all sports injuries may result from overuse; the musculotendinous unit is affected most often. Functional overpronation at the ankle promotes Achilles tendinitis and other lower extremity injuries. Excessive anteversion of the femoral neck can lead to intoeing and altered vector forces on the musculotendinous units of the lower limb. The extrinsic factors related to overuse tendon injuries are chiefly training errors.

Acute treatment of overuse tendon injuries includes rest, application of ice for 72 hours, and compression bandaging. The inflammatory response is useful at first but should be limited to 1–3 days. Range-of-motion exercises are helpful in the acute phase. Heat or both heat and cold may be initiated subsequently to promote circulation and limit swelling. Strengthening exercises should include both concentric and eccentric contractions. Sports-specific exercises are indicated when an athlete is ready to resume training. Transcutaneous nerve stimulation may help to relieve pain during rehabilitation.

Proper stretching and strengthening techniques, applied during training, will counter muscular imbalance and inelastic tissues. A proper training surface is important in preventing overuse injuries; it should provide adequate impact cushioning but be firm enough to confer stability. Proper foot support also is critical for runners.

▶ This is an excellent review of the subject matter. The interested reader is referred to the original article.—J.S. Torg, M.D.

Overuse Injuries in Triathletes: A Study of the 1986 Seafair Triathlon
Collins K, Wagner M, Peterson K, Storey M (Sports Medicine Clinic, Seattle)
Am J Sports Med 17:675–680, September–October 1989   10–11

Triathlons are increasing in popularity, but few studies have evaluated their potential for overuse injuries. Triathletes were questioned to determine their overuse injuries and the relationship of these injuries to training schedules. A 3-page questionnaire was mailed to 600 finishers in the 1986 Seafair Triathlon. Questions sought demographic data, data on training and sports, medical history, and history of sports injuries. Respondents also described any injuries that occurred during the triathlon.

Forty-five percent of those surveyed responded. Of these, 49% had had a training-related injury during the preceding year that was sufficiently serious to cause them to interrupt training, seek medical care, or take medications. Overall, 62% of overuse injuries were caused by running and another 8% were related to running plus another sport. The knee, shoulder, and ankle were the most common sites of injuries. Female triathletes and those who were older had approximately the same incidence and distribution of injuries. Elite triathletes had a slightly higher incidence of injuries than less accomplished athletes, but the difference was not significant. Neither age, sex, body mass index, mileage per week, nor other training factors affected the likelihood of injury.

Persons training for a triathlon have an approximately 50% chance of sustaining an overuse injury during the year before the event, particularly while running. Overuse injuries apparently do not correlate with training mileage or with age, sex, or other characteristics of triathletes. Prospective studies investigating other factors may identify causes of overuse injuries.

Overuse Injuries in Ultraendurance Triathletes

O'Toole ML, Hiller DB, Smith RA, Sisk TD (Univ of Tennessee, Memphis; Campbell Clinic, Memphis)
Am J Sports Med 17:514–518, July–August 1989   10–12

Overuse injuries are the most common sports-related injuries requiring medical treatment. These injuries are particularly significant in ultraendurance athletes. After the 1986 Hawaii Ironman Triathlon World Championship, investigators sent a training and medical history questionnaire to 788 competitors from the United States and Canada and to 25 competitors from elsewhere. The questionnaire included a list of common overuse injuries and asked athletes to indicate injuries they had sustained.

Of the 75 men and 20 women who responded, 91% had sustained at least 1 soft tissue overuse injury during the previous year's training. On average, each athlete sustained 2.9 injuries in the training year. The back was the single area most frequently involved, but it was common for an athlete to have injuries to all 3 areas, i.e., the back, knee/thigh, and ankle/foot. Combinations of injuries were consistent, suggesting that mechanical abnormalities (e.g., reduced shock absorptions) might have contributed to injury. Training practices varied widely and did not appear to be related to either the incidence or type of injury.

▶ Collins et al. (Abstract 10–11) reports that 49% of the questionnaire respondents sustained a training-related injury serious enough for them to stop training for at least 1 day, seek medical care, or take medicine. On the other hand, 91% of the ultraendurance triathletes reported by O'Toole et al. (Abstract 10–12) had at least 1 soft tissue overuse injury during the previous year of training. However, these authors also state that ". . . most of these conditions respond to conservative medical management if combined with a reduction of the stresses that have caused them." Also, "The majority of these overuse syndromes encountered by ultraendurance athletes lead to no permanent impairment in ability to perform." Both studies agree that training patterns of the athletes do not appear to be related to their physical problems.—J.S. Torg, M.D.

Injury Rates in a National Sample of College Football Teams: A 2-Year Prospective Study
Zemper ED (Univ of Oregon, Eugene)
Physician Sportsmed 17:100–113, November 1989   10–13

Few long-term studies of football injuries have been made on a national scale. During 1986 and 1987, data were gathered on 6,229 college football players with 445,856 athletic exposures. Time-loss injuries totaled 2,820, for an overall rate of 6.3 injuries per 1,000 athletic exposures, or 45.3 per 100 players. The injury rate during games was 8.6 times higher than that during practice. At least 1 injury was sustained by 32.1% of the players. Of the injuries, 8.3% were season ending and 8.5% required surgical intervention.

The direct cause of injury was impact from another player's helmet in 14.4% of players; in 7% from a shoulder pad, and in .3% from another player's knee brace. The site of injury usually was the knee, then the ankle; sprains and muscle strains were the most common types of injury. The most common mechanisms of injury were being tackled, blocking, and tackling. Injuries were incurred by offensive players in 50.9% of instances and by defensive players in 45.2%. Most injuries occurred during the third quarter and the fewest during the first quarter. Artificial turf was associated with a 60% higher overall injury rate than natural grass.

Rules prohibiting use of the head as initial contact point need more emphasis and enforcement. Opportunity for players to warm up and stretch before the third period may help to reduce injury. The observation of higher injury rates on artificial turf should be thoroughly investigated.

▶ The lack of knowledgeable medical input in the authorship is quite apparent in this report. Although designed to express injury rates in terms of athlete exposures and by anatomical site, the necessary and commonly accepted pathologic nomenclature has been ignored. Great danger lies in such an approach. It is stated that, "The overall injury rate was 60% higher on artificial turf than on natural grass." There is no indication, however, if the increased injury rate on Astroturf was attributable to serious knee injuries, fractures, or superficial abrasions, as reported by Grippo (1).—J.S. Torg, M.D.

Reference

1. Grippo J: *Stanford Research Report*, Menlo Park, California, 1973–1975.

The Epidemiologic, Pathologic, Biomechanical, and Cinematographic Analysis of Football-Induced Cervical Spine Trauma
Torg JS, Vegso JJ, O'Neill MJ, Sennett B (Univ of Pennsylvania)
Am J Sports Med 18:50–57, January–February 1990   10–14

Data compiled by the National Football Head and Neck Registry since 1971 were analyzed to determine the frequency of cervical spine trauma. Data were obtained through injury report forms mailed to secondary school principals and athletic trainers, as well as through a media clipping service hired to identify head and neck injuries reported in the press, radio, or on television. When possible, game films were studied.

In 1975, preliminary analysis of the data showed that most serious cervical spine football injuries resulted from axial loading (Fig 10–1). As a result of this finding the National Collegiate Athletic Association and the National Federation of High School Athletic Associations made rules changes that forbid "spearing" and the use of the top of the helmet as the initial point of contact in tackling or blocking. These changes have resulted in a dramatic decrease in both the total number of cervical spine injuries and in the number of injuries that result in quadriplegia (Fig 10–2).

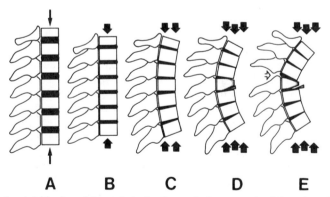

A   B   C   D   E

Fig 10–1.—Axial loading of the cervical spine first results in compressive deformation of the intervertebral disks (**A** and **B**), followed by maximum compressive deformation; angular deformation and buckling then occur. The spine fails in a flexion mode (**C**) with resulting fracture, subluxation, or dislocation. Compressive deformation (**D** and **E**) to failure with a resultant fracture, dislocation, or subluxation occurs in as little as 8.4 msec. (Courtesy of Frankel VH, Burstein AH: *Orthopaedic Biomechanics*, 1970. From Torg JS, Vegso JJ, O'Neill MJ, et al: *Am J Sports Med* 18:50–57, January–February 1990.)

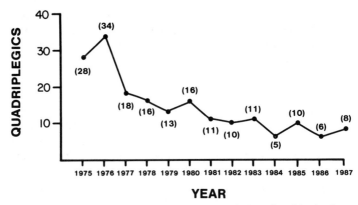

Fig 10–2.—The yearly incidence of permanent cervical quadriplegia for all levels of participation (1975 to 1987) decreased dramatically in 1977 after initiation of the rule changes prohibiting the use of head-first tackling and blocking techniques. (Courtesy of Torg JS, Vegso JJ, O'Neill MJ, et al: *Am J Sports Med* 18:50–57, January–February 1990.)

Similar studies directed toward the prevention of injuries incurred in other sports could result in decreased rates for many types of injuries in a wide variety of sports.

▶ It is said that "an ounce of prevention is worth a pound of cure." The significance of this paper is best appreciated when one understands that with regard to cervical quadriplegia, there is no cure.—J.S. Torg, M.D.

Epidemiology and Traumatology of Injuries in Soccer
Nielsen AB, Yde J (Århus County Hosp, Århus, Denmark)
Am J Sports Med 17:803–807, November–December 1989   10–15

Soccer is the most popular team sport in Europe and is responsible for most athletic injuries. A prospective study was undertaken to examine the distribution and patterns of injury in 123 soccer players; the group included 93 men older than 18 years and 30 boys aged 16–18 years. Thirty-four of the 93 adult soccer players were playing at the division level and 59 played at the lower level of the senior leagues. During the 9-month playing season, the coach of each team recorded the number of practice sessions and games for each player and noted all injuries and subsequent absences from practices and games.

At the start of the season none of the players was absent because of injuries. During the study period, 89 players incurred 109 injuries, 43 during practice and 66 during games. Thirty-eight injuries were treated at hospitals, and 6 knees were operated on. Overall, 35% of the injuries caused absences of more than 1 month's duration. The injury incidence during games was highest among players participating at the division level; injuries during practice were more common in the lower series.

Most (84%) of the injuries were of the lower extremity, with ankle sprains the most common (36%). There were 20 knee injuries, including 4 ruptured ligaments and 4 lesions of the meniscus. More than half of the knee injuries were caused by tackling. Contact injuries during tackling occurred most often in the lower and the youth divisions (45%), whereas players at the senior level had only a 30% incidence of tackling injuries. Overuse caused 37% of the injuries, and these occurred most commonly during the spring; the incidence was comparable in both age groups. At follow-up 1 year after the end of the playing season, 28% of the injured players still had problems and 5% were unable to play soccer. Prophylactive interventional measures should be designed for different skill levels of individual teams within a soccer club.

▶ This study appears to bear out the principle that with regard to contact activities, the incidence and severity of injuries increases with the age and performance level of the participants. To be noted, the findings in this study were similar to those observed by Ekstrand and Gillquist (1) who studied soccer injuries in 180 male amateur players (average age, 25 years) participating at division level.—J.S. Torg, M.D.

Reference

1. Ekstrand J, Gillquist J: *Med Sci Sports Exerc* 15:267, 1983.

Surface-Related Injuries in Soccer
Ekstrand J, Nigg BM (Univ Hosp, Linköping, Sweden; Univ of Calgary, Alta)
Sports Med 8:56–62, 1989   10–16

More than 60 million registered persons in 150 countries play soccer and undoubtedly many more play who are not registered. The most frequent injuries are sprains and strains of the ankles and knees. There is some evidence that the type of playing surface, especially natural grass vs. artificial turf, influences the type and frequency of injuries.

Although the stiffness of a surface may influnce some chronic overuse injuries, there is no definitive evidence that stiffness is related to acute soccer injuries. Overuse injuries may be minimized by adequate training, gradual adaptation to a new surface, and the use of appropriate insoles in soccer shoes. Ligament sprains often occur when a player is tackled with the loaded leg fixed to the ground. Long cleats may lower the risk of such injuries. High friction between the shoe and surface may produce excessive force on the knee or ankle, but too little friction can lead to slipping, which itself can cause injury.

▶ This is an excellent review of the subject matter. The interested reader is referred to the original article.—J.S. Torg, M.D.

Mountaineering and Rock-Climbing Injuries in US National Parks

Addiss DG, Baker SP (Johns Hopkins Univ)
Ann Emerg Med 18:975–979, September 1989   10–17

Despite advances in safety equipment, the American Alpine Club has reported an increase in the number of deaths and injuries related to mountaineering and rock climbing. Investigators analyzed mountain-climbing injuries reported to the National Park Service in 1981 and 1982 and prepared a model of the factors involved in these injuries. Data were extracted from a computer printout for 127 climbing-related injuries. Chi-square and Mann-Whitney rank sum tests were used for statistical analyses.

Twenty-eight percent of the injuries were fatal. The mean age of injured persons was 27 years. Ninety-one percent of those injured were men and boys, and 88% of injuries occurred from May through August. Falls were responsible for 75% of all climbing-related injuries. Four national parks were associated with 58% of reported injuries, and 67% of fatalities occurred in either Grand Teton Park or Mount Rainier Park. Further, 63% of the injuries occurred on rock and 37% on snow or ice. The latter were significantly more likely to be fatal. Of 44 injuries on snow or ice, 25% were caused by rockfall, icefall, or avalanche. Sixty-nine percent of injuries occurred during ascent.

The median length of fall for fatal injuries was 91 m; for nonfatal injuries, it was 9 m. Avalanche or icefall caused only 9% of all injuries but 28% of deaths. Seven percent of injuries were caused by exposure to cold or high altitude; equipment failure or misuse caused 6% of all injuries. A third of the victims had multiple injuries; of 38 climbers with multiple injuries, 21 died. Fractures comprised 29% of the injuries, 10% were sprains, and 5% were frostbite.

It may be that traditional safety principles are now inadequate to prevent the occurrence of additional injuries. Models can be used to evaluate specific climbs or climbing areas.

▶ The authors develop a "basic model" adopted from Blumenthal (1) comprised of 2 curves, one representing the difficulty or demands of the climb and the other representing the climber's performance. They point out that an accident occurs when the demands of the task exceed the capabilities of the individual. The prevention of injuries is possible by reducing the demands on the climber and improving climber performance. However, this appears to be at odds with the author's observation that, "Those who climb in the Himalayas are among the most experienced and skillful mountaineers, yet the Himalayan climbing mortality rate is probably the highest in the world."—J.S. Torg, M.D.

Reference

1. Blumenthal M, cited in Baker SP: Injury control, in Sartwell PE (ed): *Preventive Medicine and Public Health,* ed 10. New York, Appleton-Century-Crofts, 1973, pp 987–1005.

Personal and Environmental Factors in Relation to Injury Risk in Downhill Skiing
Bouter LM, Knipschild PG, Volovics A (Univ of Limburg, Maastricht, The Netherlands)
Int J Sports Med 10:298–301, August 1989   10–18

Many potential risk factors associated with downhill skiing have been evaluated. A case-control study was conducted among Dutch downhill skiers to assess the circumstances and the personal and environmental factors associated with injury risk of downhill skiing. The data were obtained from the records of an insurance company that writes ski insurance for approximately one third of all skiers who take out such policies. Cases were those who had filed claims for ski injuries. Controls were selected from uninjured skiers who filed claims for other reasons (e.g., loss or theft of property).

The 572 cases had a mean age of 32 years, and the 576 controls, 32.6 years. Forty-six percent of the cases and 67% of the controls were men. Because of selection bias caused by the way the controls were chosen, risks associated with age and gender could not be estimated, and odds ratios were adjusted for confounding by age and gender.

Most accidents (84%) happened on hard-packed ski trails. Ski lifts were involved in about 6% of the accidents. Only 2% of the injured skiers collided with an object, but 4% of the men and 8% of the women collided with another skier. Premature release of bindings was not a direct cause of accidents. Poor condition of the ski run (30%) and lost balance (24%) were the 2 most frequently cited direct causes of accidents. Risk did not vary significantly by day of week or time of day, but the injury risk appeared to be increased with increasing duration of exposure. A relatively low risk was observed for skiers who were only moderately rested, and for skiers who admitted a certain fear of having a ski accident. The presence of icy sports was associated with a relatively high injury risk, whereas poor visibility, the presence of clouds, and perceived coldness were associated with a relatively low risk of injury.

Because most of the personal and environmental risk factors assessed in this case-control study are not open to manipulation, the results cannot be used to formulate recommendations for the prevention of ski injury. Prospectively controlled trials are needed to quantify the risks associated with skiing injuries.

Parachuting Injuries During Training Descents
Lowdon IMR, Wetherill MH (John Radcliffe Hosp, Oxford, England)
Injury 20:257–258, September 1989   10–19

Previous reports have discussed injuries sustained during recreational or military parachuting. Injuries incurred in a 6-year period of parachute training. Major injuries included fractures, dislocations, and head injuries; minor injuries included bruises, strains, and sprains.

During the 6-year study period there were 51,828 descents, and the overall casualty rate was .4%. The casualty rate associated with major injuries was .22%, with 117 major injuries being sustained by 109 parachutists (4 deaths). The most commopn lower extremity injury was ankle fracture; more than half of these were isolated lateral malleolar fractures. All 5 patients who had multiple injuries had fractures of 1 leg or foot in association with other injuries. In 95 of 104 single injuries the cause was a hard or awkward landing.

Entanglement of 2 parachutes and air stealing caused more serious injuries: 4 spinal fractures, 3 multiple injuries, and 2 deaths. The other 2 deaths resulted from problems on exiting the aircraft, which prevented correct use of the parachute. There were no parachute failures. Until the fourth jump the incidence of injuries to parachutists declined as they gained experience; the incidence of injuries rose again as conditions became more difficult.

The conditions for parachute descents in military training are far more exacting than those for sports descents, but the injury rate associated with military descents is lower, which suggests that military ground instruction is effective in reducing the frequency of injuries.

▶ Another way of looking at the data is to determine the major casualty and death rates in terms of those per number of participants per basic military course. The paper appears to indicate that the median number of descents completed by the trainees was 10. Thus if each trainee averaged 10 descents and there was a total of 52,000 descents, it appears that 5,200 individuals were exposed. In other words, 109 (2%) of the parachuters sustained a major injury. There was 1 death per 2,500 participants, or 61.5/100,000 participants.—J.S. Torg, M.D.

Snowboard Injuries
Pino EC, Colville MR (Oregon Health Sciences Univ, Portland)
Am J Sports Med 17:778–781, November–December 1989   10–20

Snowboarding has become increasingly popular during the past 5 years. A snowboard is a laminated wood or fiberglass board similar to a short wide ski, and snowboard riding techniques are similar to those of surfing and skateboarding. Because little is known about injury rates, risks, and liabilities associated with this sport, most ski area operators do not allow snowboarding.

Snowboard riders participating in racing events were interviewed in person and asked to complete a comprehensive questionnaire. A total of 267 snowboard riders provided the data for analysis. This group included 239 male riders and 28 female riders aged 12–48 years (average, 21 years). Of these, 257 considered themselves to be in average or above average physical condition; 49% perceived themselves as intermediate riders and 36% as expert riders, with 71% of those surveyed having more than 20 days' experience. Also, 84% skied, 28% surfed, 67%

skateboarded, and 23% were board sailors. Some method to increase ankle support and foot control was used by 126 riders (47%) and knee, shin, or elbow pads were used by 16%. None wore a helmet.

A total of 110 injuries required a visit to a physician. Most of the injuries were ligament sprains, fractures, and contusions, and 92 occurred among those who were most active in the sport. Half of the injuries were to the lower extremities, with ankle injuries the most common. Those who used ankle supports sustained half the number of ankle injuries compared to those who wore only soft boots. Injuries to the lower extremity were concentrated in the forward limb, probably because of the unequal weight distribution that occurs in turning.

The injury pattern associated with snowboarding accidents differed from that associated with downhill skiing in that impact, rather than torsion, was the major mechanism of injury. This resulted in a comparatively increased incidence of ankle injuries and upper extremity injuries and a decreased incidence of knee injuries. Because of the frequency of impact injuries in snowboard riding accidents, safety equipment for this sport should include helmets and padding.

▶ This paper represents the first published report dealing with snowboard injuries. In view of what are, in the eyes of this observer, increased numbers of snowboarders on the ski trails, it is important that injury data be collected and analyzed. Also, another question to be answered is whether or not the presence of snowboards on the downhill ski trails contributes to injuries to Alpine skiers. The fact that the authors have identified a distinct injury pattern resulting from snowboarding that is different from that of downhill skiing is noteworthy.—J.S. Torg, M.D.

Shoulder Injuries in Archery

Mann DL, Littke N (McMahon/Saddledome Sports Medicine Clinics, Calgary, Alta)

Can J Sports Sci 14:85–92, June 1989   10–21

To study the injury rate, the structures involved, and causative factors in shoulder injuries, 21 elite-caliber archers were studied using a questionnaire and physical examination. The 12 men had a mean age of 32.5 years and the women, 34 years.

Significant shoulder injuries had been incurred by 3 men during a mean 13.5-year career and by 5 women during a mean of 10.9 years. Shoulder asymmetry and decreased internal and external rotation of the drawing arm were frequent. Palpable tenderness was evident over the distal third of the infraspinatus and teres minor areas. Isometric testing revealed weakness or pain in more than half of the drawing arm shoulders in women. Results of the impingement test were positive in 3 bowing arm and 6 drawing arm shoulders, often with posterolateral pain. Results of the supraspinatus test were seldom positive. Cadaver prosection showed that the supraspinatus tendon is impinged beneath the lateral coracoacromial arch during horizontal extension toward full draw.

The causes of drawing arm shoulder injuries in archers are probably supraspinatus impingement and tendinitis, and infraspinatus and teres minor traction tendinitis, which are most effectively mangaed by prevention. Keeping the drawing arm elbow stationary at full draw to prevent elbow-shoulder movement, conditioning of the shoulder girdle muscles, and participating in a weight program, are recommended, especially for women.

▶ This article represents one of the first, if not the first, study dealing with shoulder problems in archers. By suggesting that most problems are caused by supraspinatus impingement/tendinitis and infraspinatus/teres minor traction tendinitis, the authors recommend implementation of preventive measures. However, other than suggesting several minor faults in technique and "muscular conditioning," this aspect is rather vague.—J.S. Torg, M.D.

Injuries in Elite Pair Skaters and Ice Dancers

Smith AD, Ludington R (Alfred I duPont Inst, Wilmington, Del)
Am J Sports Med 17:482–488, July–August 1989   10–22

The incidence, severity, and causes of injuries in a group of elite pair skaters and ice dancers were examined prospectively. Sixteen teams of pair skaters and 8 teams of ice dancers were studied for a 9-month competitive season. Skaters were encouraged to report all injuries. Injuries causing a skater to miss at least 1 week of training were classified as serious. Less serious injuries included short-term injuries that markedly limited the skater's training program and chronic injuries that limited the skater's training to a lesser degree.

There were 33 serious injuries during the study period. Female senior pair skaters reported an average of 1.4 serious injuries; other groups averaged more than .5 serious injuries per skater. Injuries to the lower extremities were most common; 7 serious injuries were directly related to the skating boot. Eleven serious injuries occurred during lifts.

Few serious injuries in this study appeared to be preventable, but changes in boot design and training for lifting movements should be attempted and studied prospectively. At present, the injury rate is unacceptably high among elite pair skaters and ice dancers.

▶ The authors' definition of a "serious injury" being one that causes the skater to miss at least 1 week of training is at odds with the AMA nomenclature and other more comprehensive definitions. Specifically, a mild injury is one that sidelines the participant for 1–7 days, a moderate injury is one in which the participant misses 7–21 days, and a severe injury is one that causes the particpiant to miss 3 or more weeks. It appears that a more comprehensive injury grading system would have been more meaningful. Also, it is interesting to note that, "All skaters were offered a 1 day symposium on injury prevention and training methods, but only three skaters attended." It should be noted that with the exception of the lift-related injuries, these acute and overuse injuries were comparable to those reported by Garrick (1) and Brock and Striowski (2).—J.S. Torg, M.D.

References

1. Garrick JG: *Med Sci Sports Exerc* 14:141, 1982.
2. Brock RM, Striowski CC: *Physician Sports Med* 14:111, 1986.

Injuries to Dancers: Prevalence, Treatment, and Perceptions of Causes
Bowling A (London School of Hygiene and Tropical Medicine)
Br Med J 298:731–734, March 18, 1989   10–23

Injury is the most common medical problem among classical ballet and modern dancers. When the British National Organisation of Dance and Mime commissioned a survey of injuries to dancers, 141 dancers from 7 professional ballet and modern dance troups responded to a questionnaire.

Nearly half of the dancers (47%) had a chronic injury, and 42% had sustained an injury within the previous 6 months. About 80% of the dancers reported at least 1 injury at some time that affected dancing. Twenty-three dancers had 2 or 3 chronic injuries. The back, neck, or both, and the ankle were the most frequently reported sites of injury. Muscular injuries were the most common chronic injuries, followed by fractures and dislocations. Injuries to the feet and toes were reported by some dancers. Most dancers thought their injuries were caused by being overtired and/or overworked. Other perceived causes were dancing on unsuitable flooring, dancing in cold or drafty environments, not being properly warmed up, difficulty of the choreography, and continued repetition of difficult movements. Most dancers who consulted professionals after injury saw a physiotherapist; less than half of all dancers consulted medically qualified practitioners. Many injuries to soft tissues had not responded to treatment.

Dancers experience a high rate of injuries, but most are aware of preventive procedures. Dancers suggested learning good technique was most important. As other preventive measures they also suggested being aware of body limitations, warming up, dancing in warmer studios and theaters, having less exposure to pressure and overwork, dancing on better flooring, following a proper diet, and engaging a resident physiotherapist.

▶ The author has failed to either define or establish the criteria for "injury" on the basis of prevailing pathoanatomical nomenclature. Also, although the data are presented in terms of chronic and recent injuries, they are not expressed in terms of severity and duration of disability.—J.S. Torg, M.D.

Degenerative Joint Disease in Ballet Dancers

Andersson S, Nilsson B, Hessel T, Saraste M, Noren A, Stevens-Andersson A, Rydholm D (Malmö Gen Hosp, Lund Univ, Malmö, Sweden)
Clin Orthop 238:233–236, January 1989   10–24

Ballet dancers subject their joints, especially their first metatarsopha-langeal joint, to heavy weight-bearing and repeated trauma. Forty-four retired dancers who had long careers were examined to determine whether they had a higher incidence of lower limb arthrosis than found in the general population.

Six had coxarthrosis (3 men, 3 women). One woman also had signs of segmental collapse of the femoral head that indicated possible osteone-crosis. Three dancers had undergone total hip arthroplasty. The duration of the dancing careers of these 6 dancers was longer than average. The incidence of coxarthrosis among the dancers was significantly higher than in the general population.

Four dancers (9%) had tibiofemoral arthrosis or gonarthrosis. All 4 were symptomatic and had required either nonsteroidal anti-inflamma-tory drugs or intra-articular steroid injections. Bilateral ankle arthrosis not preceded by fracture was found in a 64-year-old woman. Twenty-four dancers (54%) had radiographic signs of arthrosis in the first meta-tarsophalangeal joint; all were asymptomatic. This prevalence is very high, even higher than in a previous study of younger dancers. The prev-alence in the general population is not known.

These observations comprise the first real evidence that extreme physi-cal activity can cause coxarthrosis. Load, or at least load under extreme conditions (e.g., those in classical choreography), may lead to coxarthro-sis. If this proves true, coxarthrosis may also be caused by other extreme, repeated loads and thus may be classified as a worker's compensation in-jury.

▶ The author's observation of an apparent increased incidence of osteoarthro-sis is interesting. However, the conclusion that this is produced by "extreme physical activity" is not supported by the data. Specifically, appropriate data from the history with regard to other possible inciting incidents (e.g., direct blow trauma, infection, or associated medical diseases) were not excluded.— J.S. Torg, M.D.

Head and Neck

Boxing-Related Injuries in the US Army, 1980 Through 1985

Enzenauer RW, Montrey JS, Enzenauer RJ, Mauldin WM (Fitzsimons Army Med Ctr, Aurora, Colo)
JAMA 261:1463–1466, March 10, 1989   10–25

Competitive boxing is currently promoted in the United States military. Interunit matches are common on most large installations, and interser-vice competition is typical at many overseas duty stations. The extent of morbidity and mortality directly related to participation in military boxing was assessed.

The records of hospitalization for boxing-related injuries in U.S. Army medical treatment facilities around the world from 1980 through 1985 were reviewed. An average of 67 hospitalizations attributable to military boxing matches occurred annually. The injured men spent an average of 5 days in bed and almost 9 days disabled and unfit for duty. One man died of a serious head injury; another sustained unilateral blindness from ocular trauma, requiring enucleation. Of all injuries, 68% were to the head, occurring most commonly in the younger and presumably less experienced boxers.

Evidence that boxing can result in irreversible brain damage is now as indisputable as the link between cigarette smoking and lung cancer. Serious head and eye injuries can be especially devastating sequelae of this competitive sport. Although any sport can result in injury, the main goal of boxing is to cause potentially life-threatening damage. The advisability of continuing to promote boxing in the U.S. military should be addressed.

▶ So military boxing takes a toll on our own soldiers. Is it worth the price? Many medical associations urge that boxing be banned. For more on the dangers of boxing, and on the public debate over boxing, see recent issues of YEAR BOOK OF SPORTS MEDICINE: 1986, pp 227–228, and 1987, p 217, and pp 331–332.—E.R. Eichner, M.D.

Eye Injury in Sport
Jones NP (Manchester Royal Eye Hosp, Manchester, England)
Sports Med 7:163–181, 1989   10–26

Sports participation accounts for an increasing number of ocular injuries, especially severe ones. Racquet sports, mainly squash, are of particular concern and at some centers are responsible for the bulk of accidents that occur. At the same time, ocular protection for racquet sports is relatively simple and inexpensive.

A contusional injury is caused by a blow from a blunt object, e.g., a ball. Apart from anterior segment injuries, rapid distortion of the globe places the retinal periphery under stress. Vitreous hemorrhage frequently is seen. Adnexal injuries also are encountered.

Each sport has its own requirements for ocular protection. Accumulation of data on types of injury can support rational recommendations for protective measures appropriate for individual sports activities. Changes may be voluntary or imposed by rules. The ideal eye protector should dissipate force onto a wide area without reducing the visual field and without converting potential oculofacial injury into intracranial injury. The protector should be safe, convenient, cosmetically acceptable, and as inexpensive as possible. It is unfortunate that some measure of conflict exists between optimal safety and the acceptability of a protector. Sacrificing some safety to assure more widespread use of a lightweight protector sometimes may be necessary. Polycarbonate is the best material for all sports protectors used when impact is a risk, but it is not a panacea.

► This is an excellent review of the subject matter. The interested reader is referred to the original article.—J.S. Torg, M.D.

Auricular Injury and the Use of Headgear in Wrestlers

Schuller DE, Dankle SK, Martin M, Strauss RH (Ohio State Univ; Med College of Wisconsin, Milwaukee)
Arch Otolaryngol Head Neck Surg 115:714–717, June 1989   10–27

In both high school and collegiate wrestlers, auricular injuries are commonplace. If the injury goes untreated, the so-called cauliflower deformity results. The treatment for this deformity is both inconvenient and associated with a high degree of noncompliance by the wrestler. Prevention consists of a variety of different types of headgear that are required to be worn; however, during practice there is no headgear requirement. In any event, auricular injury can occur with or without the use of headgear. A total of 537 division I collegiate wrestlers completed questionnaires designed to assess attitudes and the use of headgear.

Only 189 wrestlers (35%) always wore headgear during practice, but 496 (92%) always wore it during team competition. This is a statistically significant difference. The most common reason given by 35% of respondents for not wearing headgear was discomfort. Of the 537 respondents, 208 (39%) reported that 1 or both of the auricles were permanently deformed by injuries occurring in 11% with and in 27% without headgear. Thus there is a high frequency of permanent auricular deformities in wrestlers not only because nonuse of headgear is widespread, but also because it is only partially protective.

► The fact that 40% of those interviewed admitted to having a permanent auricular deformity clearly identifies this as a problem. However, the data presented do not necessarily establish that wearing protective headgear will appreciably decrease this incidence. Perhaps the lack of compliance by both the players and their coaches reflects this phenomenon.—J.S. Torg, M.D.

Preventing Cauliflower Ear With a Modified Tie-Through Technique

Dimeff RJ, Hough DO (Rush Presbyterian St Luke's Med Ctr, Chicago; Michigan State Univ)
Physician Sportsmed 17:169–173, March 1989   10–28

An auricular hematoma forms after a direct blow to, or fall on, the ear, when blood and serum accumulate between the perichondrium and external ear cartilage. If not treated effectively, a "cauliflower" or wrestler's ear can develop. After evacuating the hematoma by aspiration or incision-drainage, it is necessary to compress the auricle to prevent fluid from reaccumulating. The best means is a tie-through suture in which a contoured collodion packing is secured to the auricle with buttons.

Technique.—Under local 1% lidocaine anesthesia, the hematoma is aspirated with a sterile needle; 2 buttons are then sewn loosely to the auricle using a tie-through technique, 1 on either side. A contoured packing is wedged tightly beneath the anterior button. Collodion-impregnated Webril is used in the helix and white wool is used in the concha. A mastoid dressing then is applied. The patint can return to full activity using ear protectors. Antibiotics are given orally for 1 week.

This rapid, simple method has few complications. If a hematoma is infected secondarily the area must be incised and drained and the exudate cultured. Surgical débridement may be required to check the spread of infection. Chondritis is managed by débridement of infected cartilage and intravenously administered antibiotics.

▶ This is a technique paper not supported by data as to results and complications. As a method, it is clearly investigational and cannot be recommended for general use. A randomized study using this technique and the more conventional repeated aspiration/incision and drainage would be most helpful.—J.S. Torg, M.D.

A Survey of Oral Injuries in Female College and University Athletes

Morrow RM, Bonci T (Univ of Texas, San Antonio; Univ of Texas, Austin)
Athletic Training 24:236–237, Fall 1989   10–29

Women's athletic trainers at 389 colleges and universities participated in a program to record oral injuries, including lip laceration, chin-tongue laceration, fractured jaw, and chipped, displaced, broken, or lost teeth throughout the year. Total injury information was requested at the end of the academic year. Trainers were also asked to list the sports in which participants would benefit from wearing mouthguards. Data were received on 21,564 female college and university athletes for the academic year 1987–1988.

More than 90% of the athletes wore mouthguards while playing lacrosse and field hockey, but less than 10% wore them for basketball, soccer, softball, and volleyball. The highest oral injury rate, 7.5% occurred in basketball; the lowest rate, 1.6%, occurred in softball and volleyball. However, softball players incurred some of the more serious injuries.

Seventy-eight percent of trainers believe that mouthguards would be beneficial for field hockey. The percentage of trainers who indicated that mouthguards would be beneficial in other sports included 74% for lacrosse, 62% for basketball, 46% for soccer, 9% for volleyball, 3% for ice hockey, 3% for rugby, 2% for softball, and 1% for water polo.

The oral injury rate of 7.5% in female basketball players represents a significant risk. Even after soft tissue injuries were excluded, the dental injury rate was 2%, which is greater than that reported for football players, who wear mouthguards. The wearing of mouthguards is recommended for sports participants, whether or not they are mandated by the rules of the game.

▶ A recent communication with one of the authors (T. Bonci) indicates that a newly designed mouthpiece that is more acceptable from the standpoint of comfort as well as cosmetic appearance has resulted in higher compliance by athletes. It should be interesting to see what effect this will have on the relatively high incidence of oral and dental injuries among those basketball players wearing it.—J.S. Torg, M.D.

Anterior Neck Trauma
Storey MD, Schatz CF, Brown KW (Sports Med Clinic, Seattle)
Physician Sportsmed 17:85–96, September 1989   10–30

Anterior neck trauma can occur in hockey, football, softball, wrestling, field hockey, soccer, and gymnastics. Anterior neck trauma occurred in a lacrosse player, whose laryngeal injury resulted in severe respiratory distress.

Man, 33, was hit in the left side of the neck with a ball thrown about 10 ft. The patient was a recreational lacrosse defenseman. After being hit, he fell to the ground and was unable to exchange air or speak, although he was alert enough to remove some tobacco from his mouth. Within 30 seconds he was able to cough and subsequently to exchange air. The trainer described the patient's respiration as labored, with inspiratory and expiratory stridor and periodic obstruction. Each obstructive episode was cleared by coughing, which produced bright red blood. In the hospital the patient was treated initially with oxygen 4 L min delivered by nasal prongs, which provided significant relief. Soft tissue neck roentgenograms showed edema and/or hemorrhage of the left glottis and associated retropharyngeal swelling. On indirect laryngoscopy the vocal cords were found to be intact and moving normally. On day 2 CT showed a fractured right lamina of the thyroid cartilage lateral to the thyroid angle with good apposition of the 3 fragments; edema and/or hemorrhage of both true and false cords, with a mucosal tear on the left false cord; submucosal air; intact true cords; and edema and hemorrhage of the left subglottic region into the left supraglottic region. About 24 hours after the injury the patient was discharged; he was still hoarse but had excellent respiratory exchange. By 1 week after injury, the glottic edema had decreased significantly and the patient's voice was normal. He returned to lacrosse playing 3 weeks after the injury wearing a special neck guard suspended from his face mask.

Acute laryngeal injuries are life-threatening and must be managed carefully. Field management of anterior neck trauma includes several options for reestablishing the airway. Signs such as aphonia, hemoptysis, tracheal deviation, or palpable crepitus indicate that immediate transport to the hospital is necessary. To prevent such injury, all players who use their body to block high-speed shots should wear beardlike anterior neck protectors.

▶ The clues here to major laryngeal trauma were acute respiratory distress and aphonia, followed by stridorous respirations, cough, hemoptysis, and prolonged hoarseness. This article presents a thoughtful, practical approach to sports-related injuries of the anterior neck, with useful tips on diagnosis, management, and prevention. Presented at the 1990 annual meeting of the American College of Sports Medicine was another clinical problem caused by blunt trauma to the neck. A high-school hockey goalie was struck in the neck by a puck. He asked to stay in the game, but his mother took him to the doctor. He had mild neck swelling and bruising, a normal neurologic finding, and a bruit in the area of the bruise. Arteriography showed an intimal tear and 50% narrowing of the common carotid artery. The artery was repaired surgically, and the patient recovered smoothly (1).—E.R. Eichner, M.D.

Reference

1. Troop B, Hurley J: *Med Sci Sports Exerc* 22:118, 1990. (abstr)

Infarction of the Medulla and Cervical Cord After Fitness Exercises
Pryse-Phillips W (Meml Univ of Newfoundland, St John's)
Stroke 20:292–294, February 1989   10–31

Manipulation of the neck, minor falls, prolonged hyperextension of the neck, and abrupt head turning have all been implicated in the etiology of occlusion of a vertebral artery, which can lead to brain stem or spinal cord ischemia or infarction, although this is rare. In 1 case fitness exercises were the relevant preceding event.

Woman, 32, complained of discomfort in her neck with difficulty in turning her head to the right for 2 weeks. On day of admission she awoke with paresthesias and numbness in her left arm and leg and left side of her face. Her voice had changed and swallowing was difficult. She vomited and had a brief episode of vertigo. She could not walk, even with assistance, and her left arm was grossly incoordinate. Examination showed left-sided Horner's syndrome, reduced light touch and pinprick sensations on the left side of her face, weakness of the left palate, and a pyramidal syndrome in her left arm and leg. She had obvious left cerebellar dysmetria. She was not taking oral contraceptives and there had been no recent trauma. She was attending fitness classes that required maxillary turning the neck to either side and holding the head in the rotated position for 1–2 minutes. Left brachial angiography revealed a threadlike left vertebral artery, with a long segment of narrowing in the midcervical area, indicating dissection. Ischemic damage to the left lower medulla and upper segments of the cervical cord on the left was diagnosed. Anticoagulants and later antiaggregant agents were given. She made a slow and incomplete recovery, being left with diminished coordination on the left side and an altered voice. For 6 years she has continued to have markedly abnormal dysesthetic sensations throughout her left side.

In this case prolonged head turning to the right apparently damaged and perhaps predisposed to dissection of the left vertebral artery, causing ischemic damage to the left lateral medulla and left side of the upper cervical cord. Sustained rotation of the neck has no documented benefits but has potential harmful effects; thus it is doubtful whether this exercise should be recommended.

▶ A rare cause of stroke. Angiography research suggests that, even in normal persons, when the head is turned and kept maximally to one side, the vertebral artery can be compressed enough at the level of the first cervical vertebra to cause brain stem ischemia. Although in most case reports vertebral artery damage has been incurred from cervical manipulation, including chiropractic, other "sports medicine" causes have included yoga, bow hunting, and head-turning while driving an automobile or leading a parade. Another hidden cause of stroke in women is "conjugal disharmony," i.e., occlusion of the internal carotid artery from attempted strangulation by the husband (1).—E.R. Eichner, M.D.

Reference

1. Milligan N, Anderson M: *Br Med J* 282:421, 1980.

Spine Fracture in Winter Sports
Reid DC, Saboe L (Univ of Alberta, Edmonton)
Sports Med 7:393–399, June 1989   10–32

Although most winter sports involve high-speed activities, until recently the incidence of spine fractures has been low. However, the popularity of snowmobiling has added to the incidence, and there have been reports that cervical spine injuries are becoming more common in hockey players. The data on winter sports and recreationally acquired spine fractures were analyzed to document trends. In a 7-year review, there were 202 spine fractures resulting from recreational activity. Investigators tabulated demographic data, events leading to the injury, mechanism of injury, methods of treatment, and patient outcomes. Injured individuals were contacted and reexamined at 1 and 2 years.

Sports-related spine fractures accounted for 14% of all spine fractures, and sports injury was the fourth leading cause of spine fracture. It was the second most common cause of spine fracture resulting in paralysis. Snowmobiling, tobogganing, Alpine skiing, and ice hockey accounted for 24% of recreationally acquired fractures. Injuries incurred in tobogganning appear to be declining, whereas those associated with Alpine skiing, ice hockey, and snowmobiling are increasing. Men were 3 times as likely to be injured as women. In 44% of spine injuries, patients had associated major injury; 21% had multiple trauma. The most common associated injury was a long bone fracture, followed by chest trauma and head injury.

The principal factors contributing to the increase in snowmobiling injuries were use of alcohol, poor lighting, young age, and terrain inappropriate for the activity. Cervical fractures, most of which were compression injuries, received during ice hockey were often secondary to collision with the boards after being hit from behind.

Measures should be introduced to reduce the likelihood of sports-related injuries, especially during ice hockey, as 67% of those injuries were associated with permanent paralysis. Equipment, training methods, rules, and officiating standards should all be examined carefully to identify correctable problems.

▶ This paper brings out several interesting points. Although one would expect otherwise, there was an absence of spinal fractures resulting from ski jumping, which reflects the overall low injury incidence in this series. Snowmobile injuries are clearly identified as a significant problem, comprising 10% of the spine fractures incurred during sports and recreational activities. With regard to cervical injuries resulting from ice hockey, the observations in this study coincide with those of Tator and Edmonds (1). Specifically, "While the helmet protected the head from concussion, it had little effect in dispersing the axial load, leading to fracture and quadriplegia."—J.S. Torg, M.D.

Reference

1. Tator CH, Edmonds VE: *Physician Sports Med* 14:157, 1986.

Upper Extremity and Shoulder

A Biomechanical Evaluation of the Restraints to Posterior Shoulder Dislocation
Weber SC, Caspari RB (Univ of California, Davis; Sacramento Knee and Sports Medicine; Orthopedic Research of Virginia, Richmond)
Arthroscopy 5:115–121, 1989   10–33

The biomechanics of posterior shoulder dislocation were studied in 9 cadaver shoulders using a testing machine to generate force displacement. Each shoulder was examined arthroscopically and roentgenographically before force displacement data were collected. Posttest arthroscopy and open dissection followed.

Mild acromioclavicular arthritis was present in 3 shoulders. Displacement of the humerus to the diameter of the humeral head consistently led to instability, but force displacement curves showed no inflection point, which implies a continuum between subluxation and dislocation. A posterior Bankart lesion or posterior capsular lesion was invariable, but there was no anterior pathology. The rotator cuff was not damaged. Open dissection confirmed all arthroscopic findings.

The findings in this reproducible model of posterior instability suggest that such instability probably is a continuous process from subluxation to dislocation in which the posterior capsule and its attachments are progressively damaged.

Glenoid Labrum: Preliminary Work With Use of Radial-Sequence MR Imaging

Munk PL, Holt RG, Helms CA, Genant HK (Univ of California, San Francisco)
Radiology 173:751–753, December 1989   10–34

Although the glenoid labrum is only a minor contributor to glenohumeral joint stability, it is an important source of persistent symptoms when damaged. Most recent studies of the utility of MR shoulder imaging have assessed the rotator cuff and sought the shoulder impingement syndrome. Another method of visualizing the glenoid labrum of the shoulder joint was developed that involves a radial sequence using fast-imaging, gradient-recalled acquisition in steady-state (GRASS).

Three healthy men aged 30–42 years underwent imaging of 5 normal shoulders. Two patients, a 26-year-old man with symptoms of shoulder impingement syndrome but no suspicion of a glenoid labrum lesion, and a 36-year-old man with symptoms of recurrent anterior shoulder dislocation and surgical confirmation of an extensive glenoid labrum tear, each had 1 shoulder imaged.

The glenoid labrum was well visualized in all 7 shoulders examined by the GRASS technique. In normal shoulders it appeared as a discrete triangular structure. However, the radial-sequence images of the patient who was operated on showed extensive areas of increased signal intensity, suggesting a complex tear and loss of the normal triangular shape. Standard axial MR images confirmed the presence of an extensively torn glenoid labrum. At operation the anterior and anteroinferior portions of the labrum were seen to be detached and extensively macerated. The GRASS technique for imaging the glenoid labrum is still in its early stages of development, and its future role in the routine evaluation of the shoulder dysfunction cannot yet be predicted.

▶ As the authors state, this work is extremely preliminary. The study reports on 7 shoulders, 5 in 3 healthy asymptomatic patients, 1 in a symptomatic patient, and 1 in a recurrent shoulder dislocator. Surgical confirmation was available only for the patient with a history of dislocation in whom a labrum lesion was identified on MR and confirmed at surgery. The GRASS technique images the labrum in a radial sequence similar to the arthrographic method of evaluating knee menisci. A much larger series is necessary to evaluate this radial sequence method for accuracy and cost effectiveness.—J.S. Torg, M.D.

Rotator Cuff Tears: Diagnostic Performance of MR Imaging

Zlatkin MB, Iannotti JP, Roberts MC, Esterhai JL, Dalinka MK, Kressel HY, Schwartz JS, Lenkinski RE (Hosp of the Univ of Pennsylvania)
Radiology 172:223–229, July 1989   10–35

Recent studies have shown that MR imaging is a promising technique for evaluating disorders of the rotator cuff. The results of MR imaging and arthrographic study of the shoulder were compared in patients with suspected rotator cuff injuries who subsequently underwent shoulder surgery.

Thirty-two consecutive patients with a diagnosis of rotator cuff tendinopathy were evaluated before operation by orthopedic history, clinical examination, and MR imaging of the affected shoulder. All patients had positive impingement tests and conservative treatment had failed in all. Eight asymptomatic volunteers also had MR imaging. A scoring system was developed for the imaging studies. Twenty-four of the 32 patients underwent arthrographic study within a short interval after MR imaging. Results of arthrographic studies and MR imaging were reviewed without knowledge of surgical results.

For all rotator cuff tears MR imaging had a sensitivity of .91 and a specificity of .88, whereas arthrography had both a sensitivity and a specificity of .71. When the scoring system was used, the sensitivity of MR imaging improved to 1 and the specificity to .92. There was excellent correlation between preoperative assessment of the size of the rotator cuff tears and the actual measurement of the tears at surgery.

Magnetic resonance imaging had excellent sensitivity and specificity in detecting rotator cuff injuries. In this series MR imaging was superior to arthrography, and it provided useful information about the size and site of tears and the quality of torn tendon edges (Fig 10–3). When used in

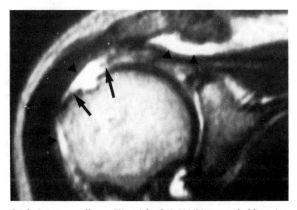

Fig 10–3.—Grade 3 rotator cuff tear; T2-weighted (2,500/80) coronal oblique image at level of acromioclavicular joint shows disruption of supraspinatus tendon as it is outlined by high-signal intensity fluid *(arrows)*. Large amount of fluid is seen in subacromial and subdeltoid bursae *(arrowheads)*. Increased signal intensity is seen in edges of proximal retracted tendon. (Courtesy of Zlatkin MB, Iannotti JP, Roberts MC, et al: *Radiology* 172:223–229, July 1989.)

conjunction with plain radiography and clinical evaluation, MR imaging should obviate the need for other invasive or noninvasive studies in most cases.

▶ As the authors clearly point out, "There were several limitations to this study . . . which must be considered in the interpretation of [the] findings." The patients were not fully representative of the spectrum of patients with suspected rotator cuff tears in whom MR imaging might be useful clinically. Rather, because surgery was needed to determine the true condition, the patients represented a group whose symptoms or disability were such that surgery was performed. Conversely, 14 of the 24 patients (58%) without cuff tears represented asymptomatic volunteers. Such subjects would not be included in a population with suspected rotator cuff tears in routine clinical practice. Although such spectrum bias is often unavoidable in the early stages of evaluated diagnostic tests, one should recognize the impact of this bias and the inflation of both test sensitivity and specificity. As noted, a selection bias also occurs among patients being considered for surgery to the extent that the results of available diagnostic information influence the decision as to whether or not to proceed to surgery. The impact of available diagnostic information is to reduce the specificity of the tests used to select surgical patients. Thus, although this study presents exciting results, the findings must be confirmed in a larger study of a broader range of patients."—J.S. Torg, M.D.

Rotator Cuff Tears: Prospective Comparison of MR Imaging With Arthrography, Sonography, and Surgery
Burk DL Jr, Karasick D, Kurtz AB, Mitchell DG, Rifkin MD, Miller CL, Levy DW, Fenlin JM, Bartolozzi AR (Thomas Jefferson Univ Hosp, Philadelphia)
AJR 153:87–92, July 1989   10–36

Arthrography is a highly accurate method of detecting rotator cuff tears. However, the procedure is invasive and relies on indirect visualization of the cuff. To assess the relative accuracy and role of MR imaging in the diagnostic evaluation of rotator cuff tears, the MR findings in 38 patients with suspected rotator cuff tears were compared prospectively in a blind fashion with the results of double-contrast arthrography in all 38 patients, high-resolution sonography in 23 patients, and surgery in 16.

Magnetic resonance imaging showed all 22 rotator cuff tears and 14 of 16 cuffs seen as intact on arthrography. In the 16 patients with surgically proved tears, both MR and arthrography correctly showed 11 of 12 cuff tears and 4 of 4 intact tears, for a sensitivity of 92% and specificity of 100% for both procedures. The 1 tear missed by both procedures measured less than 1 cm^2. In a subgroup of 23 patients sonography detected 9 of 15 tears and 7 of 8 intact cuffs as determined by arthrography. In the 10 surgically proved tears that included sonography in evaluation of the rotator cuff, the sensitivity was 63% for sonography, 88% for MR, and 88% for arthrography, and the specificities were 60%, 90%, and 90%, respectively.

Magnetic resonance imaging is as accurate as arthrography in the diagnosis of rotator cuff tears. Large rotator cuff tears can be detected reliably with MR, but small tears may be missed. Sonography is not as accurate as MR and arthrography in the diagnosis of rotator cuff tears. Magnetic resonance imaging should be the preferred noninvasive test for evaluation of rotator cuff disease.

▶ Arthrography, sonography, surgery, and MR are all operator-dependent techniques. The accuracy of these techniques is influenced by the interest and experience of the individual performing and interpreting the study. Magnetic resonance has potential for evaluating rotator cuff disease because the entire cuff can be seen. Tears on the bursal side of the cuff, which are not evident with arthrography, may be detected with sonography and MR. At present, it is too soon to say which study is best, and the diagnostic imaging modality requested by the referring surgeon should be dependent on the expertise and accuracy of interpretation available.—J.S. Torg, M.D.

Rotator Cuff Sonography: A Reassessment
Brandt TD, Cardone BW, Grant TH, Post M, Weiss CA (Michael Reese Hosp, Chicago)
Radiology 172:323–327, November 1989   10–37

Sonography has been suggested as an alternative to double-contrast arthrography for evaluating shoulder diseases, but lack of agreement on what constitute reliable sonographic signs hinders its acceptance. The usefulness of this method in detecting rotator cuff injury was studied in 62 patients undergoing sonography and double-contrast arthrography and 38 patients subjected to operation after sonography.

When 7 published criteria for defining rotator cuff injury were used, sonography as compared with arthrography had a sensitivity of 75% and a specificity of 43%. When the central echogenic band and echogenic foci in the rotator cuff were eliminated as criteria because of their unreliability, the sensitivity was 68% and the specificity was 90%. Assessment of sonography with the reduced number of criteria vs. surgery revealed a sensitivity of 57% and a specificity of 76%.

Focal discontinuity of the rotator cuff is considered a reliable sonographic sign, yet false positive results were encountered. Also, various anatomical features, (e.g., impingement of the acromion on the supraspinatus), can cause a false negative diagnosis.

Shoulder sonography has low sensitivity and is hindered by technical and methodologic difficulties. Sonographic examination cannot be recommended at this time for evaluating rotator cuff injuries.

▶ The accuracy of shoulder sonography depends on the examiner's experience and interest, and the equipment available. This report demonstrating that shoulder sonography is less reliable than reported elsewhere is as valid as the studies indicating higher accuracies. Referring physicians will have to determine from their own experience the accuracy of available studies. Early reports have shown that MR has the potential for demonstrating rotator cuff disease, and it is replacing sonography as a noninvasive method of evaluation—J.S. Torg, M.D.

Spontaneous Atraumatic Anterior Subluxation of the Sternoclavicular Joint

Rockwood CA Jr, Odor JM (Univ of Texas, San Antonio)
J Bone Joint Surg 71-A:1280–1288, October 1989   10–38

Little research has been done on atraumatic spontaneous anterior subluxation or dislocation of the sternoclavicular joint. Untreated spontaneous atraumatic anterior subluxation of the sternoclavicular joint may have a benign course.

Thirty-seven patients aged 10–36 years sustained spontaneous atraumatic anterior subluxation of the sternoclavicular joint. Twenty-nine patients were managed conservatively with observation and rehabilitation. Eight others had been treated initially at another center; in these patients operative reconstruction of the sternoclavicular joint or resection arthroplasty was attempted. On follow-up an average of 8 years later, the conservatively treated patients had excellent results with no limitations on activity. The patients treated surgically had several problems, including scars, persistent instability, pain, or limitation of activity resulting in a change in life-style.

Spontaneous atraumatic anterior subluxation of the sternoclavicular joint, a rare problem occurring mostly in teenagers and young adults with general ligamentous laxity, has a benign natural course and should not be treated surgically. Therapy should include education and reassurance.

▶ This is an excellent and important article that is required reading for all those who would attempt to operate on patients with spontaneous atraumatic anterior subluxation of the sternoclavicular joint.—J.S. Torg, M.D.

Clinical Presentation of Complete Tears of the Rotator Cuff

Norwood LA, Barrack R, Jacobson KE (Hughston Orthopaedic Clinic, Columbus)
J Bone Joint Surg 71-A:499–505, April 1989   10–39

The diagnosis of tears of the rotator cuff, one of the most serious pathologic conditions of the shoulder requiring surgery, is often missed or delayed. Some authors believe that acute trauma plays an important role in most tears of the rotator cuff, whereas others think a specific traumatic episode occurs in a few such patients. Some authors believe that a decreased active range of shoulder motion is correlated with the extent of tears of the rotator cuff. Radiographs may or may not be helpful.

To determine what factors in the patient's history, clinical features, physical examination, and radiographs are most useful in diagnosing the presence and extent of a complete tear of the rotator cuff of the shoulder, data on 103 patients were analyzed. An age-matched control group of 51 patients with similar symptoms but normal arthrograms was used for comparison.

Two groups of patients with tears of the rotator cuff were identified. Twenty-eight patients, or 27%, had a tear of a single tendon. The histories and physical and radiographic findings in these patients were consistent with a symptomatic local mechanical impingement process in the shoulder. Sixty (80%) of the 75 patients comprising the second group had a history of acute trauma. The latter patients were older and not athletic. Previously, they had not had symptoms severe enough to require treatment. These patients were found subsequently to have a complete tear of more than 1 tendon. Multiple radiographic findings in the shoulder and other coexisting orthopedic conditions were more common in the second group. In the second group, acute trauma in a shoulder that had chronic degenerative changes, rather than localized mechanical impingement, probably caused the tendons to rupture.

▶ This is an excellent paper. Rotator cuff tears have been classified as (1) small, less than 1 cm; (2) moderate, 1–3 cm; and (3) large, 3–5 cm. The authors point out that such grading by size alone is modified by the size of tendon, orientation of the tear, and size of the patient. Thus they propose a grading system based on the tendon(s) involved. By their classification, tears are categorized as (1) small and confined to the supraspinatus tendon; (2) moderate when involving 2 tendons and; or (3) large or massive when 3 to 4 tendons are involved. What is most appreciated is the fact that this classification can be applied clinically by use of an adequate history and physical without such high tech and expensive studies as pneumotomoarthrography, magnetic resonance imaging, or CT scan.—J.S. Torg, M.D.

The Management of Acute Acromioclavicular Dislocation: A Randomised Prospective Controlled Trial
Bannister GC, Wallace WA, Stableforth PG, Hutson MA (Bristol Royal Infirmary, Bristol; Queen's Med Ctr, Nottingham, England)
J Bone Joint Surg 71-B:848–850, November 1989   10–40

Conservative and operative managements of acute acromioclavicular dislocation were computed in a prospective study of 61 consecutive patients who were assigned to treatment in a broad arm sling or to reduction and fixation with a coracoclavicular screw. Surgery was performed under general anesthesia within 10 days of injury. The sling was worn for 2 weeks. Rehabilitation was similar in the 2 treatment groups.

A sling was used in the treatment of 33 patients, and 27 patients were operated on. Manual workers treated conservatively returned to work af ter 4 weeks on average, and those treated surgically returned to work in 11 weeks. Surgery also delayed clerical workers and prolonged the time to return to sports activities. After 1 year, 88% of conservatively treated patients and 77% of those operated on had good to excellent results. Half of the patients in each group had a perfect result at this time. After 4 years about 60% of both groups had a perfect outcome; 4 patients treatd with a sling eventually required surgery, and 2 surgically treated patients required reoperation for subluxation. The mean reduction of acromioclavicular separation was 12 mm with surgery and 8 mm with conservative management.

Closed treatment of acute acromioclavicular dislocation is preferable to early open reduction and screw fixation in most dislocations. Younger patients with marked displacement, however, are more likely to have an excellent outcome if the injury is stabilized at an early stage.

▶ The observations and conclusions of the authors are in keeping with my own clinical experience.—J.S. Torg, M.D.

Biomechanical Evaluation of Rotator Cuff Fixation Methods
France EP, Paulos LE, Harner CD, Straight CB (LDS Hosp, Salt Lake City)
Am J Sports Med 17:176–181, March–April 1989   10–41

The most common techniques for tendon reattachment to the humeral head include suturing the tendon into a bony trough through the cortical surface of the greater tuberosity. Initial fixation strength and failure mode for various rotator cuff reattachment methods—variations of the McLaughlin technique—were assessed (Fig 10–4).

Repair techniques included standard suture in the control group, reinforced suture with expanded polytetrafluoroethylene patch and polydiox

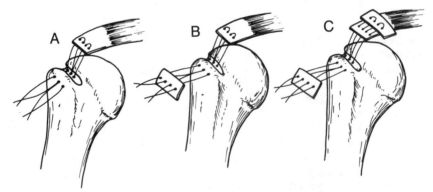

Fig 10–4.—Rotator cuff repairs: **A,** trough-in-bone rotator cuff repair; **B,** trough-in-bone repair with bone augmentation under suture; and **C,** trough-in-bone repair with bone and tendon augmentation under suture. (Courtesy of France EP, Paulos LE, Harner CD, et al: *Am J Sports Med* 17:176–181, March–April 1989.)

anone tape augmentation, and stapling with nonarthroscopic and arthroscopic soft tissue staples. The different repairs were done on fresh-frozen cadaver shoulder pairs. Repairs were tested to failure in pure tension; the shoulder was fixed at 60 degrees of abduction. Load and displacement results were normalized to controls, grouped according to failure modes, and analyzed.

The 2 basic failure modes were bone failure, or suture tearing through the bone, that indicated weak bone stock, and tendon failure, or suture tearing of the rotator cuff. Gross comparisons of intact and repaired tendons showed that the intact tendon was 2–3 times stronger than the repaired tendon. Based on mode of failure and lack of increased strength after the repair, the use of staples for cuff attachment was discouraged. Polydioxanone tape suture reinforcement did not raise fixation strength. Polytetrafluoroethylene patch suture augmentation, however, showed significantly higher initial failure loads than did the control and was of specific benefit in shoulders with weak bone stock.

There was no significant difference between the initial strength of staple repairs and suture repairs. In vivo testing of patch augmentation is needed to determine its effects on postoperative strength and tissue healing.

▶ The authors discourage the use of staples to repair rotator cuff lesions. With regard to those methods described that use synthetic substances and patch bone augmentation, the question arises regarding their use in vivo resulting in increased subacromial debris and the increased propensity for impingement symptoms.—J.S. Torg, M.D.

. **Arthroscopic Anatomy of the Shoulder**
Blachut PA, Day B (Univ of British Columbia, Vancouver)
Arthroscopy 5:1–10, 1989   10–42

Because many arthroscopists have problems becoming oriented in the glenohumeral joint, a systematic approach to examination of this articulation was developed using 20 cadaver shoulders. The arthroscopic anatomy of the shoulders was evaluated in the lateral decubitus position. Posterior and anterior portals were used. The joint was inflated with 30–50 cc of saline.

Technique.—The tendon of the long head of the biceps is useful for starting the examination. Elevating the arm laterally and viewing it superiorly allows assessment of the undersurface of the rotator cuff. If the scope is withdrawn slightly and the shoulder rotated externally and extended, the posterior humeral head and posterior synovial reflection are seen. Medially, the posterior labrum is observed at its attachment to the glenoid. Moving superiorly, the anteroinferior labrum is visualized. The anterior labrum is followed superiorly by viewing across the glenoid surface with the glenohumeral joint distracted. The glenohumeral ligaments are then examined sequentially. Changing from the posterior to the anterior portal, the labrum and posterior rotator cuff are viewed to complete evaluation of the shoulder.

▶ This is a beautifully illustrated presentation of the intra-articular anatomy of the glenohumeral joint.—J.S. Torg, M.D.

Rotator Cuff Tears: A Shoulder Arthroscopy Complication
Norwood LA, Fowler HL (Hughston Orthopaedic Clinic, Columbus, Ga)
Am J Sports Med 17:837–841, November–December 1989   10–43

The selection of portals for performing arthroscopic surgery on the shoulder has been well examined. The cephalic vein, brachial plexus, and long head of the biceps tendon pose anatomical limitations to anterior access. Because there appear to be no specific limitations on use of the posterior portal, that access is now most commonly used for insertion and orientation of the arthroscope. Four patients experienced iatrogenic rotator cuff tears, however, caused by insertion of the arthroscope into the glenohumeral joint via the posterior arthroscopic portal. This particular complication has not previously been reported.

All 4 patients were athletes aged 19–37 years who underwent arthroscopic resection of a torn anterior labrum. After operation the patients continued to have shoulder pain that interfered with their sport activities. Follow-up arthrographic examination performed 7 months to 2 years after arthroscopic surgery revealed incomplete rotator cuff tears in all 4 shoulders. Two shoulders actually had 2 separate rotator cuff tears each. It was assumed that these tears had occurred while the trocar was redirected after the initial arthroscopic examination. All 4 men required surgical repair and rehabilitation. After regaining shoulder motion and strength, 3 patients were able to return to normal preoperative athletic activities, but the fourth remained symptomatic despite normal motion, stability, and strength in the treated shoulder.

When a shoulder fails to improve after arthroscopic resection of a glenoid labrum tear and all common causes of failure have been ruled out, a partial or complete iatrogenic rotator cuff tear should be considered.

▶ The authors describe a previously unreported but important complication of shoulder arthroscopy. It is my belief that the sharp trocar is an instrument of the devil and has no place in arthroscopic procedures. When the dull trocar is used both to locate and penetrate the descended glenohumeral joint capsule, it follows the path of least resistance and enters the interval between the infraspinatus and teres minor tendons. We have not had a problem entering a well-distended glenohumeral joint with the blunt trocar, thus presumably avoiding the described complication.—J.S. Torg, M.D.

Arthroscopic Versus Nonoperative Treatment of Acute Shoulder Dislocations in Young Athletes

Wheeler JH, Ryan JB, Arciero RA, Molinari RN (United States Military Academy, West Point, NY)
Arthroscopy 5:213–217, 1989   10–44

Anterior shoulder dislocation is a common athletic injury. Because of the high rate of recurrent instability after dislocation in West Point cadets, conventional nonoperative management was compared with early arthroscopic treatment, by either staple capsulorrhaphy or anterior glenoid abrasion.

Of 38 cadets who were treated by immobilization, supervised physical therapy, and limited activity, 35 had recurrent instability. All recurrences developed within 14 months of initial injury. Arthroscopic treatment succeeded in 7 of 9 cadets who were followed for 14 months or longer. One of 6 patients having a staple repair and 1 of 3 others had recurrent instability.

Because recurrent instability is so frequent after nonoperative treatment of acute shoulder dislocations in young athletes, arthroscopic surgery is indicated. This approach can lower the recurrence rate significantly. If a Bankart type lesion is present, the glenoid labrum or glenohumeral ligaments may be reattached to the anterior glenoid with a suture, screw, or staple technique. In patients with acute shoulder dislocations it may suffice to abrade the anterior glenoid and débride the torn labrum or glenohumeral ligament attachments.

▶ This report presents a small series with relatively short follow-up in which 22% had recurrence of instability after arthroscopic management. Although I would agree that conservative management of acute anterior glenohumeral dislocation in the young athlete has an unacceptable dislocation rate, I would not agree that a 22% recurrent instability rate is acceptable in view of the 4% redislocation rate reported by Rowe for the Bankart procedure (1) and the 4% rate for the Bristow procedure that I reported (2).—J.S. Torg, M.D.

References

1. Rowe CR: *J Bone Joint Surg* 60-A:1, 1978.
2. Torg JS: *J Bone Joint Surg* 69-A:904, 1987.

The Prevention and Treatment of Injuries to the Shoulder in Swimming

Ciullo JV, Stevens GG (Sports Medicine Ctr of Metro Detroit)
Sports Med 7:182–204, March 1989   10–45

Swimming causes stress on the shoulder that can be aggravated by improper stretching or training techniques. There is evidence of an interrelationship among many shoulder structures that leads to the so-called swimmer's shoulder.

The average age at referral for complaints of shoulder pain associated with swimming is 18 years. More males report shoulder pain than females. Freestyle is the most common stroke used by patients reporting shoulder pain, but complaints are also reported with use of the butterfly and the backstroke.

The performance of repetitive overhead strokes places the rotator cuff and supraspinatus tendon at risk. Arthritis in the shoulder is focused primarily at the acromioclavicular joint. Degeneration may be caused by overuse, leverage of the scapuloclavicular mechanism, or motion associated with upward pressure at the undersurface of the acromion caused by subluxation or instability of the glenohumeral joint. Instability of the glenohumeral joint can be a major problem alone or in combination with rotator cuff tendinitis. Fragments of labral tissue mechanically wedged into the joint can lead to symptoms of subluxation. If the humeral head is wedged or slips out of joint as a result of capsular incompetency, secondary rotator cuff impingement may occur; this injury is especially difficult to manage. The patient can often pull his or her own arm down at the side, creating a "sulcus sign" at the lateral inferior acromion, substantiating the component of inferior subluxation; this test is definitive for multiaxial instability.

Prevention is the most important factor in managing swimmer's shoulder. Stretching and strengthening, and avoiding overuse, are the best preventive measures. In training, proper technique should be emphasized rather than performance time. If injury does occur, treatment consists of cutting training to half the previous level along with emphasis on stretching, strengthening, fundamentals, and the use of anti-inflammatory medication. As pain decreases, activity can be increased.

▶ We still see a number of swimmers who relate a history of improper stretching techniques in their youth swim programs (see the 1988 YEAR BOOK OF SPORTS MEDICINE, Abstracts 4–39 and 4–40, pp 242–244 for related articles on this subject). Improper stretching, especially at a young age, may lead to capsular incompetency. As in the treatment of all injuries, the authors stress the importance of prevention through proper stretching and strengthening techniques.—F.J. George, ATC, PT

Posterior Shoulder Instability: Approach to Rehabilitation
Engle RP, Canner GC (Ctr for Sports Physical Therapy, Berwyn, Pa; Berkshire Orthopaedic Associates, Wyomissing, Pa)
J Orthop Sports Phys Ther 10:488–494, June 1989   10–46

Posterior instability of the glenohumeral joint is a commonly occurring and recurring problem among athletes. Posterior dislocations are much less frequent than subluxation in this joint, but both conditions are difficult to treat and can result in significant dysfunction and limited levels of performance.

After posterior subluxation has been diagnosed, conservative management is usually best initially. Rehabilitation, particularly proprioceptive neuromuscular facilitation exercises, can help to stabilize the shoulder complex and decrease symptoms and keep the patient functioning. Ongoing examinations are needed for a successful outcome. Rehabilitation centers on the posterior rotator cuff. Glenoid labrum tears, partial rotator cuff tears, and chronic impingement syndromes may cause treatment failure and necessitate surgery.

Patients with posterior shoulder instability depend on the neuromuscular system for functional support and require proper rehabilitation. Many cases of shoulder instability are improperly diagnosed and as a result are improperly treated.

▶ The author describes a number of exercises for the scapula and shoulder rotator muscles, among them the traditional patterns of proprioceptive neuromuscular facilitation (PNF). There is progression from manual resistance to the use of pulleys to exercise these muscles. We have discontinued the use of pulleys and now use the multiaxial shoulder exerciser to perform PNF patterns and specific rotator cuff exercises.

In the 1988 YEAR BOOK OF SPORTS MEDICINE, Abstract 7–7, p 406, there is a description of the use of biofeedback to treat this problem.—F.J. George, ATC, PT

Comparison of Midazolam and Diazepam for the Reduction of Shoulder Dislocations and Colles' Fractures in Skiers on an Outpatient Basis
Sherry E, Henderson A, Cotton J (Prince of Wales Hosp, Randwick, NSW; Univ of New South Wales; Roche Products Pty Ltd, Dee Why, NSW)
Aust J Sci Med Sport 21:23–27, June 1989   10–47

To avoid hospitalization it is necessary to develop safe and effective treatments for non-life-threatening injuries such as shoulder dislocations and Colles' fractures, which are common in skiers. Treatment with midazolam and diazepam for sedation and muscle relaxation during reduction of these injuries was evaluated.

After initial examination and roentgenography 49 skiers with shoulder dislocations and 15 with Colles' fractures were randomized to receive either 2.5 mg of midazolam or 5 mg of diazepam intravenously along with equal parts of nitrous oxide and oxygen. Shoulder reduction was attempted by using the Hippocratic technique. Reduction of Colles' fractures was attempted by using longitudinal traction with the wrist in slight palmar flexion and ulnar deviation. After 2 unsuccessful attempts at reduction, patients received a second dose of the treatment drug. After 5 unsuccessful attempts, patients were hospitalized for reduction under general anesthesia.

The integrity of the axillary nerve and the palpability of the radial pulse were evaluated for all shoulder dislocations before reduction was attempted. The Trieger test of psychomotor performance was used to assess recovery.

The mean number of manipulations required was similar with either drug treatment. The success rate in the midazolam-treated shoulder group was 100% after an average of 1.4 attempted reductions. In the diazepam-treated shoulder group the success rate was 92% after 1.7 attempted reductions. In the shoulder groups, the probability of needing a second dose was similar regardless of the drug used. However, 43% of midazolam-treated patients with a Colles' fracture required a second dose, compared with none of the diazepam-treated group. The values for all vital signs decreased with time in both groups.

After the procedure scores on the Trieger test were lower on average than before the procedure or on discharge. Patients had similar recall of the treatments 24 hours later, but midazolam-treated patients in the shoulder group had less recall of the initial Trieger test than did those treated with diazepam.

Diazepam and midazolam in combination with nitrous oxide were similarly effective in providing muscle relaxation and sedation in patients who required reduction of a shoulder dislocation or a Colles' fracture. Midazolam provided a greater degree of retrograde amnesia, but a second dose was more likely to be required to reduce Colles' fractures when this drug was used.

▶ The ability of intravenous sedative supplements to facilitate the variety of surgical procedures performed on an outpatient basis deserves study, both with regard to the therapeutic efficacy as well as contribution toward cost-containment goals. We have used such agents successfully in the routine performance of surgical arthroscopy with local anesthesia (1). The question I would raise with regard to this study reported by Sherry et al. is why nitrous oxide was necessary!—J.S. Torg, M.D.

Reference

1. Yacobucci G, et al: *Arthroscopy.* In press.

Arthroscopic Stapling Repair for Shoulder Instability: A Retrospective Study of 50 Cases
Hawkins RB (John Fitch Orthopaedic Associates, Fitchburg, Mass)
Arthroscopy 5:122–128, 1989   10–48

The results of arthroscopic stapling of the detached glenoid labrum were reviewed in 50 shoulders of 47 patients with chronic shoulder dislocation or subluxation. No arthrotomies were performed. Repair begins with débridement of the joint. All procedures were performed under general anesthesia on an outpatient basis. Physical therapy was initiated 3 weeks after stapling; range of motion usually returned almost to normal within 6 weeks.

During an average follow-up of 39 months, 8 shoulders of 7 patients sustained additional trauma causing recurrent dislocation or subluxation.

These failures were ascribed to lack of immobilization of the shoulder for 3 weeks after surgery, either because of lack of instruction or inadequate patient compliance. Hardware complications were managed without difficulty and did not affect the outcome adversely.

Longer follow-up is needed to learn whether stapling is an effective permanent solution to this problem. It is important that the patient be willing to make initial adjustments and accept temporary changes in lifestyle. The affected arm should be immobilized in a sling for 3 weeks after the operation.

▶ The reported redislocation/resubluxation rate of 16% in this group is worrisome. It should be noted, however, that most of these apparently occurred early in the learning curve and before institution of 3 weeks of sling immobilization postoperatively. The authors have presented a candid study with good long-term follow-up. However, it would appear that the jury is still out regarding this procedure.—J.S. Torg, M.D.

An Approach to the Repair of Avulsion of the Glenohumeral Ligaments in the Management of Traumatic Anterior Glenohumeral Instability

Thomas SC, Matsen FA III (Univ of Washington)
J Bone Joint Surg 71-A:506–513, April 1989   10–49

Many patients with recurrent anterior glenohumeral instability have a history of specific trauma that initiated the unidirectional instability. The shoulders in these patients usually have a rupture of the glenohumeral ligament at the point of glenoid attachment, called a Bankart lesion. Several surgical procedures are available for stabilizing this type of lesion, but many complications have been reported with use of screws and staples around the glenohumeral joint. A new approach was developed for the surgical repair of recurrent traumatic anterior glenohumeral instability (Fig 10–5).

During a 9-year period, 49 men and 12 women (average age, 26 years) underwent surgery for recurrent traumatic anterior glenohumeral instability. Patients with atraumatic anterior instability or multidirectional instability were excluded. Operation involved direct repair of the structural defect of the capsular liagment using a drilling and suturing technique similar to that described by Rowe in 1978. Although the technique causes some minimal limitation of motion, it eliminates the need for any tendon or bone transfer, or the use of hardware. After an average follow-up of 5.5 years, 39 shoulders in 37 patients were available for evaluation.

Based on the Rowe rating scale, excellent results were obtained in 34 shoulders, good results in 4, and poor results in 1. Patients evaluated the results as excellent in 33 shoulders, good in 1, fair in 3, and poor in 2. Thus excellent or good results by the Rowe criteria were obtained in 97% and by the patients' own evaluations in 87%. One patient had a redislocation 4 years after operation while doing karate. No reoperations have been required. The average range of motion was 171 degrees of for-

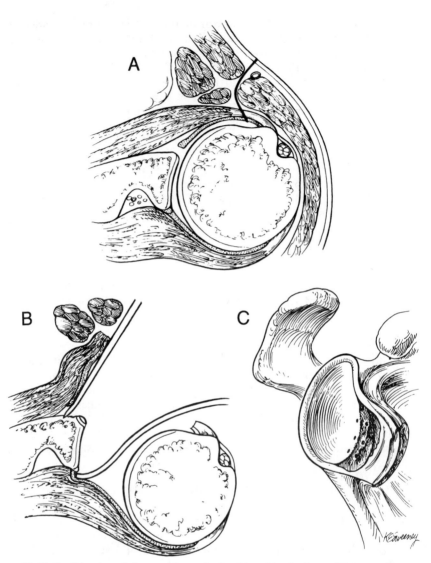

Fig 10–5.—Operative technique used for repair of avulsion of the glenohumeral ligaments. **A,** transverse plane section shows incision and plane for exposure. Note use of the deltopectoral interval. The subscapularis tendon and the underlying joint capsule are incised, as a unit, 1.0 cm medial to insertion. **B,** transverse plane section showing placement of retractors and location of drill holes. Note area roughened by the curet along the anterior part of the glenoid neck, and position of the drill hole relative to the anterior aspect of the glenoid rim. **C,** anteroinferior part of the glenoid rim with holes drilled. The nonarticular edge has been curetted and the holes placed 4.0 mm from glenoid rim to afford strong fixation. Note reflection of the capsule in the typical location of the Bankart lesion (3–6 o'clock).

(Continued.)

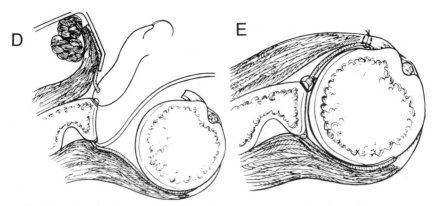

Fig 10–5 (cont.).—**D**, transverse plane section showing passage of no. 5 nonabsorbable suture through drill hole and into capsule. Note use of a deep right angle retractor of the subscapularis and superficial aspect of the capsule to afford the necessary exposure for proper placement of the suture. **E**, transverse plane section showing completed repair of the incision through the subscapularis and capsule. (Courtesy of Thomas SC, Matsen FA III: *J Bone Joint Surg* 71-A:506–513, April 1989.)

ward elevation, and 84 degrees of external rotation in abduction. Direct repair of an avulsed glenohumeral ligament as used in this group of patients leaves the healthy tissues intact, minimizes unnecessary dissection, and yields a high success rate.

▶ An interesting approach to the problem of anterior glenohumeral instability. Although the authors do not claim "originality" for the technique, this description apparently has not been previously published. Contrary to the observations of Blasier et al. (see Abstract 10–51), who point out that the Bankart repair does not precisely restore premorbid anatomy, it appears that the approach of Thomas and Matsen does reconstitute the anatomy.—J.S. Torg, M.D.

Comparative Functional Analysis of the Bristow, Magnuson-Stack, and Putti-Platt Procedures for Recurrent Dislocation of the Shoulder
Regan WD Jr, Webster-Bogaert S, Hawkins RJ, Fowler PJ (Univ Hosp, London, Ont.)
Am J Sports Med 17:42–48, January–February 1989   10–50

The resultant dynamic shoulder function after the Magnuson-Stack, Bristow, and Putti-Platt operative procedures for recurrent anterior dislocation was compared in a retrospective review of 27 patients, 9 in each surgical group. The subjective function, loss of motion, and shoulder strength after these procedures were analyzed. All patients were right-hand-dominant men who had dominant extremity surgery, and no postoperative dislocation or ongoing pain. The average follow-up was 6.75 years (range, 4.2–10.3 years). Nine right-hand-dominant normal men matched for age and recreational activity served as controls.

Overall, 60% of the patients returned to sports involving throwing. One patient each in the Magnuson-Stack and Bristow groups had full functional return to preinjury level. Whereas 3 patients each from both of these groups returned to unmodified throwing in sports activities, none of the Putti-Platt patients attained this level. The external rotation deficit of the operative side vs. the nonoperative side with the shoulder in 90 degrees of abduction favored the Magnuson-Stack over the Bristow procedure, but the difference was not significant. In contrast, the Putti-Platt procedure resulted in significantly greater deficit in external rotation compared with the other groups. With the shoulder in neutral position, patients having the Magnuson-Stack procedure had less external rotation deficit than those having the Bristow procedure, who in turn had less deficit than those having Putti-Platt procedure. The operative groups as a whole vs. controls demonstrated significant weakness of external rotation at shoulder neutral position and 90 degrees of abduction. No flexion weakness was found in the group having the Bristow procedure.

It appears that patients with weak shoulder musculature in the functional throwing position may compromise their ability and reinjure their shoulder. Significant deficits of external rotation strength with the shoulder in neutral position and in 90 degrees of abduction are apparent, particularly after a Putti-Platt procedure. This weakness should be addressed more aggressively in the postoperative rehabilitation of these patients.

▶ The authors report a 60% return to a throwing sport. However, there is no clear delineation of what the specific throwing activities were, or to which level of performance the participant returned. The observation made on the basis of isokinetic testing revealed the operative groups' dominant shoulder to be significantly weaker in external rotation both at neutral and 90 degrees of abduction. It is suggested that this problem can be overcome by addressing this weakness in postoperative rehabilitation more aggressively. We recently reported the results of 250 modified Bristow procedures (1), in which it was observed that in addition to limited external rotation at 90 degrees of abduction, a concomitant isokinetic test demonstrated weakness in both external and internal rotation at the crossover phase of the cocking act. We believe that this weakness both contributes to difficulty in pitching and is a function of the altered mechanics produced by the operative procedure rather than failure of postoperative rehabilitation.—J.S. Torg, M.D.

Reference

1. Torg JS, et al: *J Bone Joint Surg* 69-A:904, 1987.

The Bankart Repair Illustrated in Cross-Section: Some Anatomical Considerations
Blasier RB, Bruckner JD, Janda DH, Alexander AH (Univ of Michigan; Naval Hosp, Oakland, Calif)
Am J Sports Med 17:630–637, September–October 1989   10–51

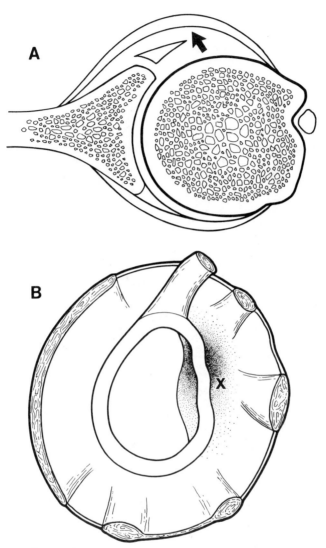

Fig 10–6.—**A,** diagram of cross-section of capsule and labrum separated from glenoid rim showing labrum pushed medially and dislocation occurring over the labrum and into the overly capacious capsule. **B,** diagram looking into the shoulder socket as if from the humeral head showing where the dislocation occurs over the injured labrum and into the capacious capsule. (Courtesy of Blasier RB, Bruckner JD, Janda DH, et al: *Am J Sports Med* 17:630–637, September–October 1989.)

The Bankart procedure for repairing chronic anterior shoulder instability addresses the lesions that cause it. The complex surgical anatomy can be illustrated by cross-sectional dissections and double-contrast CT. The so-called Bankart lesion comprises 5 main patterns: (1) the labrum and capsule are separated from the glenoid rim; (2) the capsule is detached from the scapular neck and the labrum is separated from the glenoid rim

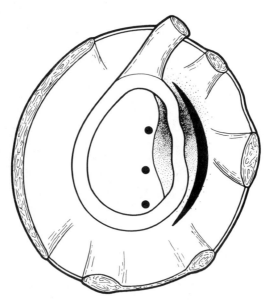

Fig 10–7.—Treating this view into the glenoid cavity as the face of a clock, the suture fixation holes are seen at 2, 4, and 6 o'clock. For patients in whom inferior instability is especially prominent, the inferior hole may be carried around posteriorly toward 7 o'clock. (Courtesy of Blasier RB, Bruckner JD, Janda DH, et al: *Am J Sports Med* 17:630–637, September–October 1989.)

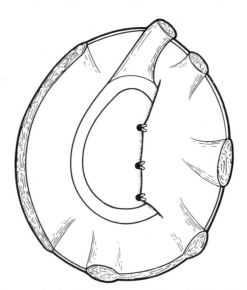

Fig 10–8.—Looking into the shoulder socket showing the medial edge of the lateral capsular flap being secured to the holes in the glenoid rim deep to and lateral to the cartilagenous labrum. The labrum is thus excluded from the anteroinferior aspect of the joint. This routine feature of the Bankart repair has not been emphasized in the past. (Courtesy of Blasier RB, Bruckner JD, Janda DH, et al: *Am J Sports Med* 17:630–637, September–October 1989.)

by being pushed medially so that the head of the humerus moves over it into the capsule (Fig 10–6); (3) the capsule is torn from the neck of the scapula and the labrum is stripped from the glenoid rim separately; (4) the anteroinferior part of the labrum is abraded away; (5) a rim fracture is united medial to the anatomical position.

Technique.—After the deltopectoral interval is opened and the cephalic vein taken medially or laterally, a plane is developed between the subscapular muscle and tendon and the capsule underneath by sharp and blunt dissection. The capsule is opened vertically parallel to and lateral to the rim of the glenoid cavity. Sutures are threaded through holes placed in the glenoid rim at the 2, 4, and 6 o'clock positions (Fig 10–7). Securing the medial edge of the lateral capsular flap to the roughened glenoid rim leaves the labrum in an extracapsular position (Fig 10–8). The lateral edge of the medial capsule is secured into the same suture line. The subscapular insertion is then repaired anatomically and the deltopectoral interval closed.

An essential feature of this procedure is its attachment of the fibrous capsule directly to bone. Also, the labrum is moved to an extra-articular position to protect the head of the humerus from anterior translation.

▶ This is a beautifully illustrated presentation of the authors' proposed patterns of the Bankart lesion. Combining CT scans, pathologic specimens, and line drawings has resulted in a clear, concise presentation. Also pointed out, contrary to popular belief, is that the Bankart repair does not precisely restore the premorbid anatomy. "The capsule is reattached to the bone rim of the anteroinferior glenoid deep to and lateral to the torn cartilagenous labrum, thus excluding the labrum from the joint anteriorly."—J.S. Torg, M.D.

Rotator Cuff Function in the Impingement Syndrome
Watson M (Guy's Hosp, London)
J Bone Joint Surg 71-B:361–366, May 1989   10–52

The rotator cuff stabilizes the glenohumeral joint while the deltoid elevates the arm. Patients with impingement syndrome have normal rotator cuff function. An attempt was made to observe intraoperatively the normal excursion of the rotator cuff in such patients during surgery.

Thirty-three patients aged 41–64 years underwent operation for impingement syndrome that had failed to respond to conservative treatment. All patients had normal shoulder mobility without weakness. The indication for operation was pain during arm elevation experienced as tenderness over the humeral head. None of the patients had gross glenohumeral disorders, and all had normal arthrographic findings. Radiographs were taken perpendicular to the scapular plane with the arm in the neutral position, in mid-elevation, and in full elevation. Palpable bony points on the scapula and humerus were used as landmarks for providing measurements from which the angular excursion of the glenohumeral joint was calculated.

Elevation of the arm is achieved with 2 distinct cuff movements: early glenohumeral abduction and continuous flexion and external rotation. The rotator cuff lengthens and twists as the arm is elevated. About 60 degrees of the abduction occurs during the first half of arm elevation. As elevation progresses, the range of free rotation at the glenohumeral joint decreases progressively. Comparison of operative and preoperative radiographs showed that the amounts of passive abduction, flexion, and external rotation during operation were similar to the active amounts.

▶ Perhaps the most valuable observation from the clinical standpoint is that, "Excision arthroplasty of the acromioclavicular joint and anterior acromioplasty is highly effective for impingement under the acromium, but only moderately effective where impingement is under the acromioclavicular joint."—J.S. Torg, M.D.

Shoulder Pain in the Overhand or Throwing Athlete: The Relationship of Anterior Instability and Rotator Cuff Impingement
Jobe FW, Kvitne RS (Kerlan-Jobe Orthopaedic Clinic, Inglewood, Calif)
Orthop Rev 18:963–975, September 1989   10–53

Repetitive high-velocity throwing motions can result in chronic microtrauma to the stabilizing mechanisms of the glenohumeral joint, which in turn can lead to anterior subluxation of the humeral head. Secondary impingement involving the rotator cuff and biceps tendon may occur and, eventually, the rotator cuff may tear.

At diagnosis, pain on late-cocking and acceleration in the throwing athlete are often clues to secondary impingement and rotator cuff tears. The clinician should identify localized areas of tenderness, crepitus, lost range of motion, muscle atrophy, bony deformity, or shoulder asymmetry. Muscular strength should be assessed by manually testing the muscles or using an isokinetic system. Impingement signs are usually obvious on physical examination, but subluxation signs may be subtle. The Apprehension Test and the Relocation Test are the most sensitive means of detecting occult anterior glenohumeral subluxation. When subluxation is suspected, examination under anesthesia and arthroscopy are helpful.

Results of examination should permit classification of throwing athletes into 1 of 4 groups: (1) patients with pure impingement and no instability, (2) patients with primary instability resulting from chronic labral microtrauma with secondary impingement, (3) patients with instability caused by hyperelasticity and subsequent impingement, and (4) patients with subluxation without impingement. Conservative treatment should be tried first. However, if the patient does not improve, surgery should be considered.

▶ This is a well-written paper in which the authors clearly delineate their concepts regarding the etiology of shoulder pain in the overhand-throwing athlete.

Also, anterior capsular labral reconstruction and a rehabilitation program are defined. Basically, the report relates the experience of the authors and is lacking in supporting data. However, the concepts expressed are sound, and the original paper is recommended for the interested reader.—J.S. Torg, M.D.

Rupture of the Pectoralis Major Muscle

Kretzler HH Jr, Richardson AB (Seattle)
Am J Sports Med 17:453–458, July–August 1989   10–54

Rupture of the pectoralis major muscle may occur with trauma or as a consequence of performing the bench press. Some authorities report full recovery of motion and strength without surgery, but most report full recovery only after repair. The anatomy of the insertion of the pectoralis major was studied. Cadaver dissections showed the insertion of the pec-

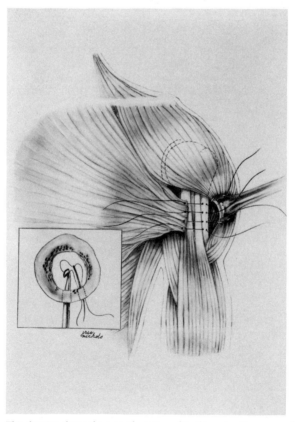

Fig 10–9.—This drawing shows the type of repair used in this series. Two rows of drill holes are made in the humerus just lateral to the biceps tendon. Sutures are passed down 1 hole and out the other, aided by the use of a crochet hook. (Courtesy of Kretzler HH Jr, Richardson AB: *Am J Sports Med* 17:453–458, July–August 1989.)

toralis major just lateral to the biciptial groove. The tendon was thin and appeared more like a coalescence of the anterior and posterior investing fascia than a true tendon.

Repaired ruptures in 16 patients and nonrepaired ruptures in 3 were evaluated. The principal cause of rupture in 19 patients was the bench press. In 11 patients the nondominant arm was injured. All patients complained of weakness, pain, and deformity. Those with acute tears had swelling and ecchymosis of the anterior axillary chest wall and upper arm. The technique and results of surgery were reviewed.

Technique.—At surgery the deltoid is retracted to reveal the site of insertion on the humerus. Two rows of drill holes are made in the humerus just lateral to the long head of the biceps tendon. Sutures are passed through these holes with the aid of a crochet hook (Fig 10–9) and then are passed through the free end of the muscle. The sutures are tied with the arm held in adduction and internal rotation to return the muscle to its original position (Fig 10–10).

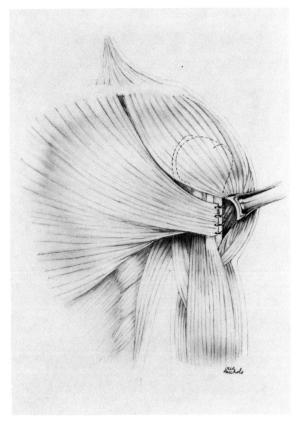

Fig 10–10.—Drawing of the completed repair. (Courtesy of Kretzler HH Jr, Richardson AB: *Am J Sports Med* 17:453–458, July–August 1989.)

All 16 patients had relief of pain and correction of deformity. One had slightly limited abduction, whereas 15 recovered full motion. Thirteen patients had return to full strength. Two patients who had late repair (5½ years after injury) did not return to full strength but had significant improvement.

Ruptures of the pectoralis major muscle occur under tension tear near the insertion on the humerus. Distal tears can be repaired even after a lapse in time. Most patients who undergo repair experience relief of pain, recovery of strength, correction of the deformity, and maintenance of range of motion.

▶ This paper not only supports the desirability of surgical repair of acute rupture of the pectoralis major muscle but also reports good results after late repair. Specifically, 5 of the patients were operated on between 4 and 12 months and 2 more than a year after injury. In view of the fact that most of the patients were injured while weight lifting, an interesting question not addressed in this paper is what effect, if any, anabolic steroids may have had in contributing to the problem.—J.S. Torg, M.D.

Upper Extremity Arterial Injury in Athletes
McCarthy WJ, Yao JST, Schafer MF, Nuber G, Flinn WR, Blackburn D, Suker JR (Northwestern Univ)
J Vasc Surg 9:317–327, February 1989   10–55

The rigorous repetitive shoulder motion required in certain athletic activities may lead to thoracic outlet syndrome and ischemia of the upper extremities in conditioned athletes. During a 5-year period 21 men and 2 women aged 18–47 years were evaluated for arm and hand complaints. Nine of the 12 men were professional baseball catchers. Seven of the 11 athletes with symptoms suggestive of compression of a subclavian or axillary artery were baseball pitchers.

Hand complaints included cold hypersensitivity, numbness, coolness, and blanching of the fingers. Chronic arm complaints included severe fatigue and heaviness in the throwing arm, severe finger ischemia from emboli, and coldness of the hand. Noninvasive testing included Doppler ultrasound, duplex scanning, and cold immersion. Arteriography in the 11 athletes with arm complaints confirmed compression of a subclavian, axillary, or posterior humeral circumflex artery and 2 subclavian aneurysms. Arteriography also confirmed a thrombosis in the ulnar artery in a first baseman and occlusion of the palmar arch in a frisbee player. Both patients required hospitalization, during which they were treated with infusions of a vasodilator followed by infusions of heparin and dextran for 2–4 days. Both returned to competitive athletics. The other patients with hand ischemia were managed without operation.

Two patients with subclavian artery aneurysms were treated with saphenous vein bypass and cervical rib resection. Eight athletes with muscular compression of an artery underwent standard surgical decompression of the thoracic outlet with resection of the anterior scalene or pectoralis minor muscle. A pitcher with distal embolization and circumflex humeral branch thrombus did not have an operation. All athletes were able to continue their professional or recreational activities.

Repetitive blunt hand trauma or violent shoulder motion may compromise the arterial system of an upper extremity in athletes. Early noninvasive arterial examination can prevent the sequelae of arterial thrombosis.

▶ This is a timely and comprehensive clinical compilation and review of the presentations, diagnosis, and treatment of sports-related causes of the thoracic outlet syndrome, as well as other arterial causes of hand ischemia in athletes. The outlines of both conservative and operative management are followed by a useful discussion and perspective by experts.—E.R. Eichner, M.D.

Tenodesis of the Long Head of the Biceps Brachii for Chronic Bicipital Tendinitis: Long-Term Results
Becker DA, Cofield RH (Mayo Clinic and Found, Rochester, Minn)
J Bone Joint Surg 71-A:376–381, March 1989   10–56

Surgical tenodesis of the long head of the biceps has been a recommended treatment for chronic bicipital tendinitis for about 50 years. Reports based on short-term results were favorable. To evaluate the long-term effectiveness of this procedure, data on 51 patients (54 shoulders) followed for an average of 13 years were reviewed. Only 50% had a long-lasting satisfactory outcome.

Thirty patients were men, and the median age at the time of surgery was 51 years. In 19 patients shoulder symptoms were traced to a notable injury. Most of the patients had reported severe pain for an average duration of 2.6 years. Various conservative measures brought only short-term relief. Preoperative radiographs of 43 shoulders were normal.

One of 3 techniques was used to accomplish a tenodesis (Fig 10–11). Intraoperative findings were recorded for 38 shoulders. The biceps ten

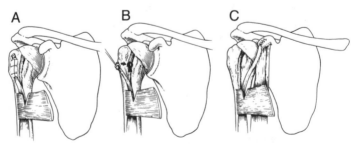

Fig 10–11.—Surgical techniques for fixation of the tendon. **A,** tenodesis of Hitchcock and Bechtol, performed in 30 shoulders (56%); **B,** tenodesis of Froimson and Oh, performed in 14 shoulders (26%); and **C,** tenodesis of DePalma and Callery, performed in 10 shoulders (19%). (Courtesy of Becker DA, Cofield RH: *J Bone Joint Surg* 71-A:376–381, March 1989.)

don was described as grossly abnormal in 32 shoulders, inflamed in 15, with adhesions in 12, and degenerated in 5. Complications occurred in 6 patients, and 29 required additional treatment, (e.g., injections or a later operation).

At early follow-up (averaging 6 months), all but 3 patients reported no or only slight pain. But at the latest follow-up, 16 shoulders were moderately painful and 10 continued to be severely painful. Physical findings, however, were normal or nearly normal. Active abduction of the shoulder measured more than 150 degrees in all but 1 patient.

Tenodesis of the long head of the biceps achieved a satisfactory result in only 28 of the 54 shoulders in this series. Thus the procedure is not recommended as the primary component in surgical treatment of chronic bicipital tendinitis.

▶ This paper vividly demonstrates the necessity for adequate long-term follow-up to evaluate any given procedure. In this instance in which tenodesis of the long head of the biceps was performed for chronic bicipital tendinitis, there were uniformly good results at 6 months post surgery. However, a repeat examination at an average of 7 years (range, 1–22 years) post surgery revealed a satisfactory result in only 50% of the group. Also, to be noted is the 12% rate of significant complications, which included 2 patients with reflex sympathetic dystrophy and 4 with postoperative stiffness requiring manipulation under anesthesia. The authors conclude that tenodesis of the long head of the triceps tendon is not an effective treatment for tendinitis over the long term.—J.S. Torg, M.D.

Acute Brachial Neuropathy in Athletes
Hershman EB, Wilbourn AJ, Bergfeld JA (Cleveland Clinic Found)
Am J Sports Med 17:655–659, September–October 1989   10–57

In the sports literature, acute brachial neuropathy has been overlooked as a cause of shoulder pain and weakness. However, it is important to distinguish this entity from other sports-related shoulder conditions.

Five athletes complained of shoulder soreness and/or weakness. A complete neurologic history was taken and physical examination performed. Physicians made nerve conduction studies on both upper extremities and performed needle electrode examinations of the involved limbs, ipsilateral cervical paraspinal muscles, and contralateral muscles for comparison. Electrodiagnostic studies were also done at follow-up.

Onset of acute brachial neuropathy occurred in both noncontact and contact sports. All symptoms developed acutely or subacutely during or after sporting activity, but patients could not relate the onset to any specific trauma. Pain continued after cessation of activity, and patients soon became weak. The dominant arm was involved in all 5 patients. Both electromyographic (EMG) studies and physical examination revealed a variety of findings. Various combinations of nerve fibers were involved.

The athletes refrained from sports participation for 1 week to 9 months. After resolution of symptoms, all 5 patients were enrolled in a rehabilitation program. Initial scapula winging persisted in 3 patients. Four patients had residual weakness, but the deficit was pronounced in only 1. At follow-up EMG disclosed abnormalities in 3 of the 5 athletes.

Nerve conduction studies and EMG can often confirm suspected acute brachial neuropathy. Rest is the initial treatment, followed by rehabilitation. Weakness may persist in the affected muscles.

Isolated Infraspinatus Atrophy: A Common Cause of Posterior Shoulder Pain and Weakness in Throwing Athletes?

Bryan WJ, Wild JJ Jr (Houston; Tucson)
Am J Sports Med 17:130–131, January–February, 1989   10–58

Disabling posterior shoulder pain may develop in the athlete whose sport involves throwing. It may be that isolated infraspinatus muscle atrophy is responsible for shoulder pain and weakness.

Man, 24, professional baseball outfielder, experienced sudden pain in his posterior right throwing shoulder after a long hard throw from center field. The pain abated over several days but returned with repetitive long hard throws in ensuing weeks. Clinical examination revealed pain and decreased muscle bulk on palpation of the right infraspinatus muscle. The patient also had pain and weakness on resistance to external shoulder rotation. The patient was advised to avoid throwing for 1 month, after which he began as gradual return to play and a concomitant low-weight, high-repetition, rotator cuff strengthening program. This regimen was only marginally successful. Complete evaluation showed frank absence of the right infraspinatus mass and gross infraspinatus weakness. The ipsilateral supraspinatus was intact. Plain radiographs were normal, but electromyographic nerve conduction studies indicated complete denervation of the right infraspina-

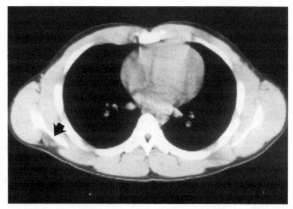

Fig 10–12.—Computed axial tomographic scan of both shoulders 6 months after acute onset of posterior right shoulder pain. Note complete loss of infraspinatus mass when compared with opposite normal side. (Courtesy of Bryan WJ, Wild JJ Jr: *Am J Sports Med* 17:130–131, January–February 1989.)

tus muscle. A CT scan showed almost complete replacement of the infraspinatus muscle with fatty tissue (Fig 10–12). The patient began a rigorous posterior shoulder strengthening program to build teres minor strength. During the ensuing 3 baseball seasons, the athlete has thrown without shoulder pain, instability, or weakness.

This condition seems to have been caused by a single traumatic incident that irreversibly denervated the infraspinatus muscle. Rotator cuff muscle strengthening programs may prevent such incidents. In this case, rotator cuff muscle strengthening allowed the athlete to resume his career.

▶ Hershman et al. (Abstract 10–57) clearly differentiate acute brachial neuropathy from the more commonly shoulder disorders seen in athletes, including impingement syndrome, rotator cuff tear, glenoid humeral instability, tendinitis, nerve entrapment syndrome, and "burner syndrome," as well as a variety of acute fractures. They fail, however, to answer the one important question: what is the etiology of the problem? Nor is the exact site of the lesions in acute brachial neuropathy determined. The fact that there is involvement of muscles not innervated via the brachial plexus, as well as the observation of severe denervation limited to muscles innervated by a single peripheral nerve, have led many investigators to consider acute brachial neuropathy a multiple axon loss mononeuropathy, not a brachial plexopathy.

The phenomenon appears to be characterized by severe pain that continues despite rest, associated with a day or so required for complete recovery of motor function. In view of this, the case reported by Bryan and Wild (Abstract 10–58) appears to fit the pattern.—J.S. Torg, M.D.

Osteochondritis in the Female Gymnast's Elbow

Jackson DW, Silvino N, Reiman P (Southern California Ctr for Sports Medicine, Long Beach; Northeast Ohio Sports Medicine Inst, Akron)
Arthroscopy 5:129–136, 1989   10–59

Data were reviewed concerning 7 high-performance female gymnasts with osteochondritis dissecans of the humeral capitellum. Ten extremities were affected in the 7 patients, whose average age was 13 years. In most of them activity was restricted for several months before surgery was performed. Eleven operations were necessary, including arthroscopy and/or arthrotomy with antegrade drilling of a cyst or curettage of a defect in the capitellar articular surface. Loose bodies were removed when present.

No postoperative complications developed. On follow-up for 3 years on average, all patients reported aching in the elbow, and all 4 with unilateral involvement had some limitation of both flexion and extension compared with the uninvolved limb. Tenderness of the radiocapitellar joint was persistent in 2 patients, and 4 had palpable crepitus. Only 1 patient still trains actively and competes in gymnastics.

Early detection is the key to treating osteochondritis of the elbow in young female gymnasts. Arthroscopy is of value in symptomatic patients, but once disease becomes symptomatic, the clinical results have been guarded.

▶ The findings in this report dealing with osteochondritis dissecans of the humeral capitellum in female gymnasts closely parallels the report of Brown et al. (1) dealing with osteochondritis of the capitellum in Little League pitchers. Of 18 pitchers who underwent elbow arthrotomy for loose bodies, only 1 was able to return to "repetitive hard throwing without symptoms." Brown et al. also stated that, "Our series does not reflect the possibility of healing of these lesions if they are diagnosed early and the inciting activity is discontinued." Jackson et al. point out that, once radiographs are positive and conservative management fails, a return to competitive gymnastics is unlikely. Although I would agree with their conclusion that measures are needed to prevent the lesion and its sequelae, the suggestion that with early detection conservative treatment is indicated is not consistent with the data on either Brown et al. or my own personal experience. Perhaps a more effective approach would be early detection and early surgical retrograde drilling of the lesion.—J.S. Torg, M.D.

Reference

1. Brown R, et al: *J Sports Med* 2:27, 1974.

Decompression of the Posterior Interosseous Nerve for Tennis Elbow
Jalovaara P, Lindholm RV (Univ of Oulu, Finland)
Arch Orthop Trauma Surg 108:243–245, 1989   10–60

Pain involving the lateral elbow may stem from a variety of causes. Usually, tennis elbow can be relieved with conservative treatment; in about 10% of patients, however, surgery is required.

Entrapment of the posterior interosseous nerve (PIN) was presumed to be the predominant cause of tennis elbow in 107 patients who underwent PIN decompression. Most were manual workers whose jobs required repetitive tasks using the arms. They experienced local tenderness, pain at rest, and pain during exertion. None had improved with conservative treatment or previous operations.

During surgery, all sites of compression along the PIN were identified and released. Procedures were repeated in 6 patients. The overall rate of improvement, including all reoperations, was 89%. Primary decompression resulted in complete healing in 30% of patients.

Previous studies have reported various rates of success when surgery is directed at entrapment of the PIN. Reported excellent results ranged from 47% to 71%. The role of PIN in tennis elbow is not fully understood, and decompression may prove effective for other causes of this condition.

▶ In a review of the literature the authors found that 3 different surgical procedures—(1) decompression of posterior interosseous nerve, (2) lengthening of the extensor carpi radialis breves tendon, and (3) lateral release—provided equally effective results for resistant tennis elbow. Their explanation is that the etiology is "multifactorial," and that these various procedures address pain arising from posterior interosseous nerve entrapment or being epicondyle in origin. They also conclude that the remaining question is to how to differentiate this problem from others that contribute to tennis elbow symptoms preoperatively.

Peripheral Nerve Entrapments of the Forearm
Herring SA (Puget Sound Sports Medicine Physicians Inc, Seattle)
Sports Training Med Rehab 1:135–139, 1989   10–61

Athletes may incur a variety of injuries to the elbow and other forearm structures. Throwing, racquet sports, and weight lifting may place the athlete at particular risk for such injuries. The ulnar nerve can be injured by traction, or the nerve may be trapped in abnormal tissue around the elbow or under a thickened arcuate ligament. Symptoms include intermittent paresthesias in the fourth and fifth digits, aggravated by elbow flexion; early true sensory loss may occur in the dorsoulnar aspect of the hand. Forearm numbness is rare, but a feeling of clumsiness is common.

The posterior interosseous nerve is subject to entrapment neuropathies, usually at the proximal aspect of the supinator under the rigid arcade of Frohse or through the midsubstance or distal end of the supinator muscle. Muscular hypertrophy in weight lifters and other upper-extremity athletes has been associated with entrapment of this nerve. Symptoms include deep, aching, forearm pain that proceeds to weakness. Patients with resistant "tennis elbow" should be evaluated for possible of entrapment of the adjacent posterior interosseous nerve.

The pronator syndromes, ligament of Struthers, and lacertus fibrosis are frequently involved in median nerve entrapment in the forearm, as are the pronator teres muscle and the fibrous arch within the pronator region. It is important to differentiate median nerve entrapment from other syndromes such as carpal tunnel syndrome. The musculocutaneous nerve is subject to entrapment between the biceps tendon and the brachialis fascia, especially with hyperextension of the elbow associated with pronation. Symptoms include a dysesthetic sensation in the distribution of the lateral cutaneous nerve of the forearm.

Repetitive motion and secondary muscular hypertrophy during upper-extremity sports participation can cause entrapment of the ulnar nerve, radial nerve, median nerve, or musculocutaneous nerve tissue. Peripheral nerve entrapment or injury should be considered in the differential diagnosis when patients have sensory or motor changes or chronic aching pain in the forearm.

▶ The author's description of the variety of nerve entrapment possibilities in the forearm is not accompanied by relevant clinical data. As a result, suggested treatment alternatives are also lacking.—J.S. Torg, M.D.

Wrist Pain Syndrome in the Gymnast: Pathogenetic, Diagnostic, and Therapeutic Considerations

Mandelbaum BR, Bartolozzi AR, Davis CA, Teurlings L, Bragonier B (Univ of California, Los Angeles)
Am J Sports Med 17:305–317, May–June 1989   10–62

Wrist pain in the gymnast is often a difficult diagnostic and therapeutic challenge. To define and characterize the factors that contribute to such pain and to develop a protocol for evaluation and treatment, 38 collegiate gymnasts had radiographic and magnetic resonance imaging (MRI) studies on 1 or both wrists.

Group I consisted of 11 male and 9 female members of a championship collegiate gymnastics team; the group included 5 individual men's champions. Group II included 18 randomly selected male gymnasts competing in a national competition; none was a top finisher. Both groups also completed a questionnaire to characterize the nature of the wrist problem. Wrist arthroscopy was performed in selected subjects. Cadaver wrists were studied histologically and the findings were compared with those at MRI.

Overall, 75% of the male and 33% of the female gymnasts had wrist pain for at least 4 months. All gymnasts complained of pain during compression and impaction but not during distraction. Male members of group I had significantly greater ulnar variance than male members of group II. Female members of group I had a significantly greater ulnar variance than controls. Among male gymnasts the pommel horse routine was consistently responsible for wrist pain.

Magnetic resonance imaging differentiated the complex transitions between cortical and trabecular bone, ligaments, articular surfaces, and the triangular fibrocartilage complex of the wrist. From the findings a therapeutic algorithm was developed to assist in the evaluation and management of wrist pain in gymnasts. Arthroscopic surgery of the wrist was successful, and arthroscopic findings correlated well with those of MRI and arthrography.

Wrist pain in the competitive gymnast results from repetitive compressive impact of significant duration, frequency, and intensity. Certain routines (e g, pommel horse exercise) may have a cumulative negative effect on normal growth. Further studies of younger gymnasts may delineate when and how these changes in normal growth may occur.

▶ This is a beautifully illustrated presentation that includes graphics, illustrations of anatomical specimens, MRI appearances, and histologic sections, as well as line drawings, arthroscopic photographs, and roentgenograms. To be noted, the authors were the recipients of the American Orthopaedic Society for Sports Medicine 1987 Young Investigator Award.—J.S. Torg, M.D.

Wrist Pain and Distal Growth Plate Closure of the Radius in Gymnasts

Albanese SA, Palmer AK, Kerr DR, Carpenter CW, Lisi D, Levinsohn EM (State Univ of New York, Syracuse and Binghamton)
J Pediatr Orthop 9:23–28, Janauary–February 1989   10–63

The skeletal system appears to respond to the stresses of intense athletic training by adaptive structural changes. However, the occurrence of stress fractures related to athletic activities suggests that the skeletal system's ability to respond to chronic stress is limited. Furthermore, intense athletic training in children may damage the growth plates in these skeletally immature individuals.

Three girls aged 12–14 years complained of wrist pain. All 3 had been active participants in competitive gymnastics before the pain developed, but none had experienced acute gymnastic injuries. Radiographic findings were suggestive of premature growth plate closure, which had resulted in shortening of the radius and alterations in the normal distal radioulnar articulation. One patient underwent successful ulnar-shortening osteotomy and plate fixation. At follow-up she was asymptomatic with a full range of motion and was able to return to competitive gymnastics. The other 2 patients did not follow suggestions of activity modification and eventually had to leave the sport.

Chronic overuse in skeletally immature children can cause wrist pain associated with premature fusion of the distal radial growth plate. A growth plate's structure and function may be altered by repetitive subfracture loading. To maintain the normal anatomical relationship between the distal portions of the radius and ulna, both bones need to grow at the same rate during a given time period. Closure of the distal ulnar growth plate should precede that of the distal radial growth plate. A reversal in the sequence of the closure of the growth plates probably contributed to alteration of the ulnar variance.

▶ The findings reported in this paper, distal growth plate closure of the radius, form an interesting contrast with the reports of Carter et al. (1) and Yong-Hing et al. (2), who both noted widening of the radial growth plate with regularity of the metaphaseal margin in adolescent gymnasts.—J.S. Torg, M.D.

References

1. Carter SR, et al: *Br J Radiol* 61:109, 1988.
2. Yong-Hing K, et al: *J Bone Joint Surg* A-70:1087, 1988.

Fracture of the Hook of the Hamate

Stark HH, Chao E-K, Zemel NP, Rickard TA, Ashworth CR (Orthopaedic Hosp; California Hosp Med Ctr; Hosp of the Good Samaritan, Los Angeles)
J Bone Joint Surg 71-A:1202–1207, September 1989   10–64

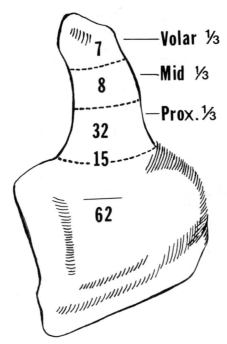

Fig 10–13.—Locations of 62 fractures of the hook of the hamate. (Courtesy of Stark HH, Chao E-K, Zemel NP, et al: *J Bone Joint Surg* 71-A:1202–1207, September 1989.)

Sixty-two patients aged 11–67 years were treated for an isolated fracture of the hook of the hamate. Forty-five were younger than age 40 years. Fifty-nine patients were males. All had pain on the ulnar side of the wrist or over the hook of the hamate in the proximal part of the palm. Pain was intense on grasping and swinging an implement with the injured hand. Grip strength, however, averaged only 20% less than that of the uninjured hand.

Fifty-four patients were injured during athletic activity; in all but 4 the fracture occurred while the patient swung a baseball bat, golf club, or tennis racquet. Three patients fell on the outstretched hand, and 1 struck the wrist on a basketball hoop. Twenty-eight of the 54 were professional athletes. Among the nonathletes, 2 had work-related crush injuries, 4 struck the palm on fixed objects, and 2 fell on the hand.

In most cases the fracture was diagnosed conclusively on a carpal tunnel roentgenogram or on an oblique roentgenogram of the supinated wrist, or both. In some cases CT scans were required. Fifteen fractures were through the base of the hamulus (Fig 10–13) 20 fractures were displaced.

Three of 10 fractures diagnosed within 2 weeks of injury and therefore considered to be acute were treated with short casts. All failed to heal and required removal of the fracture fragment. Three patients refused surgery. The others were treated initially by removal of the fragment and segmental tendon grafting. There were no surgical complications, and all but 2 patients, who had crush injuries, returned to regular sporting and work activities. Computed axial tomography is now considered the best imaging method for demonstrating an isolated fracture of the hook of the hamate. Surgical excision of the fragment should provide a satisfactory outcome.

Fractures of the Hook of the Hamate
Gupta A, Risitano G, Crawford R, Burke F (Derbyshire Royal Infirmary, Derby, England)
Injury 20:284–286, September 1989   10–65

Fracture of the hook of the hamate were diagnosed and treated between 1982 and 1988 in 3 patients. Two patients sustained injuries while playing squash and 1 was injured while playing golf. All injuries were diagnosed some months after they were incurred.

Fracture of the hook of the hamate was diagnosed conclusively by oblique radiographs in each case. After excision of the fragments all 3 patients were able to resume normal activities without further symptoms.

Because the hook of the hamate is a fairly deep structure, well covered on the volar aspect by the palmaris brevis, the transverse carpal ligament, fibrofatty tissue, subcutaneous tissue, and thick skin, it seems unlikely that direct pressure of a racquet or golf club would cause the hook to fracture. It may be that a sudden application of force through the tendon of the flexor digitorum profundus causes it to break. The same mechanism may be responsible for the nonunion that follows.

Fracture of the hook of the hamate may be more common than reported. Oblique radiographic views are recommended for the definitive diagnosis. Excision of the hook provides the most reliable treatment.

▶ The 2 articles reviewed in Abstracts 10–64 and 10–65 clearly delineate the diagnostic parameters for this particular lesion. Of note, Stark et al. report that the interval between injury and correct diagnosis in their series averaged 5.8 months, thus indicating the necessity of a high index of suspicion for the lesion. Also, Stark's group noted that, "When the fracture had occurred at or near the base of the hamulus, both pain and tenderness often were most pronounced on the dorsal ulnar aspect of the wrist."—J.S. Torg, M.D.

Metacarpo-Phalangeal Thumb Sprains: Based on Experience With More Than 1000 Cases
Moutet F, Guinard D, Lebrun C, Bello-Champel P, Massart P (Hôp A Michallon CHU, Grenoble; Hôp Sud CHU de Grenoble, Echirolles, France)
Ann Chir Main 8:99–109, October 1989   10–66

Since 1980 more than 1,000 patients have been treated at Grenoble for sports-related injuries of the metacarpophalangeal (MCP) joint of the thumb. Data on the first 1,000 case histories were reviewed.

The study population comprised 596 males and 404 females aged 6–83 years, but 62% were younger than 30 years of age. Skiing mishaps accounted for 75.4% of the thumb injuries, 19% of injuries were incurred while playing ball, 4.1% during practicing martial arts, 1% while mountain climbing, and 5% from other causes. Most (86%) of the patients had ulnar collateral ligament (UCL) injuries; the others had radial collateral ligament injuries. Snow quality rather than ski pole straps was directly responsible for most of the injuries.

All thumbs were assessed by physical and radiographic examination; arthrography was not used. Thirty percent of the patients had only mild MCP ligament sprains that were treated with active mobilization for 21 days, with or without protective taping. Moderately severe MCP sprains, diagnosed in 39% of the patients, were treated by rigid immobilization for 4 weeks. Thirty-one percent were severe injuries and required operation. Limpness felt toward the end of the range of motion was always an indication of severe injury. A hematoma on the dorsal side of the interphalangeal thumb was a sign of total UCL rupture. Displaced proximal bone fragments and torn or ruptured ligaments were always operated on, as these injuries never heal spontaneously (Fig 10–14).

All operations were done under local or regional anesthesia. Large displaced bone fragments, accounting for 23% of the treated injuries, were repaired with microscrews or K wire. Uncomplicated ligament injuries comprised the other 77%. Mid-ligament ruptures (20%) were repaired by suturing. Small bone fragments (28%) were always removed. Torn ligaments (29%) were reinserted with either a transosseous or a subperiosteal suture. Nonhealing conservatively treated lesions or postoperative instability were treated with secondary ligamentoplasty. Arthrodesis was not used because of the patients' young age. Ligamentoplasties were done with either woven Dacron or polytetrafluoroethylene suture, using either the Verdan-Simonetta (Fig 10–15) or the Littler procedure, always followed by physiotherapy for at least 15 days. Forty-nine patients (5%) un-

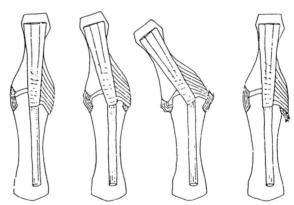

Fig 10–14.—Stener lesion. (Courtesy of Moutet F, Guinard D, Lebrun C: *Ann Chir Main* 8:99–109, October 1989.)

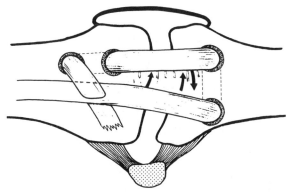

Fig 10–15.—Verdan-Simonetta assembly permits reconstructing a lateral triangular ligament, the proximal end of which should be located slightly above the center of the metacarpal head so that the ligament can be recreated as physiologically as possible. (Courtesy of Moutet F, Guinard D, Lebrun C: *Ann Chir Main* 8:99–109, October 1989.)

derwent secondary ligamentoplasties. The overall outcome was rated good or very good in 90% of the patients.

▶ The authors have reported an extraordinarily extensive experience with what is also known as "gamekeeper's thumb." On the basis of this experience, they point out what they describe as 2 symptoms of great diagnostic value. First, more than the amplitude of laxity measured, they believe it is the "limpness" toward the end of the range of motion that indicates a severe ligamentous lesion. Second, the presence of a discrete hematoma on the dorsal aspect of the thumb interphalangeal joint signifies capsuloligamentous rupture and hemarthrosis diffusion along the thumb extensor pollicis longus, indicating a severe injury requiring surgery. Also, they believe that when in doubt between a grade II and grade III sprain, it should be remembered that sequelae of a primary repair are always simpler and heal faster than those of a secondary ligamentoplasty.—J.S. Torg, M.D.

Metacarpal Fractures in the Athlete
Rettig AC, Ryan R, Shelbourne KD, McCarroll JR, Johnson F Jr, Ahlfeld SK (Methodist Sports Medicine Ctr, Indianapolis)
Am J Sports Med 17:567–572, July–August 1989   10–67

Fifty-six fractures of the metacarpal occurring in 53 athletes were reviewed to assess the mechanism of injury, type of fracture, treatment, and time lost from sport. The patients were aged 8–28 years (average, 16); 77% were 14–18 years. Twenty-nine fractures occurred in football, 14 in basketball, and 13 in other sports. Most of the injuries were caused by falls or by hitting an object, such as a helmet or another player. Fractures were evenly divided regarding which digit was involved in football, whereas most basketball injuries involved the fourth and fifth metacarpals. Nearly 50% were diaphyseal fractures.

Forty-six fractures that were minimally displaced or undisplaced were treated by simple casting or splinting. Of the 10 displaced fractures, 2 underwent closed reduction and casting, 3 had closed reduction and percutaneous pin fixation, and 5 underwent open reduction internal fixation using AO type plates and screws. All fractures healed primarily and radiographically.

The average time lost from sport was 13.7 days (range, 0–56), and was significantly higher in basketball (19.7 days) than in football (10.63 days). The average time lost from sport for patients with stable fractures treated with casting or splinting was 12.3 days. Those who underwent open reduction internal fixation with plate and screws lost an average of 13.6 days. The more unusual unstable fracture should be treated by stable internal fixation to allow early range of motion and early return to sports.

▶ The observations and conclusions of the authors are in keeping with my own clinical experience.—J.S. Torg, M.D.

Boxer's Knuckle: Dorsal Capsular Rupture of the Metacarpophalangeal Joint of a Finger
Posner MA, Ambrose L (Hand Services Hosp for Joint Diseases Orthopaedic Inst; Lenox Hill Hosp, New York)
J Hand Surg 14A:229–236, March 1989   10–68

An injury to the dorsal aspect of the metacarpophalangeal joint of a finger usually damages the sagittal fibers of the extensor tendon mechanism. A more severe injury may result in rupture of the underlying joint capsule, which may not be recognized because the extensor tendon may remain in its normal midline position. Six patients had ruptures of the dorsal capsule in 8 joints after severe blunt trauma; 4 of the patients were professional boxers.

Examination showed that the extensor tendon was in its correct midline position in 4 patients, and was subluxated ulnarly in 2 and radially in the other 2. Tenderness over the joint varied depending on the location of the site of capsular injury. A palpable defect over the joint that represented the tear in the dorsal capsule was evident. At surgery all patients had extensive scarring over the extensor tendon. A longitudinal or slightly oblique tear in the dorsal capsule was present in all patients. The capsule was repaired.

This study underlies the potential deleterious effects of severe blunt injuries to the knuckles, particularly in boxers. There is a need to differentiate a capsular rupture from the less severe dorsal hood injuries, as the latter may respond to nonoperative treatment whereas the former requires surgical repair, particularly in athletes.

▶ It should be pointed out that injury to a boxer's knuckles occurs frequently, but unfortunately it rarely receives immediate medical attention. A concern of the authors is that, in a boxer with chronic pain and swelling involving a meta-carpophalangeal joint, it is not unusual for the condition simply to be passed off as "bursitis," "water on the joint," or "brittle hands."—J.S. Torg, M.D.

Lower Extremity and Knee

Proprioception in the Anterior Cruciate Deficient Knee

Barrack RL, Skinner HB, Buckley SL (US Naval Hosp, Oakland, Calif; Univ of California, San Francisco)
Am J Sports Med 17:1–6, January–February 1989   10–69

A high percentage of patients with tears of the anterior cruciate ligament (ACL) experience progressive instability and disability. It has been hypothesized that loss of proprioceptive feedback from disrupted ligaments contributes to this decline. Previous studies have not quantified joint position sense in persons with and without a functioning ACL.

Eleven patients with complete midsubstance ACL tears at arthroscopy were studied. All patients had at least a grade II Lachman test and a positive pivot shift test. Investigators performed proprioception testing 3 months after injury. Testing was done with the knee in 30 to 40 degrees of flexion. Patients were blindfolded, and the normal and injured knees tested in random sequence, with the normal knee serving as a control. An age-matched control group was tested in the same manner. Potentially significant variables, such as time from injury, degree of rehabilitation, and age, were included in multivariate analysis.

The mean variation in threshold values between the knees in controls was less than 2%. In the test group, however, there was a significant higher mean threshold value for the injured knee as compared to the non-injured knee. The mean variation exceeded 25%. Multivariate analysis showed that changes in the proprioception of the injured knee resulted from loss of the ACL and not from other variables.

Patients with complete ACL tears and moderate to severe rotatory instability may also experience deteriorating proprioceptive function in injured knee. Investigators using a larger sample might be able to correlate symptom level with proprioceptive measurements.

▶ An interesting and well-designed study that was awarded the American Orthopaedic Society for Sports Medicine 1988 Excellence in Research Award. One might ask whether or not the observed increase in proprioception threshold was the cause rather than the result of injury to the ACL. Also, determination of proprioception threshold in patients who had ACL reconstruction would certainly be interesting.—J.S. Torg, M.D.

Reflex Inhibition of Thigh Muscles in Knee Injury: Causes and Treatment

Morrissey MC (Boston Univ)
Sports Med 7:263–276, 1989   10–70

Reflex inhibition of a muscle occurs when sensory stimuli impede its voluntary activation. The stimuli usually arise from injury of the joint in which the muscle functions. In a knee injury, reflex inhibition can affect all of the muscles traversing the knee. Reflex inhibition may be measured directly by electromyography, or its physical sequelae can be measured by estimating muscle size or torque production.

Methods of reducing knee pain immediately include transcutaneous electrical nerve stimulation, cold, iontophoresis, joint mobilization, and rest. If effusion produces quadriceps reflex inhibition, this particular cause can be approached directly. Knee immobility also may cause quadriceps reflex inhibition.

Electromyostimulation is a means of rehabilitating weakened muscle through increasing its activation. It usually requires that there be some advantage of a contraction caused by an external source compared with one resulting from voluntary activation. Electromyographic biofeedback is an alternative means of eliciting independent muscle contractions. The more traditional approach is resistance training of voluntary muscle contraction. If possible, active range-of-motion exercises should be performed in the more extended range of quadriceps motion, both concentrically and eccentrically.

▶ This is an excellent review of the subject matter. The interested reader is referred to the original article.—J.S. Torg, M.D.

Prone Examination for Anterior Cruciate Ligament Insufficiency
Feagin JA, Cooke TDV (Jackson, Wyo; Queen's Univ, Kingston, Ont)
J Bone Joint Surg 71-B:863, November 1989   10–71

Two tests that make the clinical diagnosis of anterior cruciate ligament (ACL) insufficiency easier and more reliable, conducted with the patient prone, were evaluated.

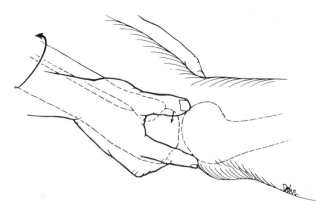

Fig 10–16.—The knee is held 20 or 30 degrees flexed and the examiner's hands grasp the tibia; the fingers are positioned on the joint line. (Courtesy of Feagin JA, Cooke TDV: *J Bone Joint Surg* 71-B:863, November 1989.)

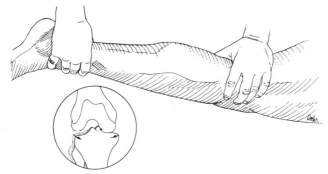

Fig 10-17.— The knee is flexed 20-30 degrees; with 1 hand, the examiner moves the tibia; the hypothenar eminence of the other hand stabilizes the femur while the fingers and thumb serve as an arthrometer at the joint line. (Courtesy of Feagin JA, Cooke TDV: *J Bone Joint Surg* 71-B:863, November 1989.)

Procedure.—The Lachman test is more easily performed if the patient is prone, especially for the examiner with small hands. While the examiner's hands hold the patient's tibia and the fingers are placed on the joint line, the knee is flexed 20-30 degrees (Fig 10-16). Anteroposterior tibiofemoral movement and the quality of the end point are then interpreted. The prone position facilitates foreward movement of the tibia, stabilization of the femur, and relaxation.

The medial translation test also requires the patient to be prone. As the patient's knee is flexed 20-30 degrees, the examiner moves the tibia with one hand while stabilizing the femur with the other, so that the fingers and thumb can perform the test at the joint line (Fig 10-17). Laxity is readily evaluated in the coronal plane. The test is specific for ACL problems. Insufficiency of this ligament is demonstrated by an increase in medial translation and varus angulation, with a gliding and rocking shift. If the ligament is absent, the lateral collateral ligament and iliotibial band should limit medial excursion; if they do not, they are also compromised.

The requirement that the patient be prone makes the medial translation and Lachman tests more effective. Performed in this way, the tests have the virtues of reliability, sensitivity, and simplicity.

▶ It is gratifying to see that the authors have overcome the bane of some orthopedic surgeons—small hands—by improvising what might be better termed the upside-down Lachman test. However, the principle remains the same, the knee is examined in subterminal extension, and, of course, "the proof is in the pudding."—J.S. Torg, M.D.

The Pivot Shift Phenomenon: Results and Description of a Modified Clinical Test for Anterior Cruciate Ligament Insufficiency

Bach BR Jr, Warren RF, Wickiewicz TL (New York Hosp-Cornell Univ Med Ctr, New York)
Am J Sports Med 16:571-576, November-December 1988   10-72

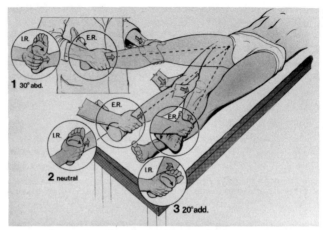

Fig 10–18.—Testing positions include 30 degrees of hip abduction, neutral, and 20 degrees of hip adduction. In each position the tibia is rotated externally about 20 degrees, and the pivot shift test is performed. The test is repeated in all 3 hip positions with the tibia internally rotated approximately 15 degrees. (Courtesy of Bach BR Jr, Warren RF, Wickiewicz TL: *Am J Sports Med* 16:571–576, November–December 1988.)

Because clinical tests of knee instability are not consistently reproducible, 37 patients with surgically documented injury of the anterior cruciate ligament (ACL) were studied to determine the effects of hip position and tibial rotation on test results. The patients were examined under anesthesia in hip abduction, neutral position, and hip adduction and with the tibia externally and internally rotated (Fig 10–18).

Hip position related closely to the degree of pivot shift independently of tibial rotation. Abduction produced the most marked pivot shift, followed by neutral position and then adduction. External tibial rotation increased pivot shift in abduction and neutral, but not in adduction. The combination of abduction and external rotation produced the highest pivot shift scores. Nine of 20 patients with a 3+ pivot shift test under these conditions were negative under conditions of adduction and internal rotation.

It appears that the iliotibial band has an important role in determining the degree of pivot shift observed on clinical testing. The band is relaxed in hip abduction and is tightened in adduction. Leg position should be taken into account when examining a patient for ACL insufficiency.

► With increased reliance on the presence or absence of the pivot shift phenomena in the surgical/nonsurgical decision-making process, the importance of the authors' observations becomes evident. Specifically, "When examining a knee for ACL insufficiency, it is critical to pay attention to the position of the leg because variations in hip position and tibia rotation affect the gradation of the pivot shift sign and a false negative test may be elicited."—J.S. Torg, M.D.

Dynamic Posterior Shift Test: An Adjuvant in Evaluation of Posterior Tibial Subluxation

Shelbourne KD, Benedict F, McCarroll JR, Rettig AC (Methodist Sports Medicine Ctr, Indianapolis)
Am J Sports Med 17:275–277, March–April 1989   10–73

Injury of the posterior cruciate ligament (PCL) and posterolateral structures leads to posterior tibial subluxation, with straight posterior instability or posterolateral rotatory instability (PLRI). The dynamic posterior shift test is a simple and reliable means of evaluating both straight posterior instability and PLRI. It is similar to the reversed pivot shift test but controls rotation of the femur; in addition, it tightens the hamstring, which provide axial loading across the knee.

Procedure.—With the patient supine, the examiner flexes the hip and knee to 90 degrees, keeping the thigh in neutral position. Supporting the distal calf or heel, the examiner's other hand extends the knee slowly (Fig 10–19). If the PCL

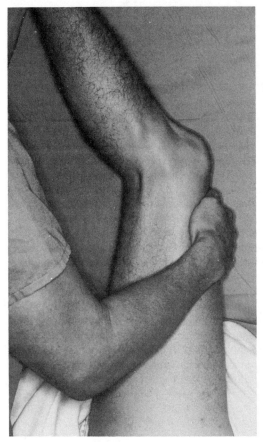

Fig 10–19.—Tibia subluxated posteriorly by pull of tightened hamstring tendons. (Courtesy of Shelbourne KD, Benedict F, McCarroll JR, et al: *Am J Sports Med* 17:275–277, March–April 1989.)

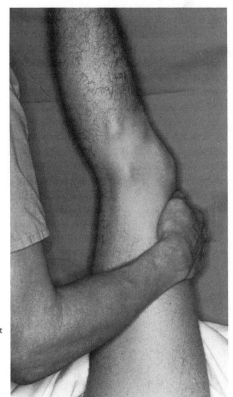

Fig 10–20.—Tibia dynamically reduced as knee nears full extension. (Courtesy of Shelbourne KD, Benedict F, McCarroll JR, et al: *Am J Sports Med* 17:275–277, March–April 1989.)

is injured, the posterior subluxated tibia reduces with a visible and palpable jerk as the knee nears full extension (Fig 10–20). In straight posterior instability, both tibial plateaus come forward equally. With PLRI, the lateral plateau is pulled back further by the tightened hamstrings, and reduction is accompanied by increased tibial rotation.

This is the most sensitive test for assessing the posterior knee structures. It is usually possible to distinguish between straight posterior instability and PLRI using the dynamic posterior shift test.

▶ The authors have described an inexpensive and noninvasive clinical test to assist in the diagnosis of both straight posterior and posterior lateral rotatory instability. They note that the pathomechanics of the dynamic posterior shift test was first described by Cain and Schwab (1) using high-speed cinematography and electromyographic gait studies.—J.S. Torg, M.D.

Reference

1. Cain TE, Schwab GH: *Am J Sports Med* 9:203, 1981.

Three-Dimensional Motion Analysis of Clinical Stress Tests for Anterior Knee Subluxations
Noyes FR, Grood ES, Suntay WJ (Univ of Cincinnati; Deaconess Hosp, Cincinnati)
Acta Orthop Scand 60:308–318, 1989   10–74

The specific abnormalities of anterior tibial translation and internal tibial rotation that follow anterior cruciate ligament (ACL) injury are not clear. The 3-dimensional motions occurring during the usual stress tests were examined for anterior subluxation of the knee, using whole lower extremities from cadavers. The studies employed a 6-degree-of-freedom electrogoniometer.

When the ACL only was sectioned, anterior displacement of both the medial and lateral tibial condyles increased markedly during the flexion rotation drawer test and the pivot shift test. Total anterior-posterior displacement doubled at 30 degrees of knee flexion, but internal-external tibial rotation increased by only 15%. In none of the anterior displacement type tests was there true rigid coupling of knee motions, because the examiner controlled the degree of internal tibial rotation and anterior tibial translation. Sectioning of the medial structures led to additional anterior translation of the medial and lateral tibial condyles.

Subluxations of the medial and lateral tibial condyles should be separately determined during each stress test. Rotatory subluxation can be simplified by expressing the translation of each tibial condyle.

▶ Perhaps the most important point made by the authors is their conclusion that classification of ligamentous injuries should be based on which structures are disrupted rather than on the pathologic motion that can be elicited.—J.S. Torg, M.D.

Genucom, KT-1000, and Stryker Knee Laxity Measuring Device Comparisons: Device Reproducibility and Interdevice Comparison in Asymptomatic Subjects
Highgenboten CL, Jackson A, Meske NB (Orthopaedic Consultants, Dallas; North Texas State Univ, Denton)
Am J Sports Med 17:743–746, November–December 1989   10–75

There are presently 3 commercial devices on the market that can be used to obtain objective knee laxity measurements: The Stryker Knee Laxity Tester, the MEDmetric KT-1000 Arthrometer, and the Genucom Knee Analysis System. The first 2 systems are relatively simple mechanical devices that can discriminate between normal knees and knees with anterior cruciate ligament (ACL) disruption. The Genucom is a computerized system that can be used for a variety of tests that theoretically allow a total description of knee ligament stability. The reproducibility of anterior and posterior knee laxity values as measured by each of the 3 devices was compared.

The study was done with 30 asymptomatic volunteers who were given a test-retest protocol on both legs with all 3 devices. To prevent order effects in the results, the order of the devices used in testing was counterbalanced across subjects. The test administrator was proficient with each of the 3 testing devices and 3 test protocols.

Repeatability of test values within devices was variable, but all were acceptable. Each of the 3 knee laxity testing devices provided reproducible quantitative measurements of knee laxity. However, because of differences in device sensitivities and functional design, specific laxity values and results for 1 device cannot be generalized to another.

The decision on which device to buy depends on what is required for a given practice. If only measurements of anterior-posterior laxity are needed, the Stryker at an approximate cost of $900, or the KT-1000 at an approximate cost of $2,900, will suffice. However, if a more sophisticated analysis of knee ligament status is important, purchase of the Genucom system at a cost of $49,000 may be justified.

▶ In addition to the initial purchase price, the matter of operational and maintenance expenses must be considered. It is my understanding that with the Genucom this can be not inconsequential. Also, should interest wane or justification for using the device abate, it would appear that the Genucom could well become a $49,000 white elephant. Daniel et al. have demonstrated the ability of the Stryker Knee Laxity Tester and the KT-1000 to discriminate between normal and ACL-deficient knees (1,2). Apparently, there are currently no published reports supporting the ability of the Genucom to accomplish this goal.—J.S. Torg, M.D.

References

1. Daniels DM, et al: *J Bone Joint Surg* 67A:720, 1985.
2. Daniels DM, et al: *Am J Sports Med* 13:401, 1985.

Instrumental Lachman Tests for the Evaluation of Anterior Laxity After Reconstruction of the Anterior Cruciate Ligament
Harter RA, Osternig LR, Singer KM (Univ of Oregon, Eugene)
J Bone Joint Surg 71-A:975–983, August 1989   10–76

Currently available instrumentation permits clinicians to assess both anterior ligamentous laxity and the effectiveness of reconstruction procedures. The normal knee and a knee that had undergone anterior cruciate ligament (ACL) reconstruction were evaluated in 50 patients who were grouped according to type of intra-articular replacement—either the middle third of the patellar tendon or the semitendinosus tendon—used for the ACL, and also according to duration of follow-up. Lachman tests were performed using 68 and 90 newtons of force, and indices for anterior compliance were calculated.

There was significantly more anterior laxity in the ACL-reconstructed knee than in the normal knee with both 68 and 90 newtons of force. However, in 13 patients, 8 of whom could not fully extend the reconstructed knee, there was more laxity in the normal knee. Neither the type of reconstruction nor length of follow-up affected the results.

Both types of ligamentous reconstructions were equally effective in limiting anterior tibial displacement. Neither substitute elongated significantly during follow-up.

▶ It is interesting to note that Noyes et al. reported that the in vivo tensile strength of the central portion of the patella tendon is approximately 175% that of the normal ACL (1) and Lipscomb's group found that the tensile strength of semitendinosus is only 50% of that of the normal ACL (2). However, on the basis of this study, it appears that the 2 types of autogenous substitutes are equally effective in limiting anterior tibial displacement during Lachman tests with forces as great as 90 newtons. Of course, this is only one of many parameters by which success of ACL reconstruction should be measured.—J.S. Torg, M.D.

References

1. Noyes FR, et al: *Clin Orthop* 172:71, 1983.
2. Lipscomb AB, et al: *Am J Sports Med* 9:77, 1981.

New Method for Fast MR Imaging of the Knee
Harms SE, Flamig DP, Fisher CF, Fulmer JM (Baylor Univ)
Radiology 173:743–750, December 1989   10–77

Magnetic resonance imaging (MRI) is often used to diagnose internal derangements of the knee. A new 3-dimensional method was developed, 3D FASTER, an acronym for field acquisition with a short repetition time and echo reduction. This method can be used as an alternative to conventional 2-dimensional (2D) spin-echo MRI.

Thirty-five patients with clinically suspected knee injuries were imaged with both conventional 2-dimensional spin-echo MRI and 3D FASTER. The images were studied by 3 reviewers blinded to the results of arthroscopic or surgical results. The grade of meniscal signal was used to correlate 2D and 3D findings.

The 3D FASTER images had optimal contrast for demonstrating the anatomy of the knee. A 9-minute 3D FASTER data acquisition achieved nearly isotropic voxels for the calculation of any image plane without significant loss in the quality of the image. The 3D FASTER images were superior to or equal to 2D images in visualizing ligament and meniscal tears, bone marrow disease, and osteochondral flaws. In addition, 2D images took 3 times as long to acquire.

The 3D FASTER imaging technique offers improved imaging capability and faster acquisition time. For these reasons it could become a standard MRI procedure for knee imaging.

▶ As experience increases and software developments become more sophisticated, new methods of MRI are being developed. The goal of these new methods is to enhance contrast, improve the image, and increase the accuracy and the efficiency of the study. The 3-D FASTER technique, compared with the standard MRI technique, had equal sensitivity to demonstrating mensical tears with better anatomical display; ligament injuries were better seen because of thinner sections oriented along the ligament plane; osteochondral lesions were better seen because of thinner sections that decrease volume-averaging effects; and the patellar femoral joint was visualized on axial views similar to CT. In addition, almost all of the time within the MR scanner is for data acquisition; no time is needed for positioning or reconstruction of previously acquired data. Hence this study takes approximately 10 minutes of MR time, compared to approximately 45 minutes for the standard method. A larger series and additional experience are necessary to determine those musculoskeletal lesions that may be obscured by this technique; however, for the majority of MR examinations of the knee this method seems to be more than adequate and will potentially increase the efficient utilization of MR and decrease the cost of the MR examination of the knee.—J.S. Torg, M.D.

Double-Blind Assessment of the Value of Magnetic Resonance Imaging in the Diagnosis of Anterior Cruciate and Meniscal Lesions
Glashow JL, Katz R, Schneider M, Scott WN (Lenox Hill Hosp, New York)
J Bone Joint Surg 71-A:113–119, January 1989   10–78

An accurate noninvasive diagnostic test for internal derangement of the knee is needed. Magnetic resonance imaging (MRI) has many advantages, but its objective accuracy for this purpose is not known. The usefulness of MRI in the accurate interpretation of pathologic intra-articular changes in the knee was assessed in a prospective double-blind study.

A group of 47 patients scheduled to have arthroscopy and 3 who were to have arthrotomy volunteered to undergo MRI before surgery. The radiologists had no clinical or radiographic data on the patients before assessment of MR images. Radiologists' interpretations were not known to the surgeon before arthroscopy or arthrotomy was performed. Observations were limited to findings in the menisci and anterior cruciate ligament (ACL).

For pathologic findings in the menisci, MRI had a positive predictive value of 75%, a negative predictive value of 90%, a sensitivity of 83%, and a specificity of 84%. For complete tears of the ACL, it had a positive predictive value of 74%, a negative predictive value of 70%, a sensitivity of 61%, and a specificity of 82%.

When combined with clinical and radiographic examination, MRI provides the most accurate noninvasive source of information for pathologic findings in the menisci and ACL.

▶ Accuracy is dependent on the technique used, as well as on the experience and diagnostic acumen of the examiner performing the procedure. The authors state a positive predictive value for MR of 75% for meniscal pathology and re port that the low accuracy was because the radiologist who interpreted the images was "blinded," i.e., no clinical information or plain roentgenograms were available. However, in the usual clinical situation it is typical for the clinical information to be lacking. Also, the authors claim that the positive predictive value of 74% for the ACL was better than that obtained with arthrography, which they quote to be 50%. The authors failed, however, to include in their references a report by Pavlov et al. (1) in which a 95% accuracy was shown in determining whether the ACL was intact or abnormal.

The conclusion that MRI provides the most accurate noninvasive source of information for pathologic findings in the menisci and the ACL is correct in that it is the only noninvasive method available; however, the accuracy, as indicated by this report, varies and confirmatory information via arthrography or arthroscopy is necessary until MR techniques and the experience of the examiners become more uniform.—J.S. Torg, M.D.

Reference

1. Pavlov H, et al: *J Bone Joint Surg* 65A:175, 1983.

Occult Intraosseous Fracture: Magnetic Resonance Appearance Versus Age of Injury
Lee JK, Yao L (Albany Med College; Albany Med Ctr Hosp, New York)
Am J Sports Med 17:620–623, September–October 1989   10–79

The diagnosis of an occult intraosseous fracture is based on typically located findings on magnetic resonance imaging (MRI), a history of recent injury, and normal radiographic appearance. Magnetic resonance findings were correlated with the age of injury in 22 patients seen during a 15-month period in which an estimated 275 MR examinations were performed.

The history always included a solitary injury to the knee, but the mechanism varied. Magnetic resonance imaging revealed bandlike or speckled areas of decreased intensity of signal in the epiphysis, especially in T1-weighted or proton density images. The T2-weighted images of corresponding regions showed signal intensity ranging from rare or absent high signal, graded as zero to increased intensity of signal in an area slightly smaller or equal in size, grade 1, to high signal findings in a more extensive area, graded 2. Generally, as the area of high signal findings on the T2-weighted images increased, the duration of injury decreased, but the findings varied considerably.

The T2-weighted images showing high signal intensity apparently change faster than the low signal intensity on T1-weighted images, but the age of the lesion cannot be predicted only on the basis of the image. The fracture seems to be caused by direct impact or axial overloading.

Diagnosis requires interpretation of the MRI findings in light of the clinical setting of pain persisting after injury in the absence of other knee lesions.

Occult Cartilage and Bone Injuries of the Knee: Detection, Classification, and Assessment With MR Imaging
Mink JH, Deutsch AL (Cedars-Sinai Med Ctr, Los Angeles)
Radiology 170:823–829, March 1989   10–80

Magnetic resonance imaging (MRI) is capable of assessing a wide spectrum of knee abnormalities including ligament tears, loose bodies, and synovial disorders. Less attention has been paid to MRI of occult traumatic lesions of bone and cartilage about the knee. In 66 patients abnormalities were not visible on plain radiographs.

Although only 4 of the 66 were considered to be slightly suspect for fracture on plain radiographs, 4 types of fracture and 30 bone bruises were identified on MRI. Of the 30 bruises diagnosed, 7 occurred after trauma and 23 were associated with a twisting injury. Most (17) bruises were in the femur. Stress fracture was the final diagnosis in 6 patients. On T1-weighted images the lesions were amorphous in 2 patients; in the other 4 patients these images were characterized by a linear zone of decreased signal intensity surrounded by a broader, poorly defined, and lighter area.

Two patients had occult femoral fractures and 13 had plateau fractures. Among the latter, T1- and T2-weighted images revealed single or multiple linear areas of decreased signal intensity extending vertically to involve the articular surfaces. Patients with osteochondral fractures showed 2 patterns: 8 were displaced lesions and 9 were impacted lesions.

Patients who have normal plain radiographs of the knee but with persistent pain, effusion, and lateralizing symptoms may have bone and cartilage disorders that can be detected by MRI. Many of these abnormalities are characterized by an area of decreased signal intensity on T1-weighted images that becomes brighter on T2-weighted images.

▶ The spectrum of MR findings in the musculoskeletal system in expanding faster than that required for documentation of what these findings indicate. Both of these reports (Abstracts 10–79 and 10–80) on "occult" MR findings have established that MR can confirm musculoskeletal lesions, including bone bruises, stress fractures, tibial plateau fractures, femoral fractures, and osteochondral lesions, that are responsible for pain and discomfort but are not, however, evident on routine x-ray studies. The clinical significance of MR findings requires follow-up and confirmation. Histologic evaluation of the various lesions requires biopsy, which is not always warranted by the clinical presentation. The MR findings must be interpreted cautiously until the sensitivity and specificity of various patterns are recognizable and can be correlated with a specific diagnosis. At present, during the learning period associated with MRI, follow-up of the patients' symptoms and correlation of resolution with MR is critical.—J.S. Torg, M.D.

The Natural History of Conservatively Treated Partial Anterior Cruciate Ligament Tears
Buckley SL, Barrack RL, Alexander AH (Naval Hosp, Oakland, Calif)
Am J Sports Med 17:221–225, March–April 1989   10–81

The expected clinical outcome in conservatively treated partial tears of the anterior cruciate ligament (ACL) was studied in 25 patients with such tears who were followed for an average of 49 months. All patients were examined under anesthesia and arthroscopy after acute injury to a previously normal knee. The percentage of tear was estimated during arthroscopy. Patients scheduled for reconstruction of the ACL were evaluated immediately before reconstruction; those who were not candidates for reconstruction were evaluated at least 18 months later. Patients who had surgery were treated with early motion and hamstring strengthening. Both weight-bearing and quadriceps rehabilitation were delayed.

Clinical score at follow-up did not correlate significantly with length of follow-up, percentage of ligament tear, or age at injury. Thirteen patients who underwent partial meniscectomy at original arthroscopy had outcomes similar to those in patients without meniscectomies. Two patients had reconstruction of the ACL 8 months and 64 months after injury. Indications for reconstruction were episodes of giving way during daily activities and a positive pivot shift test.

Overall, 28% of patients had excellent results, 32% had good results, 24% had fair results, and 16% had poor results. Half of the patients with poor results required ligament reconstruction after injury to the knee. Of 72% with activity-related symptoms, only 44% were able to resume sports at preinjury levels.

Most patients with partial tears of the ACL have symptomatic knees but not sufficient dysfunction to warrant reconstructive surgery within 3–6 years after injury. Neither the percentage of tear nor partial meniscectomy correlates significantly with eventual outcome. Knee function after a partial tear of the ACL apparently does not deteriorate with time.

▶ The authors have presented a concise documentation of conservatively treated partial ACL tears. However, although a bias is expressed, I'm not sure that it answers the larger question, i.e., what the criteria are for surgical intervention in the face of this lesion.—J.S. Torg, M.D.

External Stabilization of the Anterior Cruciate Ligament Deficient Knee During Rehabilitation
Maltry JA, Noble PC, Woods GW, Alexander JW, Feldman GW, Tullos HS (Baylor College of Medicine, Houston)
Am J Sports Med 17:550–554, July–August 1989   10–82

The anterior cruciate ligament (ACL) is the most frequently injured ligament in the knee. Anterior subluxation in the ACL-deficient knee increases as the knee is extended from 90 degrees to 30 degrees. External tibial loading also influences the degree of subluxation. However, no previous studies have documented tibiofemoral displacements in the terminal 30 degrees of extension, nor have external load requirements for offsetting anterior subluxation been determined.

Procedure.—The effect of ACL deficiency on anterior tibial translation during extension of the knee was examined in cadaveric specimens. In 5 cadaveric knees the quadriceps tendon was isolated and sutured to a nylon cuff. During the experiments a cable attached to the cuff was loaded until flexion angles of 10, 25, 40, or 60 degrees were reached. The anterior-posterior position of the tibia was recorded with biplane radiography at each angle, both before and after division of the ACL. Posterior forces of 0 N, 45 N (10 lb), 90 N (20 lb), 135 N (30 lb), and 225 N (50 lb) were applied to the tibia at each flexion angle with a nylon strap attached to the tibial tubercle.

In all specimens the anterior tibial translation increased with the loss of the ACL and was greatest at 25 degrees of flexion. At this angle there was an average displacement of 3.3 mm. Subluxation was not significant at flexion angles exceeding 60 degrees, regardless of ACL deficiency. When the nylon band was used to restrain tibial subluxation, anterior subluxation was eliminated through application of forces that ranged from a maximum of 106 N (23.6 lb) at 10 degrees to only 13 N (2.9 lb) at 60 degrees. The necessary restraining force varies with the degree of knee flexion.

Partial Tears of the Anterior Cruciate Ligament: Progression to Complete Ligament Deficiency
Noyes FR, Mooar LA, Moorman CT III, McGinniss GH (Cincinnati Sportsmedicine Ctr; Deaconess Hosp, Cincinnati)
J Bone Joint Surg 71-B:825–833, November 1989   10–83

During a 7-year-period 38 patients were treated for arthroscopically verified partial rupture of the anterior cruciate ligament (ACL). The status of the ACL and activity levels were assessed in 32 patients followed for 24–110 months. Complete deficiency of the ACL was indicated by a grade III pivot shift test result and an increase of at least 5 mm in anteroposterior translation on a KT-1000 arthrometer.

Progression to complete deficiency was found in 38% of knees. Such progression may be expected in 50% of knees with one-half tears and in 86% of those with three fourths tears. Ligaments with one-fourth tears are less likely to become ACL deficient. Three factors were significantly related to progression to complete deficiency: estimated amount of the initial tear, an increase in anterior translation initially, and a subsequent giving-way reinjury. Reinjury occurred in 56% of knees, usually at least within 2 years after the initial injury. There was some limitation of sports activity in patients with partial tears, but it was greater if deficiency was complete. Certain patients in both groups failed to modify activities despite significant problems.

Patients with partial tears of the ligament should be advised of the risk of progression to complete deficiency and of reinjury. They should be observed for a long period. Efforts to educate them about participating in strenuous sports activities may reduce the probability of osteoarthritis developing.

▶ The observations presented in this paper regarding progression of partial tears of the ACL to complete ligament deficiency are not in keeping with those of myself or Odensten et al. (1). The conclusion of Odensten's group is that partial or incomplete disruption of the ACL follows a benign course and good long-term results may be expected. This is, as mentioned, in keeping with our own observations and experience. Credit should be given to Marshall (2) for having described the ACL to consist of 2 bands, the posterior lateral band and the anterior lateral band. Generally, in incomplete ruptures it is the anterior medial band that remains intact with the posterior lateral band being disrupted. The report of Noyes et al. does not appear to appreciate this subtlety and suggests failure to recognize injuries that were in fact complete ruptures.—J.S. Torg, M.D.

References

1. Odensten M, et al: *Am J Sports Med* 13:183, 1985.
2. Marshall JL: *Clin Orthop* 106:216, 1975.

Surgical or Non-Surgical Treatment of Acute Rupture of the Anterior Cruciate Ligament: A Randomized Study With Long-Term Follow-Up
Andersson C, Odensten M, Good L, Gillquist J (Univ of Linköping, Sweden)
J Bone Joint Surg 71-A:965–974, August 1989   10–84

Some studies have shown unsatisfactory long-term results after acute repair of ruptured anterior cruciate ligaments (ACLs). To determine whether repair with augmentation of the ACL using part of the patellar tendon might improve results, 111 patients were randomized to 3 treatment groups. One group received simple repair of all injured structures; the second group underwent repair of all injured structure and augmentation of the ACL with a strip of the iliotibial band; and the third group had repair of all injured structures except for the ACL. At 45 months or more after surgery 107 patients were available for reexamination.

At last follow-up, patients treated by repair and augmentation of the ACL were significantly more stable and had significantly fewer subsequent meniscal tears. Patients who received augmentation also required fewer reconstructions for symptoms of instability. Patients with augmented repair had better knee function and higher levels of activity than patients in either of the other treatment groups. Also, 64% of patients with ruptures of the ACL had meniscal tears. More than half of these tears required primary treatment.

In patients with rupture of the ACL, repair and augmentation of the ACL results in better function of the knee and a higher level of activity than simple repair or repair of only peripheral lesions. Because patients with this injury frequently have associated injuries requiring primary treatment, arthroscopy is recommended whenever an acute rupture of the ACL is encountered.

▶ This is a well-designed, prospective, randomized study subjected to statistical analysis that substantiates repair and augmentation as preferable in the management of injuries of the ACL. However, the conclusion that all patients with clinically diagnosed acute ruptures of the ACL should be arthroscoped to determine the existence of associated injuries can be questioned. If it is the preference of the surgeon and patient not to repair and augment an isolated tear of the ACL, perhaps magnetic resonance imaging would be a more practical, conservative, and noninvasive approach. Also, it has been our experience that in instances of acute isolated rupture of the ACL, aspiration and injection of 30 mg of triamcinolone to counteract the blood-induced synovitis resolves symptoms and, except for a positive Lachman test, other physical findings. If, however, there is an injury to a meniscus or the articular surface, the patient, when examined in a week, will have persistent effusion, perhaps joint line tenderness, and inability to extend the knee.—J.S. Torg, M.D.

Nonoperative Treatment of Grade II and III Sprains of the Lateral Ligament Compartment of the Knee
Kannus P (Tampere Univ, Finland)
Am J Sports Med 17:83–88, January–February 1989   10–85

Because injuries to the lateral ligament compartment (LAT) are somewhat rare, there is a paucity of studies on this subject. The long-term results of nonoperative treatment of grades II and III sprains of the LAT were evaluated in 27 patients treated conservatively. In all cases, the mechanism of injury was forceful adduction of the extended or flexed knee. Eleven patients with grade II sprains and 12 with grade III sprains were followed for an average of 8 years. Patients were evaluated on 4 standardized knee-scoring scales for subjective, objective, radiographic, and functional findings. Knees were also evaluated for isometric and isokinetic strength.

Patients with grade II sprains had either excellent or good results. None required surgery for chronic ligament insufficiency. In 9 patients physical activity was at least at preinjury level, and knees were asymptomatic. Two patients reinjured their knees, but conservative treatment was successful. Radiographic evaluation showed no posttraumatic osteoarthritis. Patients did have some laxity of the LAT at 30 degrees of flexion. The quadriceps deficit was 4% and the hamstring strength deficit, 1%.

Patients with grade III sprains had significantly poorer results in all categories, and mean scores were only fair. None required surgery for knee ligament insufficiency, but 2 required lateral meniscectomy. Nine patients had clearly diminished physical activity. Two patients had to change jobs and 2 received partial pensions because of their injuries. Three patients reinjured their knees, 1 twice and 2 once. Injured knees were laterally unstable and were often unstable anteriorly, anterolaterally, and partly posterolaterally as well. The average stability score was poor. The average quadricep deficit was 23% and the hamstring strength deficit, 14%. Six patients had posttraumatic osteoarthritis. Only 1 patient was asymptomatic, but even this patient had an unstable knee laterally and anterolaterally.

Grade II sprains of the LAT can be treated successfully without surgery, but conservative treatment cannot be recommended for grade III sprains. The anterior cruciate ligament is often injured in grade III sprains; damage may be missed by clinical examination alone.

▶ The observations and conclusions of the author are in keeping with our own clinical experience. Undiagnosed or conservatively treated grade III lateral ligament sprains, particularly when associated with anterior cruciate ligament disruption, are disasters that defy attempts at late repair or reconstruction.—J.S. Torg, M.D.

Patellofemoral Problems After Anterior Cruciate Ligament Reconstruction
Sachs RA, Daniel DM, Stone ML, Garfein RF (Kaiser Permanente Med Ctr, San Diego)
Am J Sports Med 17:760–765, November–December 1989   10–86

A 1982 review of patients who had undergone anterior cruciate ligament (ACL) reconstruction revealed a high incidence of signs and symptoms consistent with patellofemoral problems. To better understand these problems, a prospective study was initiated to evaluate patellofemoral function after knee ligament surgery. In addition, 50 prominent knee surgeons were queried by mail, and a MEDLINE search was performed to retrieve all papers on ACL reconstruction or complications of ACL surgery published between 1965 and 1986.

The data from the literature, the replies from knee surgeons, and the 1-year follow-up data from treated patients were reviewed to determine the presence of 13 different complications.

Between 1982 and 1986, 126 patients aged 16–47 years (mean, 24.5 years) underwent ACL reconstruction. Follow-up evaluation included a patient questionnaire, physical examination, anterior-posterior ligament laxity tests, and performance tests. Knee extension measurements, patellar crepitance, and patellar irritability were the most important parameters for analyzing patellofemoral problems.

Quadriceps weakness, flexion contracture, and patellofemoral pain were the most prevalent complications after ACL reconstruction. Sixty-five percent of the patients had quadriceps weakness. This finding correlated positively with flexion contracture, patellar irritability, and ACL reconstructions in which patellar tendon grafts had been used. The finding of flexion contractures of 5 degrees or more in 24% of the patients correlated positively with increased age and patellar irritability, and 19% had patellofemoral pain that correlated positively with flexion contracture.

Flexion contracture may cause patellofemoral irritability, and both of these factors, either alone or in combination, may cause weakness of the quadriceps. If this concept is supported in future studies, it would indicate that postoperative rehabilitation programs should be geared more toward avoiding flexion contracture by placing a high priority on the maintenance of full knee extension.

▶ The authors present a candid portrayal of the not uncommon constellation of complications associated with ACL reconstruction using an infrapatellar tendon graft. Although they describe a correlation between knee flexion contracture, patella femoral pain, and quadriceps weakness, they failed to address the question as to whether or not the initiating cause could be an overconstrained knee resulting from suboptimal graft placement.—J.S. Torg, M.D.

Analysis of Rehabilitation Techniques After Anterior Cruciate Reconstruction
Anderson AF, Lipscomb AB (St Thomas Hosp, Nashville)
Am J Sports Med 17:154–160, March–April 1989   10–87

Numerous rehabilitation techniques have been advocated for patients who have undergone anterior cruciate ligament (ACL) reconstruction. A comparison was made of the effectiveness of 5 methods of ACL rehabilitation: transcutaneous electrical nerve stimulation, immobilization in flexion, immobilization in extension, electrical muscle stimulation (EMS), and continuous passive motion. Five groups of 20 patients each who had undergone the same ACL reconstruction procedure were evaluated; each underwent 1 of the rehabilitation procedures. The patients were evaluated by clinical assessment, volumetric thigh measurements, instrumented varus-valgus stress testing, KT-1000 arthrometer measurements, and Cybex II muscle evaluation.

Patients receiving transcutaneous electrical nerve stimulation were not able to reduce the amount of the pain medication needed, nor did they have improvement in any clinically measurable parameter of performance. Those treated in extension and those treated in flexion had similar measures of stability. However, 3 patients treated in extension required manipulation, whereas no patients treated in flexion needed manipulation. Strength decrease during immobilization was minimized by EMS, but EMS did not reduce atrophy. Patients treated with EMS also had significantly greater range of motion than those treated with extension or flexion and early limited motion. Compared to all other groups, EMS patients had a significant reduction in the incidence of patellofemoral crepitation. In comparison with immobilization in extension, continuous passive motion reduced the requirement for manipulation, but it was not as effective as early limited range of motion.

The best rehabilitation program for patients after ACL reconstruction includes EMS and immobilization in flexion with early limited range of motion. Prolonged immobilization is not only unnecessary, it is detrimental.

▶ This is a well-designed, prospective, and randomized study, the results of which were subjected to appropriate statistical analysis. A major problem concerns the failure of the authors to identify the technique used for ACL reconstruction. This is important, of course, because their conclusion that "The optimal rehabilitation program included EMS and immobilization in flexion with early range of motion" can apply only to this procedure and not to all ACL reconstructive procedures.—J.S. Torg, M.D.

Arthroscopic Lateral Release for Patellar Pain or Instability

Aglietti P, Pisaneschi A, Buzzi R, Gaudenzi A, Allegra M (Univ of Florence, Italy)
Arthroscopy 5:176–183, 1989   10–88

In 1982–1985, 45 arthroscopic lateral release procedures were performed in 19 knees because of recurrent patellar instability, including recurrent dislocation, and 20 other knees because of patellar pain, which usually was poorly localized and increased with prolonged sitting or stair climbing. Isolated early patellofemoral osteoarthrosis was present in 6 knees. The operation was performed only after failure of supervised conservative therapy for 6 months. No patient had previously undergone surgery.

There were 10 excellent, 3 good, and 2 fair results in the group with patellar instability after an average follow-up of 51 months; 4 patients had a poor outcome. Half of the patients had returned to the same sport and 20% changed to a less demanding activity. On follow-up for 40 months, 8 patients had excellent and 4 had good results after surgery for patellar pain; 2 others had fair and 6 had poor results. Of these patients, 66% resumed the same sport; only 1 of 6 knees did well after surgery for patellofemoral osteoarthrosis. The other 5 patients had poor results after an average follow-up of 56 months.

Arthroscopic lateral release may be used as the first surgical method if conservative measures fail in patients with patellar pain and maltracking, as well as in selected patients with less marked instability. A complete release should be performed.

▶ As stated by the authors, the results of arthroscopic lateral releases in this series were not entirely satisfactory. The value of clinical prognosticators for the efficacy of retinacular release surgery is evident. We recently published (1) a study that attempted to identify clinical pathologic and roentgenographic factors that might serve as prognosticators for acceptable results after lateral retinacular release surgery. Our data indicated that acceptable results can be expected in patients who have what we described as a negative mal-loose sign, i.e., no evidence of patellar malalignment or hyperlaxity. Also, acceptable results correlated with the presence of a positive Sage sign, a test designed to determine of tight lateral parapatellar soft tissue structures. Poor results were predictable in the patients with patellar hypermobility.—J.S. Torg, M.D.

Reference

1. Gecha SR, Torg JS: *Clin Orthop* 253:203, 1990.

An Analysis of Complications in Lateral Retinacular Release Procedures
Small NC (Univ of Texas, Dallas)
Arthroscopy 5:282–286, December 1989   10–89

The lateral retinacular release procedure originally was only a component of a series of procedures used to treat recurrent patellar dislocation. Since 1970 lateral retinacular releases have been performed increasingly as isolated procedures. Results of the isolated lateral retinacular release procedure have been relatively good, with success rates ranging from 70% to 85%. More recently, most of the lateral retinacular releases have been performed arthroscopically. However, the procedure has the highest complication rate among all arthroscopic procedures. Data compiled from 3 published prospective studies of arthroscopic lateral retinacular release were evaluated.

Of 446 lateral retinacular release procedures reviewed, 32 were associated with complications. In 271 procedures performed with a tourniquet there were 25 complications, including hemarthrosis in 22, thrombophlebitis in 1, and infection in 2. Of 152 procedures performed without a tourniquet, 5 were associated with complications, including hemarthrosis in 4 and infection in 1. The difference was statistically significant. The technique of arthroscopically controlled subcutaneous lateral retinacular release led to a higher complication rate than a technique involving release performed entirely with arthroscopic instrumentation. The use of electrocautery did not affect the complication rate. Use of a postoperative suction drain for 24 hours in 186 procedures was associated with 25 complications, compared with only 5 complications in 219 procedures performed without a postoperative drain. The difference was statistically significant. Whether surgery was performed on an inpatient or outpatient basis did not affect the complication rate. Because for this study several variables were combined in each operative procedure, prospective studies should assess the effect of a single variable on the complication rate for lateral retinacular release procedures.

▶ To the complications reported by the authors after arthroscopic lateral retinacular release procedures that included hemarthrosis, thrombophlebitis, and infection can be added yet another: Hughston and Deese (1) reported that medial subluxation of the patella developed in 30 knees postoperatively in a group of 54 patients referred because of failure to improve or because of worsening of their preoperative symptoms after lateral retinacular release.—J.S. Torg, M.D.

Reference

1. Hughston JC, Deese M: *Am J Sports Med* 16:383, 1988.

Arthroscopic "Second Look" at the GORE-TEX Ligament
Ferkel RD, Fox JM, Wood D, Del Pizzo W, Friedman MJ, Snyder SJ (Southern California Orthopedic Inst, Van Nuys)
Am J Sports Med 17:147–153, March–April 1989   10–90

The GORE-TEX ligament is a permanent prosthesis that has been implanted in more than 1,200 patients with chronic insufficiency of the anterior cruciate ligament. An arthroscopic second-look procedure was performed in 21 knees (20 patients) with GORE-TEX grafts that were implanted arthroscopically.

Arthroscopy was performed on 8 knees at time of screw removal, on 8 with knee pain, on 2 that gave way, and on 3 with recurrent effusions. The degree of synovial joint reaction, graft rupture, and graft synovial ingrowth were graded. All biopsy specimens of the GORE-TEX ligament were examined microscopically. The average age of the 13 male and 7 female patients was 30 years; average time from implantation to review was 11 months.

In 11 knees the GORE-TEX ligament was intact. There was a 10% rupture in 6 ligaments, and 4 ligaments were completely ruptured. The number of strands ruptured did not correlate with synovial reaction, nor was there any correlation between synovial coverage of the graft and the graft's integrity. Only when the graft was ruptured were particles of the graft seen in the synovium. There was no significant change in the degree of synovitis before and after graft implantation.

An intact GORE-TEX ligament is inert and does not cause significant joint reactions. The most common cause of graft failure is impingement in the intercondylar notch. Further study is required to determine the natural history of the GORE-TEX ligament and the knee's response to the prosthetic implant. Methods of decreasing graft failure and increasing knee stability should be explored.

▶ This report of "second-look" examination of 21 GORE-TEX grafts concerned a series of 103 arthroscopically implanted devices. In this group of 21 patients, the average time interval from original implantation to a second look was 11 months (range, 2–31 months). There were 4 patients with complete rupture and another 4 with an estimated partial rupture of 50%, which indicates an overall graft failure of approximately 8%. Certainly, a detailed long-term follow-up of the 82 grafts would be most enlightening. These results do not justify encouraging the use of GORE-TEX in situations other than currently recommended by the FDA guidelines. However, on the other hand, the jury is still out on the eventual role that the GORE-TEX ligament will play in cruciate reconstructive surgery.—J.S. Torg, M.D.

Chronic Anterior Cruciate Ligament Deficiency: Long-Term Results of MacIntosh's Lateral Substitution Reconstruction
Amirault JD, Cameron JC, MacIntosh DL, Marks P (Camp Hill Hosp, Halifax, NS; Univ of Toronto; Toronto Gen Hosp)
J Bone Joint Surg 70-B:622–624, August 1988   10–91

MacIntosh's lateral substitution reconstruction for anterior cruciate ligament (ACL)-deficient knees was devised to prevent anterior subluxation of the lateral tibial plateau in extension, thus preventing the pivot shift. Data collected in the longest reported follow-up of lateral substitution reconstruction were reviewed.

Twenty-seven patients with chronic ACL deficiency of the knees were treated by MacIntosh's lateral substitution reconstruction. At an average 11.3 years (range, 8–14.4 years) after operation, these patients were assessed by a scoring system that allocated a maximum of 25 points each for function and for clinical evaluation. Emphasis was placed on giving way, as well as finding of objective evidence of a positive anterior drawer sign and a positive lateral pivot shift test.

Results were rated good to excellent in 52% of patients, fair in 26%, and poor in 22%. Patients who scored poorly had evidence of articular cartilage erosions at surgery. Despite the recorded scores, 75% of the patients were improved subjectively and maintained an active life-style.

Continued symptomatic giving way of the knees, unresponsive to conservative treatment or to modification of activity, leads to unacceptably high meniscal and articular cartilage damage. The lateral substitution reconstruction still has a place in the treatment of chronic ACL deficiency.

▶ With lesser morbidity and better results obtainable with arthroscopically assisted ACL reconstruction, this paper can only be viewed from the standpoint of historical perspective.—J.S. Torg, M.D.

Corticosteroids and Anterior Cruciate Ligament Repair
Vargas JH III, Ross DG (MidVermont Orthopaedics; Vermont Sports Medicine Ctr, Rutland)
Am J Sports Med 17:532–534, July–August 1989　　　　　　　　　10–92

No studies have shown that corticosteroid therapy reduces pain after knee surgery. With the current emphasis on shortened hospitalization to reduce costs, however, it seems appropriate to identify the relationship between the use of perioperative corticosteroids and length of hospitalization, first day of recorded ambulation, and total doses of pain medication administered in patients after anterior cruciate ligament (ACL) repair.

Thirty-one patients having ACL repair received a standard protocol of intravenous perioperative and oral postoperative corticosteroids. These patients were compared with 31 age-matched ACL-repair patients who underwent similar procedures and medical therapy but without corticosteroids.

The experimental group had a higher incidence of associated injuries of the knee. However, these patients required 50% less analgesia while hospitalized than controls. Also, hospitalization was shortened by 59% and ambulation was achieved 38% more quickly in the experimental group. There were no differences between the groups in incidence of postoperative infection or problems with wound healing after follow-up of 1 year.

These preliminary data support further study of the use of corticosteroids to control postoperative pain in patients undergoing knee surgery.

The postoperative use of these drugs may also significantly reduce the length of hospitalization and length of time to ambulation.

▶ This retrospective study suggests that patients who underwent ACL repair and received 10 mg of dexamethasone sodium phosphate intravenously when the tourniquet was released intraoperatively and then 8 mg of oral dexamethasone in divided doses on the first postoperative day required less medicine to relieve pain, ambulated more rapidly, and were discharged more quickly than patients who did not recieve the steroid. The authors state that: "Follow-up to date indicates that no postoperative infections or problems with wound healing have been identified in either group;" however, the question of what effect the steroid had on ligament reconstruction was not dealt with. This major defect in this study precludes recommending corticosteroids in association with ACL surgery.—J.S. Torg, M.D.

The Biochemical and Histological Effects of Artificial Ligament Wear Particles: In Vitro and In Vivo Studies
Olson EJ, Kang JD, Fu FH, Georgescu HI, Mason GC, Evans CH (Univ of Pittsburgh)
Am J Sports Med 16:558–570, November–December 1988   10–93

There is increasing evidence that biochemical mechanisms contribute to the development of arthritis. Cartilaginous wear particles can induce destructive enzymes and cytokines. The biocompatibility of artificial anterior cruciate ligament (ACL) replacements was assessed. The effects of wear particles from GORE-TEX, the Stryker Dacron Ligament Prosthesis, Versigraft carbon, Kennedy LAD, Xenograft, Leeds-Keio, and human patellar tendon allograft were analyzed. Ligaments were frozen and ground, and added to rabbit synovial cell cultures.

All materials caused significantly increased production of collagenase, gelatinase, and chrondrocyte activating factor by synoviocytes. The highest enzyme levels were found with Xenograft and carbon. When wear particles were injected in rabbit knees, examination at 14 weeks showed accumulation of particles in the periarticular synovial folds and varying degrees of macrophage infiltration of the synovium. Wear particles also were found in the suprapatellar bursa.

Wear particles from artificial ligaments can induce the production of neutral proteinases in vitro. Artificial ligaments should be used cautiously, and materials that minimize enzyme activation by synovial cells should be selected. Particle generation may be minimized by adequate notchplasties and by chamfering ligament drill holes.

▶ This is an excellent study that was awarded the 1988 Cabaud Award by the American Orthopaedic Society for Sports Medicine. The authors point out that, "Further research is needed to determine the effects of wear particles in humans, to investigate the relationship between wear particles and sterile effusions, and to examine the effects of particle size on tissue response."—J.S. Torg, M.D.

Biomechanical Considerations of the Menisci of the Knee
McBride ID, Reid JG (Queen's Univ, Kingston, Ont)
Can J Sport Sci 13:175–187, December 1988   10–94

The menisci of the knee are important structures for maintaining a healthy joint, absorbing shock, and preventing rotatory instability. The C-shaped menisci have firm attachments to the tibial plateaus at their anterior and posterior horns. Pressure on the superior surface of the menisci has both vertical and horizontal components, but pressure on the lower surface acts only vertically (Fig 10–21). The shape of the menisci allows the tibial plateau contact area to be 3 times greater, thus decreasing stress by up to 7 times. The medical and lateral menisci move to different extents because of the variable laxities of the adjacent ligaments.

In 1 study 69% of meniscal damage was sustained during sporting ac-

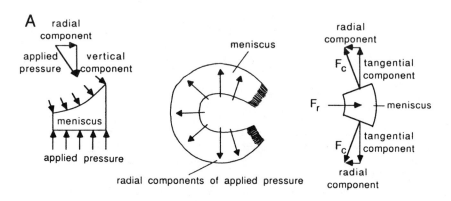

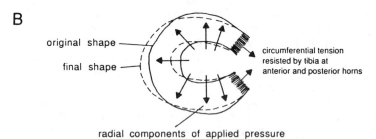

Fig 10–21.—**A**, directions of pressures that act on the meniscus. On the **left** is vertical cross-section of a meniscus indicating that the applied pressures acting on the upper surface have both radial and vertical components, whereas the pressure on the lower surface acts only in the vertical direction. The **middle** diagram shows a superior view of a meniscus and the radial components of pressure that act outwardly. The diagram on the **right** shows that the radial components acting outwardly *(F_r)* are offset by the radial components of the circumferential tension *(F_c)*, which act inwardly. The tangential components of F_c offset each other. **B**, a superior view of a meniscus showing deformation with an applied load, direction of the radial components of pressure, and resistance of the circumferential tension at the tibia. (Adapted from Shrive NG, Phil D, O'Connor JJ, et al: *J Clin Orthop* 131:279–287, March–April 1978. From McBride ID, Reid JG: *Can J Sport Sci* 13:175–187, December 1988.)

tivities. Sports with the highest risk to the menisci are those that involve twisting of the knee. Participation in football, basketball, skiing, and baseball result in relatively high incidences of meniscal damage. Approximately 25% of patients either change sports, reduce their sporting activity, or give up sports altogether after meniscectomy. Those who undergo arthroscopic partial meniscectomy tend to return to sport more quickly than those having an open partial meniscectomy. Those who have an open total meniscectomy take longest to return to sports.

The menisci are important to the normal functioning of the knee. As much of the integrity of the meniscus as possible should be maintained during partial meniscectomy. Because meniscectomy may cause adverse effects, including osteoarthritis, increased joint laxity, and other structural changes total meniscectomy should be performed only as a last resort.

▶ This is an excellent review of the subject matter and the interested reader is referred to the original article.—J.S. Torg, M.D.

Discoid Menisci of the Knee: MR Imaging Appearance

Silverman JM, Mink JH, Deutsch AL (Cedars-Sinai Med Ctr, Los Angeles)
Radiology 173:351–354, November 1989   10–95

A discoid meniscus is a symmetric or asymmetric abnormally elongated and tall meniscus. Enlarged menisci can be recognized with magnetic resonance imaging (MRI), but no criteria have been established for MRI diagnosis. Of more than 4,000 knees examined by MRI, 29 were presumed to have discoid menisci based on MRI criteria. The width of the meniscus was measured on coronal images at the midportion of the meniscus body. Coronal images were also used to measure the height of the medial and lateral menisci at the midportion of the periphery of the meniscus. A height differential of 2 mm or more was considered abnormally tall. The meniscus was considered to be discoid when 3 or more contiguous 5-mm thick sagittal sections demonstrated continuity of the meniscus between the anterior and posterior horns (Fig 10–22).

In 28 of 29 cases, the number of sagittal sections on which the anterior and posterior horns connected ranged from 3 to 5. In 27 patients a presumed discoid lateral meniscus was present according to MRI criteria. Of 10 patients who underwent subsequent knee surgery, 9 had the diagnosis confirmed at surgery. The width of the discoid meniscus ranged from 15 mm to 36 mm; 16 had widths ≥ 20 mm. Of 3 discoid menisci shown to be torn at arthroscopy, 2 were seen to be torn at MRI.

Coronal images of a discoid meniscus show a complete meniscus in all sections through the knee. However, an asymmetric discoid meniscus with an enlarged body may demonstrate a wide meniscus body on coronal images, but normal anterior and posterior horns are seen on sagittal images. For this reason it is important to have high-resolution coronal images.

▶ As MR is being used to evaluate knee pathology, criteria are being developed to document pathology. This particular manuscript describing the MR cri-

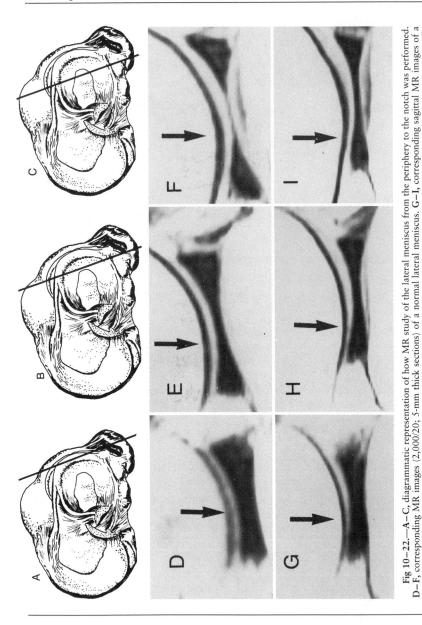

Fig 10–22.—A–C, diagrammatic representation of how MR study of the lateral meniscus from the periphery to the notch was performed. D–F, corresponding MR images (2,000/20; 5-mm thick sections) of a normal lateral meniscus. G–I, corresponding sagittal MR images of a surgically proved discoid lateral meniscus in a 35-year-old man (2,000/20; 5-mm thick sections). The normal lateral meniscus tapers rapidly from the periphery to the free edge (*arrows* in D–F), but the discoid meniscus demonstrates continuity between the anterior and posterior horns on all 3 images (*arrows* in G–I). (Courtesy of Silverman JM, Mink JH, Deutsch AL: *Radiology* 173:351–354, November 1989.)

teria for discoid menisci is extremely limited. The authors defined a discoid meniscus as present if the height differential was 2 mm or greater. In their series, all of the discoid menisci were significantly wider than normal; in fact, most were at least twice the normal width. This definition will limit identification of the discoid meniscus in which the central portion or the inner portion has undergone degeneration and has become flattened. This may explain why only 2 of the 3 discoid lateral menisci identified on MR as being torn and having surgical follow-up were confirmed to be torn. Most probably, the majority of torn degenerative discoid menisci were not recognized on the MR study as being discoid.—J.S. Torg, M.D.

Non-Operative Treatment of Meniscal Tears

Weiss CB, Lundberg M, Hamberg P, DeHaven KE, Gillquist J (Univ of Rochester Med Ctr, NY; Univ Hosp, Linköping, Sweden)
J Bone Joint Surg 71-A:811–822, July 1989   10–96

A selective approach in the treatment of meniscal tears has been adopted, preserving as much meniscal tissue as possible. To identify a subset of clinically stable meniscal tears that can be managed conservatively, the results of 3,612 arthroscopic procedures, performed in treatment of acute or chronic meniscal lesions (with or without an associated ligamentous lesion), were reviewed. Eighty meniscal tears in 75 patients were assumed stable based on clinical judgment. There were 70 longitudinal tears, including 52 lateral and 18 medial meniscal lesions. Ten were vertical radial lesions, and all involved the lateral meniscus.

Fifty-two patients were followed for 2–10 years; only 6 needed additional intervention because of symptoms unrelated to the meniscal tear. Repeat arthroscopy was performed on 32 patients at an average of 26 months after initial arthroscopy; 26 had longitudinal tears, and 6 had radial tears. Seventeen longitudinal tears healed completely. Five radial tears showed no evidence of healing and 1 had extended. Neither chronic ligamentous laxity nor a meniscal tear precluded healing of the stable longitudinal tears. No localized degenerative changes were found in the adjacent articular cartilage in any of the stable vertical longitudinal or radial meniscal lesions. Except for the 6 who had additional surgical treatment, none of the patients reported symptoms of a meniscal lesion. None of the 42 patients who were reexamined 2 years or more after the operation had signs of a meniscal lesion.

Stable vertical longitudinal tears, especially in the vascular outer area of the meniscus, have great potential for healing. The tear should be left alone unless no other lesions are present and there is sufficient disability to warrant treatment. Stable radial tears have little potential for healing, but their management could not be established.

▶ This is a excellent paper, and the authors' position that certain stable vertical tears will heal without suture is well taken. They point out that a stable knee is not necessarily a prerequisite for the healing of a torn but stable meniscus. This appears to put the horse before the cart. That is, in the face of anterior cruciate ligament instability, although healing may occur the proper mechanics are such that the meniscus remains vulnerable to reinjury. Thus a more practical point is that the peripheral vertical tear in the meniscus may be ignored when a concomitant cruciate ligament injury is restabilized.—J.S. Torg, M.D.

Arthroscopy Under Local Anaesthesia

Buckley JR, Hood GM, Macrae W (Royal Infirmary, Dundee, Scotland)
J Bone Joint Surg 71-B:126–127, January 1989   10–97

Spinal anesthesia and epidural anesthesia provide satisfactory conditions for knee operations, but they are unsuitable for outpatients. Another method that may provide satisfactory operating conditions and has high patient acceptability is anesthesia with midazolam, 2 mg administered through an intravenous cannula.

Technique.—The surgeon uses an indelible pen to mark the entry portals on the skin. After preparation with iodine, each portal is widely infiltrated from skin to synovium using 5 mL of prilocaine 0.5% with 1:200,000 epinephrine. Needle aspiration is used to withdraw any effusion. Prilocaine and epinephrine are then injected into the joint through this needle. During the 15-minute wait for the anesthesia to take effect, the knee is flexed and extended several times. During the procedure, patients are observed and pulse and blood pressure are monitored. Surgeons use the normal arthroscopic technique but without a tourniquet.

At follow-up 60 outpatients in whom the procedure was used were asked whether they would choose the same form of anesthesia again. Six donated blood for serial plasma prilocaine estimation. The view of the surgical site was satisfactory in all cases; in 3 patients blood was flushed away with saline without loss of anesthesia. There were problems when a standard portal was close to a previous arthrotomy scar. In such cases the surgeon should use an alternative portal. It was possible to examine the knee preoperatively for locking and for laxity of the cruciate ligaments but not of the collateral ligaments. It was also possible to differentiate between intracapsular and extracapsular causes of pain. Stiff or painful hips in 3 patients made manipulation of the leg difficult. Operating time ranged from 10 to 72 minutes, and the duration of anesthesia was satisfactory in all cases. Only 3 patients had unsatisfactory anesthesia and required general anesthesia; of the remainder, 53 were satisfied with the anesthetic used. Of 25 patients who previously had a general anesthetic, 24 preferred this technique.

Anesthesia with intra-articular injection of prilocaine and epinephrine is simple, safe, effective, and well tolerated by patients undergoing arthroscopy of the knee. Possible contraindications include stiff and painful hips, multiple arthrotomy, and excessive anxiety.

▶ We have reported a retrospective review of 500 cases of surgical arthroscopy performed under local anesthesia that delineates the efficacy of this technique (1). On the basis of our experience, it is concluded that all arthroscopic procedures of the knee performed under general anesthesia can be carried out successfully with lidocaine and intravenous sedation. This article stresses meticulous attention to technical details by the surgeon as well as patient relaxation and cooperation, which are maximized by some form of intravenous sedation in minimal therapeutic dosage. Also, arthroscopic surgical procedures performed in this manner allow the patient to be discharged from the ambulatory surgery facility significantly earlier than when general anesthesia is used.—J.S. Torg, M.D.

Reference

1. Yacobucci G, et al: *Arthroscopy.* In press.

Intraarticular Bupivacaine (Marcaine) After Arthroscopic Meniscectomy: A Randomized Double-Blind Controlled Study

Chirwa SS, MacLeod BA, Day B (Univ of British Columbia, Vancouver)
Arthroscopy 5:33–35, 1989   10–98

To determine whether bupivacaine can be used safely to reduce pain after arthroscopic meniscectomy, 79 otherwise healthy patients undergoing meniscectomy were given bupivacaine intra-articularly or placebo in a randomized, double-blind study. A 20-mL volume of normal saline or 0.25% bupivacaine was injected into the synovial cavity of the knee before application of the dressing.

Bupivacaine did not alter the heart rate or blood pressure. Pain was significantly reduced by the intra-articular administration of bupivacaine. The amount of supplemental morphine needed was significantly reduced, and the need for the initial dose of morphine was delayed. Acetaminophen requirements were not altered by bupivacaine administration. No adverse effects were noted.

Intra-articular administration of 0.25% bupivacaine at the end of arthroscopic meniscectomy minimizes pain without significant toxic effects.

▶ It should be pointed out that bupivacaine (Marcaine), as demonstrated in this study, is relatively benign when injected intra-articularly. However, inadvertent intravenous injection can result in cardiovascular collapse. Also to be questioned is the necessity of supplemental morphine for postoperative pain after arthroscopic meniscectomy.—J.S. Torg, M.D.

The Role of Arthroscopy in Children and Adolescents

Angel KR, Hall DJ (Adelaide Children's Hosp, North Adelaide, South Australia)
Arthroscopy 5:192–196, 1989   10–99

In the largest reported series of arthroscopies in children and adolescents, 212 procedures were performed in 192 patients who were followed for an average of 6 months. Pain was the most frequent presenting symptom, followed by swelling, giving way, locking, and inability to bear weight. Effusion was the most common clinical abnormality, followed by a restricted range of motion. Only 6 of 32 clinically normal joints were normal on arthroscopy. The activity most often responsible for injury was Australian football.

The most common arthroscopic finding in adolescents was an anterior cruciate ligament (ACL) tear. More than half of these injuries were partial tears, and most of the rest were complete midsubstance tears, followed by meniscal tears, chondromalacia patellae, and osteochondritis dissecans. A wide range of synovial disorders was encountered; 10 patients had septic arthritis. The average time until return to full activity was 4 weeks. The only complication of arthroscopy was hemarthrosis after an open lateral release.

Arthroscopy is an accurate and safe means of diagnosing and treating various disorders in children and adolescents. It is recommended when a joint is too painful to be adequately examined clinically, when ACL injury is suspected after acute patellar dislocation and in all hemarthroses. Arthroscopy also is indicated for the drainage and lavage of septic joints.

▶ This paper has 2 problems. First, the authors report an average follow-up of 6 months (range, less than 1 to 50 months). The length of follow-up in the majority of the patients appears to be too brief. Combining a population that consists of 11 patients younger than 5 years, 38 patients between 5 and 11 years, and 156 patients between 12 and 18 years appears to result in an oranges, apples, pineapples hodgepodge. This report does support Bergstrom et al. (1) Morrissy et al. (2), and Ziv and Carroll (3) in finding that arthroscopy is a ". . . safe and valuable diagnostic and therapeutic procedure for joint pathology and children and adolescents." Also to be noted, the authors found arthroscopy in children to be technically easier than in adults because of the more compliant nature of the joints. Also, procedures were performed with the standard 5-mm arthroscope as in adults.—J.S. Torg, M.D.

References

1. Bergstrom R, et al: *J Pediatr Orthop* 4:542, 1984.
2. Morrissy RT, et al: *Clin Orthop* 162:103, 1982.
3. Ziv I, Carroll NC: *J Pediatr Orthop* 2:243, 1982.

Lateral Discoid Menisci in Children
Bellier G, Dupont J-Y, Larrain M, Caudron C, Carlioz H (Marais Clinic; Trousseau Hosp, Paris)
Arthroscopy 5:52–56, 1989   10–100

Arthroscopy was used to treat 19 lateral discoid menisci in 16 children whose average age was 10.5 years. The average time from the initial symptoms to treatment was 6 months. The most frequent symptoms were a snapping or locking sensation and episodes of locking with loss of hyperextension; most patients had lateral pain. Radiographically, 12 knees were normal. Arthrography confirmed a complete lateral discoid meniscus in 4 of 5 patients. Arthroscopy was performed under general anesthesia. A 4-mm scope was used in children older than 5 years.

There were 14 complete and 5 incomplete lateral discoid menisci; 12 of the menisci were torn, 8 of them completely. Central partial meniscectomy was the usual approach to complete lateral discoid menisci. The incomplete menisci were managed by partial meniscectomy. Excellent results were obtained in all knees but 1 on observation for up to 3 years. Two second-look arthroscopies performed 1 year after treatment showed that the remaining lateral meniscus appeared normal, but hypermobility of the posterior horn persisted.

Arthroscopic treatment of meniscal malformations allows relatively rapid rehabilitation. Partial meniscectomy is appropriate for a complete discoid meniscus or a posterior megahorn. A full tear of the meniscus necessitates total lateral arthroscopic meniscectomy.

▶ The authors report 94% excellent results with a maximum follow-up of 3 years. It would have been preferable if follow-up was reported in terms of the mean and range. That is, what was minimal follow-up: a week, a month, a year? Certainly, a real long-term follow-up on this group would be most enlightening. For example, what did this group look like after a minimal follow-up of 4 years?—J.S. Torg, M.D.

Arthroscopic Treatment of the Discoid Lateral Meniscus: Results of Long-Term Follow-up
Vandermeer RD, Cunningham FK (Univ of Texas, Dallas; Baylor Univ, Dallas)
Arthroscopy 5:101–109, 1989   10–101

Arthroscopy was used to treat discoid lateral meniscus syndrome in 25 knees of 22 patients who were followed for an average of 54 months. Discoid lateral menisci were classified arthroscopically as incomplete (92%) and complete (8%) (Fig 10–23); no Wrisberg-type lesions were found. Symptomatic torn discoid menisci in 20 knees were managed by partial lateral meniscectomy using the saucerization technique; 3 knees with other significant symptomatic lesions were treated similarly, and asymptomatic intact discoid menisci in 2 knees were left alone.

An excellent or good outcome was achieved in 11 of the 20 knees with a symptomatic torn discoid lateral meniscus, whereas the outcome was poor in 3. Nearly two thirds of the patients regained their former activity level; several of these were athletes. Repeated arthroscopy in 3 patients with a good clinical result showed no lateral compartment degeneration. In all, 64% of the patients resumed a normal level of activity postoperatively.

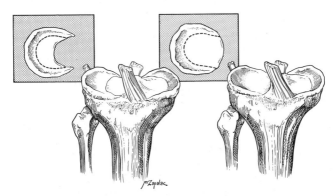

Fig 10–23.—Incomplete *(left)* and complete discoid lateral menisci. The saucerization method of partial meniscectomy removes the central portion of the discoid lesion *(inserts)*. (Courtesy of Vandermeer RD, Cunningham FK: *Arthroscopy* 5:101–109, 1989.)

Torn discoid lateral menisci and other symptomatic lesions do well with an individualized arthroscopic approach. Saucerization of a torn lateral discoid meniscus is warranted even if it does not clearly produce symptoms. If there is not tear or instability, reaction is not necessary.

▶ Although the authors report 15% poor results, it is interesting to note that 28% of the series underwent arthroscopic reevaluation for significant new or recurrent symptoms.—J.S. Torg, M.D.

Cysts of the Lateral Meniscus: Arthroscopy Versus Arthroscopy Plus Open Cystectomy
Reagan WD, McConkey JP, Loomer RL, Davidson RG (Univ of British Columbia, Vancouver)
Arthroscopy 5:274–281, 1989   10–102

Despite extensive studies, the optimal treatment for lateral meniscal cysts has not yet been defined. Furthermore, there remain some unresolved questions about the etiology of meniscal cysts and their role in the production of associated meniscal tears. A retrospective study was done to further examine the etiology and pathogenesis of lateral meniscal cysts and to define the optimal treatment for this condition.

A questionnaire was mailed to 20 men and 11 women (mean age, 28 years) who had undergone operation between 1977 and 1985 on 32 knees; all had a lateral meniscal cyst, with or without a concomitant lateral meniscal tear. Conservative treatment had failed in all 31 patients, leading to arthroscopy with or without open cystectomy. None of the patients had evidence of concomitant instability. The average time from injury to knee arthroscopy was 3 years (range, 8 months to 6 years). The average time from arthroscopy to follow-up was almost 3½ years (range, 18 to 72 months).

Diagnostic arthroscopy revealed meniscal tears in 84% of the knees. In 20 knees the cyst was removed by arthroscopic partial meniscectomy and open extra-articular cystectomy, whereas the other 12 cysts were managed by arthroscopy and partial meniscectomy without cystectomy. Subjective time to functional recovery averaged 19 weeks (range, 6 weeks to 2 years). Subjective results were rated as excellent in 13 knees (41%), good in 9 (28%), fair in 4 (12%), and poor in 6 (19%). Patients who underwent extra-articular cystectomy had an 80% good to excellent result, whereas those who did not have cystectomy had only a 50% good to excellent result.

The observed pathology ranged from large meniscal tears with minimal cyst formation to large cysts with no demonstrable meniscal tear. It is theorized that a meniscal tear begins in the meniscus and spreads through the periphery, or that the lesion starts as a compression injury to the vascular periphery and either spreads centrally, producing a meniscus tear, or spreads peripherally, producing a cyst, or both.

The recommended treatment sequence is to start by searching arthroscopically for a lateral meniscal tear, especially in the peripheral region. If no tear is found, extra-articular cystectomy is done. If a lateral meniscal tear is found, all unstable meniscal fragments should be removed, leaving a rim, if possible, especially adjacent to the popliteus recess, before proceeding to open cystectomy.

▶ The authors point out that lateral meniscal cysts present as lateral knee pain and/or a mass that may be difficult to diagnose. Interestingly, 16% of the cysts occurred without arthroscopically visible meniscal lesions. Trauma appears to be responsible for most of the lesions. When conservative treatment fails, surgical management is recommended.—J.S. Torg, M.D.

The Effect of Lateral Meniscectomy on Motion of the Knee
Levy IM, Torzilli PA, Gould JD, Warren RF (Hosp for Special Surgery, New York)
J Bone Joint Surg 71-A:401–406, March 1989   10–103

The effect of lateral meniscectomy on displacement of the tibia relative to the femur in an unloaded knee before and after section of the anterior cruciate ligament (ACL) and medial meniscectomy was studied. A 5-degrees-of-freedom mechanical testing device was used to measure translations and rotations of the knee that resulted from applied anterior and posterior forces, internal and external torques, and varus and vagus moments. Eleven intact fresh-frozen knees of cadavers were tested. After evaluation of the intact knee, either the ACL was cut or the lateral meniscus was excised, and the tests were repeated.

Lateral meniscectomy did not affect primary anterior and posterior translations. When both lateral meniscectomy and resection of the ACL were performed, anterior translation did not differ from that found after section of the ACL alone. However, when the means of the paired differences in anterior translation were compared, there was a significant difference. After excision of the medial meniscus and section of the ACL, medial meniscectomy resulted in significantly more anterior translation.

In contrast to the medial meniscus, the lateral meniscus does not serve as an efficient posterior wedge to resist anterior translation of the tibia on the femur. In knees that lack an ACL, the lateral meniscus is subject to forces different from those occurring on the medial side. These findings may explain the various patterns of injury of the lateral and the medial meniscus in knees without an ACL.

▶ The authors' apparent lack of familiarity with my initial description (1) of the "doorstopper effect" of the medial meniscus is somewhat disconcerting. We trust that they have been more diligent in laboratory efforts than they have been in their literature review.—J.S. Torg, M.D.

Reference

1. Torg JS: *Am J Sports Med* 4:84, 1976.

Review of Previous Classification Symptoms of Articular Cartilage

AUTHOR	SURFACE DESCRIPTION OF ARTICULAR CARTILAGE	DIAMETER	LOCATION
Outerbridge	I - softening and swelling II - fragmentation and fissuring III - fragmentation and fissuring IV - erosion of cartilage down to bone	I - none II - < 1/2" III - > 1/2 " IV - none	Starts most frequently on medial facet of patella; later extends to lateral facet "mirror" lesion on intercondylar area of femoral condyles; upper border medial femoral condyle.
Hungerford and Ficat	I - Closed chondromalacia. Simple softening (small blister) macroscopically, surface is intact, varying degrees of severity from simple softening to "pitting edema", loss of elasticity.	I - 1 cm² and then extends progressively in all directions.	lateral facet - 2° excessive lateral pressure

	II. Open chondromalacia.
	  a. Fissures - single or multiple, relatively superficial or extending down to subchondral bone.
	  b. Ulceration - localized loss of cartilage substance, exposes dense subchondral bone. When extensive, bone has polished appearance (eburnated).
		II - none	medial facet - 2° incongruence and combination of compression and shearing forces

	Chondrosclerosis - abnormally hard, not depressible.		
	Tuft formation - multiple deep fronds of cartilage separated from one another by deep clefts which extend to subchondral bone.	Not localized but involves entire contact zone	Centered on crest separating medial and odd facets.
	Superficial surface changes - surface fibrillation; longitudinal striations present in the axis of movement of the joint.		

	Grading	Measurement	Location
Bentley	I - fibrillation or fissuring II - fibrillation or fissuring III - fibrillation or fissuring IV - fibrillation with or without exposure of subchondral bone	I - <.5 cm II - .5 - 1.0 cm III - 1.0 - 2.0 cm IV - > 2.0 cm	Most common at junction of medial and odd facets of patella
Casscells	I - superficial area of erosion II - deeper layers of cartilage involved III - cartilage is completely eroded and bone is exposed IV - articular cartilage completely destroyed	I - < or = 1 cm II - 1 - 2 cm III - 2 - 4 cm IV - "wide area"	Patella and anterior femoral surfaces.
Insall	I - swelling and softening of cartilage (closed chondromalacia) II - deep fissures extending to subchondral bone III - fibrillation IV - erosive changes and exposures of subchondral bone (osteoarthrosis)	None	I - IV: midpoint of patellar crest with extension equally onto medial and lateral patellar facets. IV: also involves opposite or mirror surface of femur. Upper and lower 1/3 nearly always spared (patella); femur never severe.
Goodfellow	Surface degeneration - surface flaking progressing to fibrillation. Basilar degeneration - fasciculation of collagen in the middle and deep zones, without at first, affecting the surface. - fasciculation (1) - articular surface is smoothly intact; spongy consistency; exhibits "pitting edema" - blister - fasciculation (11) - rupture of tangential surface fibers.	1 cm	"Odd" facet of patella Inferior part of central ridge separating medial and lateral facets.

(Courtesy of Noyes FR, Stabler CL: *Am J Sports Med* 17:505–513, July–August 1989.)

A System for Grading Articular Cartilage Lesions at Arthroscopy

Noyes FR, Stabler CL (Cincinnati Sportsmedicine Ctr; Deaconess Hosp Ctr, Cincinnati)

Am J Sports Med 17:505–513, July–August 1989   10–104

Several systems have been devised to describe and categorize articular cartilage damage (table). However, each system has certain limitations and deficiencies that can lead to confusion. A classification system was designed based on 4 separate and distinct variables—description of the articular surface, extent (depth) of involvement, diameter of lesion, and location.

The articular surface is described as a smooth and intact, closed lesion (grade 1); damaged, open lesion (grade 2); or bone exposed (grade 3). Each grade is divided into subtypes, A or B, depending on the depth of involvement. Grade 1 is characterized as either soft (type 1A) or loss of resilience (type 1B). Grade II is based on surface damage either less than one-half thickness (type 2A) or at least one-half thickness (type 2B) of the cartilage. Grade III depends on whether the subchondral bone has a normal contour (type 3A) or shows evidence of cavitation with actual loss of bone (type 3B). The diameter of the lesion is recorded at 5-mm intervals from less than 10 mm to more than 25 mm. The location of the lesion on the femur and tibia, as well as on the patella, is noted. The degree of knee flexion also is recorded for patellofemoral lesions.

Although somewhat qualitative and subjective, the system enables the surgeon to record observed articular cartilage changes during initial and subsequent arthroscopies. The system helps to compare treatment results between different studies. For research, a point scaling system facilitates computerization and statistical analysis of data.

▶ The authors present what appears to be the most comprehensive and workable classification of articular cartilage lesions. It is difficult, however, to determine whether this newly proposed classification will clarify the matter at hand or only tend to confuse an already overcrowded field.—J.S. Torg, M.D.

The Use of the Contact Nd:YAG Laser in Arthroscopic Surgery: Effects on Articular Cartilage and Meniscal Tissue

Miller DV, O'Brien SJ, Arnoczky SS, Kelly A, Fealy SV, Warren RF (Hosp for Special Surgery, New York)

Arthroscopy 5:245–253, 1989   10–105

The technologic advances within the field of arthroscopy have generated a proliferation of new devices for cutting and dissecting. Because of its small size, safety, fiberoptic delivery, ability to function in a saline medium, and precise cutting ability, the contact neodynium:yttrium/aluminum/garnet (Nd:YAG) may be useful in arthroscopic surgery. A 3-part study compared the effects of the Nd:YAG laser, electrocautery, and the scalpel in arthroscopic procedures.

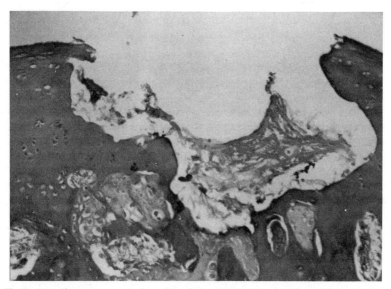

Fig 10–24.—Electrocautery articular cartilage lesion (20 W at 2 weeks). Note wide margin of necrosis along hyaline cartilage and into subchondral bone with necrotic debris and carbonized tissue remaining within the defect. (Courtesy of Miller DV, O'Brien SJ, Arnoczky SS, et al: *Arthroscopy* 5:245–253, 1989.)

The depth of damage of the Nd:YAG laser, electrocautery, and a scalpel to cartilage and menisci was compared in 6 fresh-frozen canine cadaver knees. Three knees were exposed to air and 3 knees were submerged in a saline bath during the laser cutting procedure. The depth of damage using Nd:YAG laser energy varied proportionately with power. At each wattage level the depth of damage was greater in meniscal tissue than in articular cartilage. Saline solution significantly decreased the depth of damage at each wattage level.

Bilateral knee arthrotomies were then done in 24 adult white rabbits to compare the response of articular cartilage lesions made with the Nd:YAG laser, electrocautery, and a scalpel. The Nd:YAG laser was used in 12 knees, an electrosurgical meniscal probe was used in another 12 knees, and a scalpel was used in the 24 contralateral knees. Electrocautery lesions uniformly showed significant wide margins of hyaline cartilage necrosis, which increased over time. By 12 weeks there was a limited healing response after electrocautery at wattage levels of less than 20 W (Fig 10–24). In contrast, laser articular cartilage lesions showed vigorous healing responses by 6 weeks. Scalpel defects showed only minimal response over time.

Sixteen rabbits underwent meniscectomies with the Nd:YAG laser, electrocautery, or a scalpel. Scalpel meniscectomy exhibited characteristic remodeling of the meniscus by 12 weeks. Meniscectomies by electrocautery showed wide margins of necrosis with no evidence of any remodeling. Laser meniscectomies showed an intermediate response, with 2 remodeling in 2 specimens observed after 6 weeks and viable cells in the meniscal edge in 2 other specimens. These initial findings are encouraging, as the Nd:YAG laser appears to have important biologic advantages over scalpel and electrocautery in arthroscopic surgery.

▶ It has been said that with regard to arthroscopic surgery, the laser is a treatment looking for a disease.—J.S. Torg, M.D.

Meniscus Suture Techniques: A Comparative Biomechanical Cadaver Study
Kohn D, Siebert W (Hannover Med School, Hannover, West Germany)
Arthroscopy 5:324–327, 1989   10–106

Several suture techniques are available to repair peripheral longitudinal meniscus tears. Independent of which suture technique is used, a high percentage of meniscus lesions heal properly after suturing. The primary stability of 4 different commonly used suture techniques was compared in the repair of meniscus tears.

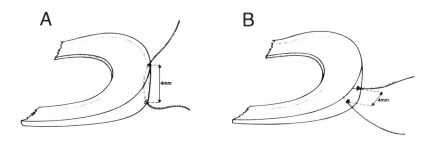

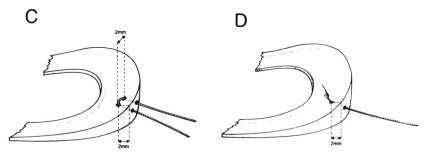

Fig 10–25.—**A,** vertical meniscus suture according to Wirth CJ, et al. **B,** horizontal suture according to Hamberg P, et al. **C,** horizontal suture involving the meniscus surface according to Jakob RP, et al. **D,** knot-end technique according to Morgan and Casscells. (Courtesy of Kohn D, Siebert W: *Arthroscopy* 5:324–327, 1989.)

The study material consisted of 20 macroscopically intact human medial menisci harvested within 24 hours of death. The specimens were randomly divided into 4 groups. Two open vertical and horizontal and 2 arthroscopic (horizontal mattress and knot end) suturing techniques were evaluated (Fig 10–25). The tensile properties of the 4 suture techniques were tested on an Instron Tensometer, Model 1122.

Primary stability differed significantly among the 4 suture techniques tested. Of the 2 open suturing techniques the vertical was more stable than the horizontal. Of the 2 arthroscopic techniques the horizontal mattress suture was superior to the knot-end technique. However, high primary stability of the suture is only 1 aspect contributing to the final outcome of meniscal repair. Nevertheless, a lower rerupture rate can be anticipated when better primary stability is achieved.

▶ In the first group of menisci a vertical suture was performed using an open technique with absorbable atraumatic suture material (2–0 Vicryl, U-R-6 needle), whereas in the second group an open horizontal technique was employed using the same suture-needle combination. However, in the third group a horizontal mattress suture using 2–0 Ethibond was used arthroscopically, and in the fourth group, O-PDS sutures were inserted arthroscopically through 18-gauge spinal needles. The authors' failure to factor the variation in the suture materials and needles into their analysis precludes any conclusion regarding the relative merits of the various techniques.—J.S. Torg, M.D.

Open Meniscus Repair: Technique and Two to Nine Year Results
DeHaven KE, Black KP, Griffiths HJ (Univ of Rochester, NY)
Am J Sports Med 17:788–795, November–December 1989   10–107

Excision rather than repair has long been the accepted treatment for a torn meniscus. Meniscectomy continues to be the primary treatment for peripheral lesions not associated with collateral ligament rupture. The intermediate-term results of open repair of acute and chronic peripheral meniscus tears were evaluated.

Between 1976 and 1983, 92 patients aged 12–40 years underwent repair of peripheral meniscus tears in 104 knees. Follow-up data were available on 80 repairs in 74 patients. Thirty-nine repairs were done in the acute stage and 41 in the chronic stage. Thirty-three of the 34 patients who underwent repair of an acute anterior cruciate ligament (ACL) tear and 21 of the 41 who underwent repair at the chronic stage had associated acute ruptures of the ACL. Forty-four patients with 49 repairs were evaluated by a return clinic visit during which they completed a questionnaire and had a physical examination including knee arthrometer measurements with the KT-1000 and radiographic examination consisting of standing anteroposterior views of both knees in extension and 45 degrees of flexion. The other 30 patients responded to the questionnaire alone.

During an average follow-up of 4.6 years, 9 of the 80 repaired menisci (11%) tore again. The interval between repair and retear ranged from 6 to 34 months. Seven retears occurred in chronic tears and 2 occurred in acute tears. Three of the 9 retears occurred through the repair zone and required meniscectomy because of extensive damage to the body of the meniscus. Retear in the other 6 cases occurred at different sites; the original repair sites were well healed at reoperation. Retears occurred in 1 of 26 isolated repairs, 2 of 38 repairs done with ACL stabilization, and 6 of 16 repairs done in ACL-deficient knees that were not stabilized. Standing radiographs showed normal compartments in 40 of the 41 repairs.

In view of the well-reported significant incidence of degenerative changes after meniscectomy in the treatment of a torn meniscus, and the satisfactory results obtained to date with open repair, retention and repair of the meniscus is highly recommended.

▶ The authors report that meniscus repair in the face of ACL deficiency results in 40% of retorn menisci. On the other hand, the failure rate in patients whose ACLs were stabilized was the same as that in those with the ligament intact. The authors note that these results have led many to state that meniscus repair must never be performed without stabilization in the ACL-deficient knee. Their position is that 62% of cases continue to do well, but each must be considered individually. My interpretation of these figures would suggest that meniscal repair of the ACL-deficient knee should not be performed unless concomitant ACL reconstruction also is done.—J.S. Torg, M.D.

The Popliteus Tendon

Tria AJ, Johnson CD, Zawadsky JP (Univ of Medicine and Dentistry of New Jersey Robert Wood Johnson Med School, New Brunswick)
J Bone Joint Surg 71-A:714–716, June 1989   10–108

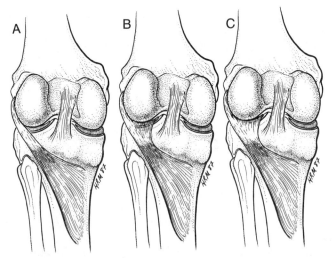

Fig 10–26.—Insertions of the popliteus tendon. **A,** isolated insertion into the lateral femoral condyle. **B,** insertion into the lateral femoral condyle, with translucent attachment to lateral meniscus. **C,** dual insertion into the lateral femoral condyle and lateral meniscus. (Courtesy of Tria AJ, Johnson CD, Zawadsky JP: *J Bone Joint Surg* 71-A:714–716, June 1989.)

The posterior aspects of 40 cadaver knees were dissected to determine the proximal insertion of the popliteus tendon, particularly its relationship to the lateral meniscus. In 45% of specimens there was an isolated insertion of the popliteus tendon to the lateral femoral condyle (Fig 10–26). Another 37.5% of specimens had both an attachment to the lateral femoral condyle and a filmy attachment to the lateral meniscus. Seven specimens (17.5%) had strong attachments to both the femoral condyle and lateral meniscus. These findings make it unlikely that the popliteus muscle helps to protect the lateral meniscus.

Anatomy of the Posterior Cruciate Ligament: A Review
Van Dommelen BA, Fowler PJ (Univ Hosp, London, Ont)
Am J Sports Med 17:24–29, January–February 1989   10–109

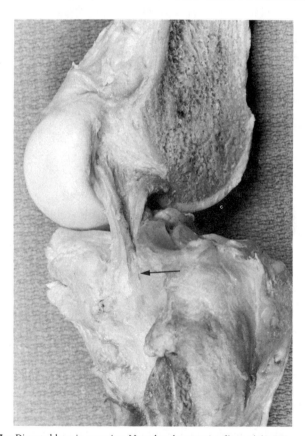

Fig 10–27.—Dissected knee in extension. Note that the posterior fibers of the PCL are taut and the anterior fibers are lax. Also, the posterior meniscofemoral ligament is originating from the tibia and not the lateral meniscus *(arrow)*. (Courtesy of Van Dommelen BA, Fowler PJ: *Am J Sports Med* 17:24–29, January–February 1989.)

Injuries to the posterior cruciate ligament (PCL) are estimated to be increasing. The anatomy of the PCL was reviewed in an attempt to determine a cause for the apparent increase in injuries to this structure and to find the best treatment approach.

The PCL attaches anteriorly in the femoral notch on the medial femoral condyle. It attaches to the tibia in a depression in the posterior tibia between the 2 tibial plateaus about 1 cm below the tibial surface. The fibers attach to the tibia in a medial to lateral direction and to the femur in a posterior to anterior direction. Medial fibers from the tibia insert posteriorly on the femur, whereas the lateral fibers insert anteriorly (Fig 10−27). The PCL provides up to 95% of the total restraint to posterior displacement of the tibia on the femur. Portions of the PCL are taut at different times between full extension and full flexion, contributing to the "screw-home mechanism" of the knee as it goes from flexion to extension. The anatomy of the meniscofemoral ligaments indicates the intimate relationship among the PCL, the popliteus muscle, and the lateral meniscus.

An understanding of PCL anatomy is important in the diagnosis and treatment of ligamentous injuries. It is also necessary in the performance of total knee arthroplasty.

► These 2 papers by Tria et al. (Abstract 10–108) and Van Dommelen et al. (Abstract 10–109) present subtle but interesting anatomical nuances that should be of interest to the knee surgeon.—J.S. Torg, M.D.

Popliteus Tendinitis, A New Perspective
Allen ME, Ray G (Simon Fraser Univ, Burnaby, BC)
Sports Training Med Rehab 1:219−226, October 1989   10−110

Diagnostic criteria for distinguishing popliteal tendinitis from the more common running injury, iliotibial band friction syndrome (TBS) are unclear. A posterior view of the knee shows the popliteus muscle having origins in the lateral condyle and the arcuate ligament, as well as in the lateral meniscus, posterior cruciate, posterior capsule, and ligaments of Winslow and Wrisburg (Fig 10−28). The popliteal muscle/tendon unit (PMTU) is active during most of flexion, with its main functions being internal rotation of the tibia, retraction of the lateral meniscus during flexion and internal rotation, prevention of forward displacement of the femur on the tibia when the foot is fixed, and tightening of the posterior capsule.

Some runners rotate the tibia externally during the swing phase, which may reflect a weak PMTU. These runners report lateral knee pain, but the problem has not previously been related to the swing phase. The injury mechanics of ITBS and popliteal tendinitis are similar. The causes include downhill running, increasing distance, overstriding, and overpronation as a result of foot malalignment or wearing improper shoes. Tenderness in the popliteal fossa or at any of the origins of the popliteus muscle may suggest a PMTU injury, but identifying the specific location

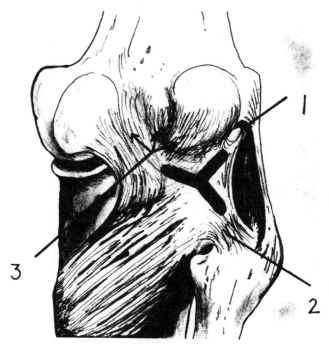

Fig 10–28.—Drawing of posterior knee showing popliteus muscle with its 3 origins: lateral condylar origin *(1)*; fibular head origin, sometimes called arcuate ligament *(2)*; and origin at lateral meniscus, posterior cruciate, posterior capsule, and ligaments of Winslow and Wrisburg *(3)*. (Courtesy of Allen ME, Ray G: *Sports Training Med Rehab* 1:219–226, October 1989.)

may be difficult in a patient with generalized knee pain. Disorders of the PMTU may also be related to elevated compartment pressure readings.

A simple test of the popliteus includes flexing the knee, resisting active internal rotation, palpation (Fig 10–29, p 390), and "listening" for discomfort. Treatment for ITBS and PMTU are similar: application of ice, modified rest, anti-inflammatory drug therapy, and ultrasound. If it can be demonstrated that PMTU disorders are related to elevated compartment pressure readings, resistant forms may be treated by surgical release of the compartment's fascia.

The etiology, clinical manifestations, and treatment of ITBS and PMTU disorders are similar and current diagnostic techniques may not clearly distinguish the pathologic diagnosis. Further research is suggested to address this problem.

▶ On the basis of my own clinical experience, I fully agree with the authors that popliteus tendinitis is in all probability a "common injury" and for the most part is misdiagnosed. The point is well taken that the diagnostic criteria are far from clear for distinguishing popliteus tendinitis from the more common injury called iliotibial band friction syndrome. This diagnosis certainly should be part of the differential when evaluating athletes with lateral knee pain.—J.S. Torg, M.D.

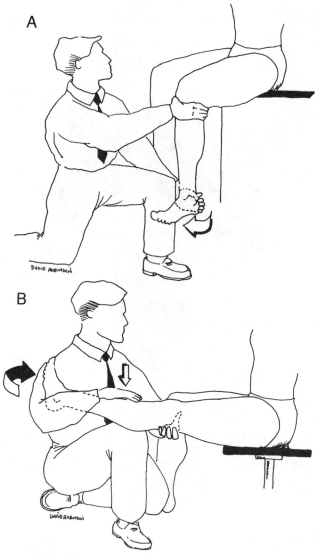

Fig 10–29.—Positions for testing PMTU. **A**, knee bent, resisted internal rotation; **B**, knee extended, resisted internal rotation, palpate for popliteus tenderness. (Courtesy of Allen ME, Ray G: *Sports Training Med Rehab* 1:219–226, October 1989.)

Popliteal Artery Entrapment: An Evolving Syndrome

Collins PS, McDonald PT, Lim RC (Uniformed Services Univ of the Health Sciences, San Francisco and Oakland; Univ of California, San Francisco)
J Vasc Surg 10:484–490, November 1989   10–111

Popliteal artery entrapment can result in calf and foot claudication and limb-threatening ischemia in otherwise healthy young adults. Preestab-

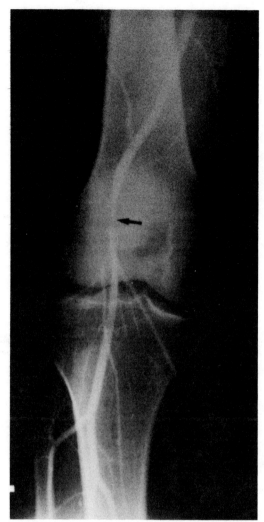

Fig 10–30.—Selective left leg arteriogram with leg in active plantar flexion. *Arrow* marks compression of popliteal artery. (Courtesy of Collins PS, McDonald PT, Lim RC: *J Vasc Surg* 10:484–490, November 1989.)

lished noninvasive and arteriographic criteria were used to establish the diagnosis of popliteal artery entrapment in symptomatic patients.

All patients were examined by Doppler ultrasonography of the posterior tibial artery and the dorsal artery of the foot at the ankle. An ankle-brachial index (ABI) was established for each patient. Patients who had normal ABIs performed a treadmill test of increasing difficulty until symptoms recurred and ABIs decreased. Patients with diminished ABIs at rest and with exercise underwent standard aortic, pelvic, and runoff arteriography. If the films showed no lesion to account for the symptoms, contrast-enhanced biplanar arteriography was obtained with the feet in a neutral position, passively dorsiflexed, and actively plantar flexed (Figs 10–30 and 10–31). Both legs were imaged to determine the incidence of bilateral disease.

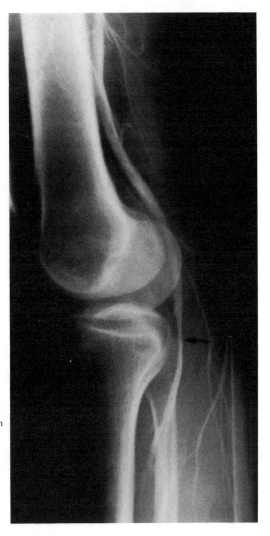

Fig 10–31.—Biplanar arteriogram (lateral view) of left leg in active plantar flexion. *Arrow* marks compression of the popliteal artery. (Courtesy of Collins PS, McDonald PT, Lim RC: *J Vasc Surg* 10:484–490, November 1989.)

Ten men and 2 women had popliteal artery entrapment. All but 1 patient was younger than age 40 years. All complained of calf pain, and 2 had foot pain on ambulation. One patient had acute occlusion of the popliteal artery limb-threatening ischemia. In 10 patients, the ankle pulse decreased with exercise. Four patients had ankle/brachial indexes less than 1. All had diminished ankle/brachial indexes after performing a treadmill test at 4.2 mph at a 10% grade for 10 minutes.

Arteriography showed abnormal extrinsic compression or occlusion of the popliteal artery in all 12 patients; 8 patients had bilateral entrapment. Thirty-seven percent of lesions were type IV, 32% were type II, and 26% were type III. There was 1 type 1 lesion and no type V lesions.

▶ Popliteal artery entrapment characteristically occurs because of a congenital anomaly of the medial head of the gastrocnemius muscle and its relationship to the popliteal artery and other structures within the popliteal fossa. In recording the results of surgery on 12 patients with this problem, it is noted that ". . . all limbs were explored by means of the posterior approach to the popliteal fossa." Other than the noting that 2 popliteal artery thromboendarterectomies and 2 saphenous vein interposition grafts were performed, no mention is made of the surgical method of dealing with the anomalous gastrocnemius muscle. Of note is the fact that in this series the anomaly was bilateral. This, coupled with the observation of Gibson et al. (1) in a cadaver study that 3.5% of the specimens demonstrated evidence of popliteal entrapment, indicates the possible existence of a higher incidence than commonly appreciated.—J.S. Torg, M.D.

Reference

1. Gibson MH, et al: *Ann Surg* 185:341, 1977.

Other Regions

Wedge Resection of the Symphysis Pubis for the Treatment of Osteitis Pubis

Grace JN, Sim FH, Shives TC, Coventry MB (Mayo Clinic and Found, Rochester, Minn)

J Bone Joint Surg 71-A:358–364, March 1989   10–112

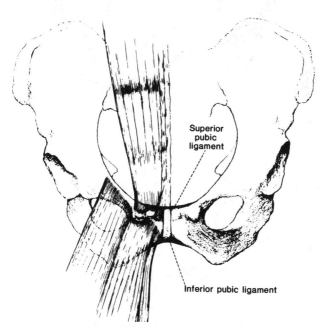

Superior pubic ligament

Inferior pubic ligament

Fig 10–32.—Superior and inferior (arcuate) pubic ligaments must be preserved. (Courtesy of Grace JN, Sim FH, Shives TC, et al: *J Bone Joint Surg* 71-A:358–364, March 1989.)

Because a variety of pathologic changes may be associated with osteitis pubis, there has been some confusion as to the cause of this disease. The signs, symptoms, and radiographic features of 10 patients with osteitis pubis who did not improve after conservative treatment were evaluated. Preoperatively, the average duration of symptoms was 32 months. Patients had not improved after nonoperative treatment of at least 6 months. Symptoms included crepitus, a waddling gait, pain, and tenderness over the symphysis pubis. Early radiographic signs of disease included rarefaction of the adjacent pubic bones and widening of the symphysis pubis. Later, radiographic signs included sclerosis and narrowing of the symphyseal joint space.

Technique.—Before surgery, an indwelling urethral catheter is inserted to decompress the bladder. Operatively, the superior and posterior aspects of the pubis are exposed subperiosteally. The anterior aspect of the symphysis pubis is not disturbed, and the integrity of the superior and inferior pubic ligaments are preserved (Fig 10–32). A trapezoidal wedge of bone is removed and the entire symphyseal joint is excised. The wedge is based cephalad and posterior, extending 1 cm on either side of the joint. The apex of the wedge, which is 5 mm wide, is caudal and anterior (Fig 10–33).

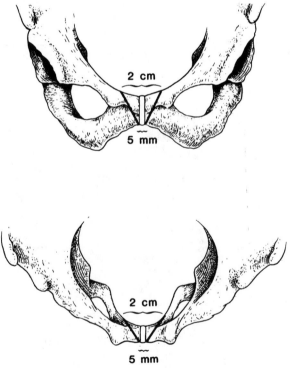

Fig 10–33.—The symphysis pubis is excised, in its entirety, with a trapezoidal wedge of bone, but the anterior aspect of the cortex is left intact. The base of the wedge is cephalad and posterior, and the apex is caudal and anterior. (Courtesy of Grace JN, Sim FH, Shives TC, et al: *J Bone Joint Surg* 71-A:358–364, March 1989.)

Pathologic examination of the resected joint revealed a chronic inflammatory reaction in all of the patients. At an average of 14 months post operatively, all patients were markedly improved and were fully active. Three patients were dissatisfied with the result at an average of 92 months postoperatively, however. One patient required bilateral sacroiliac arthrodesis for pain caused by instability.

Wedge resection of the symphysis pubis is a reliable treatment in carefully selected patients with osteitis pubis refractory to conservative treatment. If wedge resection fails or the pelvis is unstable, symphyseodesis and fixation with a compression plate can be undertaken.

▶ Groin pain in the athlete, a consistently vexing and difficult problem to manage, has been attributed to a number of causes. Such diagnoses as "pubic pain syndrome," "pubialgia," "osteitis pubis," adductor tendinitis, and symphysis pubis arthritis have been employed. Seen primarily in soccer and ice hockey players, osteitis pubis can be a career-ending affliction. To be pointed out, none of the patients in this series were athletes. However, in those required to return to strenuous physical activity, in rare situations refractory to conservative management wedge resection of the symphysis pubis could be considered. Of note, Wiley (1) coined the term "the gracilis syndrome" to describe traumatic osteitis pubis. In a case report he describes the surgical excision of an avulsion-type stress fracture, ". . . the exact site being part of the anatomical origin of the gracilis muscle. . ." in which excision of the fracture led to a satisfactory outcome. He concluded that, "Surgery seems appropriate when conservative measures fail, especially in patients with longstanding symptoms and a definite lesion."—J.S. Torg, M.D.

Reference

1. Wiley JJ: *Am J Sports Med* 11:350, 1983.

Computed Tomography of Hamstring Muscle Strains
Garrett WE Jr, Rich FR, Nikolaou PK, Vogler JB III (Duke Univ)
Med Sci Sports Exerc 21:506–514, October 1989
10–113

Disabling muscle-tendon unit injuries in the hamstring muscles are common findings in sports and occupational medicine. The anatomical location and CT characteristics of the hamstring strain injury were examined. Five cadaveric specimens were dissected to help interpret the CT findings. Ten college athletes aged 18–24 years with acute hamstring injuries were evaluated by CT, usually within 48 hours of injury. Clinical follow-up examinations were done at weekly intervals. Follow-up CT scans were obtained 1 month later for 3 of the athletes.

Eight patients had acute abnormalities observed on CT. All abnormalities appeared as regions of low density in the affected muscle (Fig 10–34). The injuries were most commonly seen proximally and laterally within the hamstring group, and probably in the long head of the biceps

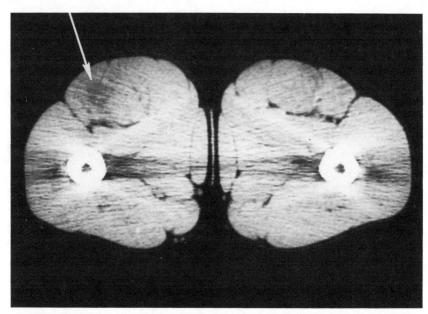

Fig 10–34.—Muscle strain of lateral hamstring region. A prone axial CT image through the midthighs in this acutely injured patient demonstrates an area of low density in the region of the lateral hamstrings on the left. The left hamstrings appear enlarged when compared to the normal right side. This most probably indicates swelling in the acutely injured tissue. (Courtesy of Garrett WE Jr, Rich FR, Nikolaou PK, et al: *Med Sci Sports Exerc* 21:506–514, October 1989.)

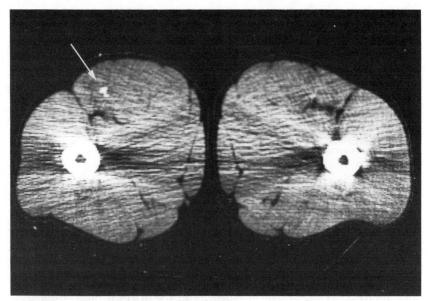

Fig 10–35.—Hamstring strain 1 month after injury in the same patient shown in **Figure 10–34.** A prone axial CT image through the midthighs demonstrates calcification in the left lateral hamstring group. On previous studies this area demonstrated the typical low-density lesion of an acute strain. (Courtesy of Garrett WE Jr, Rich FR, Nikolaou PK, et al: *Med Sci Sports Exerc* 21:506–514, October 1989.)

femoris. Two patients with no detectable acute abnormality were able to return to athletics within 1 week with mild injuries. The 8 patients with abnormalities seen on CT experienced delayed recovery.

Repeat CT scans in 2 athletes showed resolution of the low-density lesions and the appearance of small, well-defined high-density regions suggestive of calcification (Fig 10–35). The third athlete no longer had a detectable abnormality on the repeat scan.

The finding of hypodense areas on CT suggests that hamstring injuries are not acute hematomas within the muscle. Hematomas would appear as hyperdense areas on CT. The presence of hypodense areas within normal muscle tends to support inflammation or edema as the major component of muscle strain injury. Computed tomography was used in this study to characterize muscle strains. Its routine use for evaluation of muscle strains is not recommended.

▶ Data from their experimental studies have shown that biomechanical failure occurs at the muscle tendon junction and is characterized by limited tearing of the fibers and a subsequent inflammatory reaction with increased fibers or scar tissue. This work corroborates preliminary reports of magnetic resonance findings, which also demonstrated that the abnormalities were located near the insertions and/or origins of the muscles. Swelling of perimuscular connective tissues in the regions of the myotendinous junctions accounts for the restrictive range of motion of extremities observed with the postexercise muscle soreness. The major abnormality on CT was a hypodense area characteristic of edema, which can be differentiated from intramuscular hematoma and muscle strains. These findings need to be compared to preliminary findings observed on magnetic resonance in which abnormal patterns are interpreted as hemorrhage, although edema would also explain the observed changes.—J.S. Torg, M.D.

Saphenous Nerve Entrapment at the Adductor Canal

Romanoff ME, Cory PC Jr, Kalenak A, Keyser GC, Marshall WK (Pennsylvania State Univ, Hershey)
Am J Sports Med 17:478–481, July–August 1989   10–114

Saphenous nerve entrapment at the adductor canal can cause pain and discomfort in the lower extremities. The saphenous nerve, which is completely sensory in function, is distributed over the medial and inferior aspects of the lower thigh and knee, the anterior and medial portions of the lower leg, and the medial aspect of the ankle (Fig 10–36). Thirty patients who met clinical criteria were treated by a saphenous block at the adductor canal using a combination of local anesthetic (bupivacaine, .25%) and steroid (triamcinolone diacetate, 25 mg) solutions.

The patients experienced symptoms, usually anterior knee pain, an average of 36 months (range 2–156 months). After an average of 4 months of follow-up, 80% of patients responded favorably after 1 to 5 saphenous nerve blocks at the adductor canal (average 1.9 blocks). Pain level, as

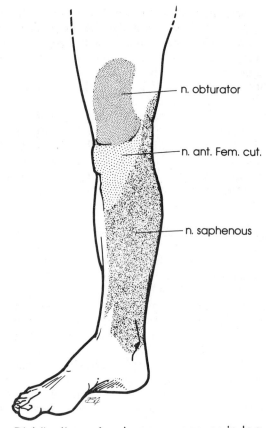

n. obturator

n. ant. Fem. cut.

n. saphenous

Distribution of cutaneous nerves in leg

Fig 10–36.—Distribution of cutaneous nerves in the leg. (Courtesy of Romanoff ME, Cory PC Jr, Kalenak A, et al: *Am J Sports Med* 17:478–481, July–August 1989.)

measured by the visual analogue scale, decreased significantly from a mean baseline level of 6.4 to 2.8. Final pain reduction correlated significantly with the length of symptoms before treatment. Age, medications taken, number of blocks performed, and length of follow-up did not correlate with the reduction.

The etiology of saphenous nerve entrapment remains unknown. Traction on the saphenous nerve as it exits the aponeurotic sheath of the adductor canal may cause inflammation, edema, and paresthesias. With longer duration of compression fibrosis may involve the nerve.

▶ With regard to response to therapy, it is pointed out that if nerve compression is transient an injection of local anesthetic may stop the pain cycle. However, compression of longer duration with inflammation and fibrosis explains the correlation between a decrease in effectiveness of the block and an increase in the length of symptoms.

Mozes et al. (1) reported a series in which only 38% of the patients had a favorable response. The authors explain that their 80% favorable response resulted from adding corticosteroids to the mixture injected in their series.—J.S. Torg, M.D.

Reference

1. Mozes M, et al: *Surgery* 77:299, 1975.

Iliotibial Band Tightness
Gose JC, Schweizer P (Blue Hen Physical Therapy, Inc, Wilmington, Del)
J Orthop Sports Phys Ther 10:399–407, April 1989   10–115

Many patients with musculoskeletal complaints have tightness of the iliotibial band (ITB), which may cause "friction syndrome" in runners. Tightness of the ITB can be a primary or secondary cause of many lower extremity complaints. The lower back, lateral hip or knee, and patella can be painful. Patients who commonly complain of tightness of the ITB include those with involvement of the nervous system, adolescents with recent growth spurts, teenaged girls with chondromalacia or subluxating patellae, and athletes, particularly long distance runners in young adulthood.

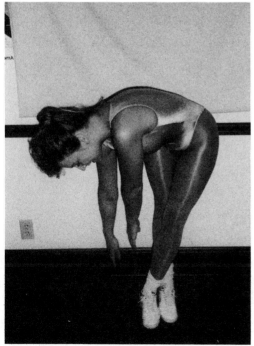

Fig 10–37.—Standing lateral fascial stretch with trunk lateral flexion-rotation contralateral to involved leg. The involved leg is crossed behind the uninvolved leg. (Courtesy of Gose JC, Schweizer P: *J Orthop Sports Ther* 10:399–407, April, 1989.)

Assessment may reveal tightness of the proximal hip flexors or contracture and a positive Ober test. The tightness can be treated by controlling acute symptoms, stretching the hip flexors and ITB (Fig 10–37), strengthening the hip musculature, and maintaining a home program. Modifying daily activities may help to alleviate the symptoms. Surgery is rarely needed.

Further study is needed to determine the frequency of tightness of the ITB or contracture in normal populations, to determine the effects of biomechanical orthotics on ITB friction syndrome, and to examine the effects of routinely adding ITB stretching to programs for patients with chondromalacia or subluxating patellae.

▶ We have traditionally done lateral retinaculum stretching with our patients who have chondromalacia and a subluxating patella. These patients may also benefit from increased flexibility of the ITB. If they are distance runners they must be cautioned about running on "crowned" roads or "banked" tracks. Distance runners who use a track should alternate directions in which they run from training session to training session.—F.J. George, ATC, PT.

Surgical Treatment of the Iliotibial Band Friction Syndrome
Martens M, Libbrecht P, Burssens A (Univ Hosp, Pellenberg, Belgium)
Am J Sports Med 17:651–654, September–October 1989   10–116

The iliotibial band friction syndrome usually responds to conservative treatment, but surgery may be necessary in refractory cases. During an 8-year-period, surgery was performed in 23 of 234 consecutive patients;

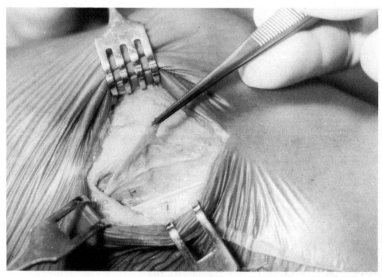

Fig 10–38.—Surgery, done with the knee in 60 degrees of flexion, consists of limited resection of a triangular piece at the dorsal part of the iliotract covering the lateral femoral epicondyle. The resected portion measured about 2 cm on its dorsal base and was approximately 1.5 cm in height to the top of the triangle. (Modified from Martens M, Libbrecht P, Burssens A: *Am J Sports Med* 17:651–654, September–October 1989.)

these 23 included football players, runners, and cyclists. The diagnosis was based on history and clinical examination performed shortly after sports activity, because the exertional pain seldom persisted. Radiography was never, and ultrasonography only rarely, useful. Surgery was performed only after conservative treatment of from 4 to 24 months failed to alleviate pain and the patient wished to continue sports participation.

The operation consisted of removal of a triangular portion containing fibrous tissue from the dorsal part of the iliotibial tract (Fig 10–38). Weight-bearing was not permitted until after splinting for 7 days with the knee in extension.

All 19 patients observed for 2–11 years had satisfactory results, with return to sports activity at the previous level within a mean of 7 weeks. The hematoma that occurred in 1 patient was evacuated. No clinical or functional abnormality was found at follow-up.

Not all patients who experience iliotibial band friction syndrome respond to conservative treatment, and the disease in athletes is not self-limited. In patients unresponsive to conservative treatment, surgery provides good results with early recovery and little morbidity.

▶ I have had no experience with this surgical approach as a means of managing the iliotibial band syndrome. However, this is certainly an interesting approach to a vexing problem. Unfortunately, the authors have not commented on the possible adverse effects of excising a segment of the iliotibial band.—J.S. Torg, M.D.

Chronic Exercise-Induced Pain in the Anterior Aspect of the Lower Leg: An Overview of Diagnosis
Styf J (Univ of Göteborg, Sweden)
Sports Med 7:331–339, 1989
10–117

It may be difficult to diagnose recurrent pain in the lower leg because of a lack of specific symptoms. In chronic anterior compartment syndrome, increased intramuscular pressure on exercise impedes blood flow and tissue function. Patients tend to have a higher level of activity than those with other forms of leg pain. Pain tends to be induced only by athletic activity and to occur only in the anterior region. Intramuscular pressure after exercise is increased and takes an inordinate time to normalize. A few patients with chronic lateral compartment syndrome have been reported.

Entrapment of the superficial peroneal nerve may be more frequent than the literature suggests. Disordered sensation over the dorsum of the foot during exercise is a characteristic finding. Other causes of pain in the anterior part of the lower leg include exercise that involves eccentric muscle contraction (e.g., downhill running) and periostitis. The medial tibial syndrome produces posteromedial lower leg pain and may occur in patients with chronic anterior compartment syndrome. Stress fractures of the tibia cause local tenderness and swelling.

▶ This is an excellent review of the subject matter. The interested reader is referred to the original article.—J.S. Torg, M.D.

Compartment Syndromes of the Lower Leg
Bourne RB, Rorabeck CH (Univ of Western Ontario, London)
Clin Orthop 240:97–104, March 1989   10–118

Increased pressure that compromises neuromuscular function within a
closed space creates a so-called compartment syndrome. In the lower leg
5 compartments have been identified: anterior, lateral, superficial poste-

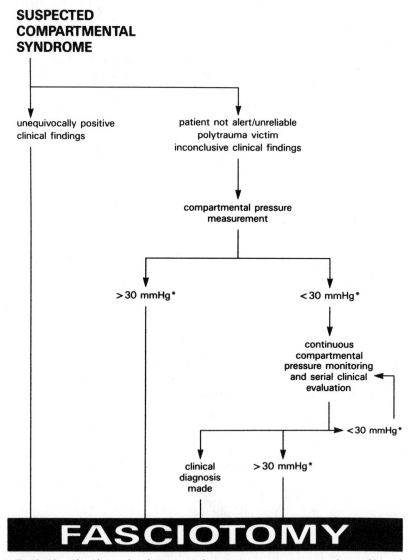

Fig 10–39.—Algorithm used in diagnosing and treating acute compartment syndrome of lower leg
secondary to tibial fracture. (Courtesy of Bourne RB, Rorabeck CH: *Clin Orthop* 240:97–104, March
1989.)

rior, deep posterior, and posterior tibial. Acute compartment syndromes are often caused by trauma, and those that are chronic are usually exercise related.

If a patient is conscious, an acute compartment syndrome usually is easily diagnosed clinically. Symptoms include increased pain, increased need for analgesics, and stretch pain referred to the compartment in question with passive movements of the toes. There are normal pulses distal to the injury. When a patient is unconscious, an intracompartmental pressure monitor may be useful. When compartmental pressures exceed 30–35 mm Hg in a normally perfused patient, there is a need for open compartment fasciotomy.

Tissue-pressure measurements form the basis of diagnosis of chronic exercise-induced compartment syndrome. However, if the patient has increased pain associated with appropriate muscle stretching and abnormal sensory or motor function in the area of the nerve that transgresses the compartment, fasciotomy should be performed without the necessity of tissue-pressure measurements. The hypothetical algorithm in Figure 10–39 was designed for a patient with a fractured tibia.

In compartment syndromes the most important parameter is increased intramuscular pressure generated by exercise, as measured immediately after exercise. In properly diagnosed cases of chronic compartment syndrome subcutaneous fasciotomy may relieve the problem (Fig 10–40).

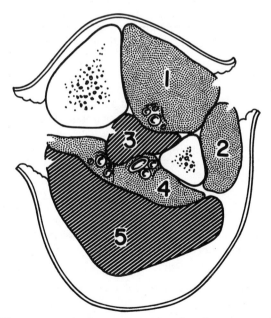

Fig 10–40.—Diagram representing 5-compartment release through separate anterolateral and medial open fasciotomy incisions. (Courtesy of Bourne RB, Rorabeck CH: *Clin Orthop* 240:97–104, March 1989.)

Posteromedial Pain in the Lower Leg

Melberg P-E, Styf J (Univ of Göteborg, Sweden)
Am J Sports Med 17:747–750, November–December 1989   10–119

Athletes commonly complain of pain along the posteromedial border of the tibial diaphysis, accounting for 60% of all lesions causing leg pain in athletes. However, there is controversy over whether this pain is caused by chronic compartment syndrome (CCS) or a non-CCS condition. History and clinical data alone are insufficient to confirm a diagnosis of CCS in the anterior compartment. The existence of CCS in the deep posterior compartment was investigated by simultaneous recording of pressure in the flexor digitorum muscle and the posterior tibial muscle during a standardized exercise test and at rest after exercise.

The study was done in 28 patients aged 19–43 years (mean, 26 years) who complained of exercise-induced posteromedial pain in the lower leg severe enough to interfere with the ability to participate in athletics. Twenty-four patients had bilateral pain. The symptoms had persisted from 6 months to 4 years. Many patients also had pain during activities of daily living. None of the conservative treatments tried provided pain relief. All patients were thought to have CCS in the deep posterior compartment. None had neurologic or circulatory diseases.

All intramuscular pressure parameters in the posterior tibial muscle and flexor digitorum longus muscle in the posteromedial part of the lower leg were within normal limits, both at rest and during exercise. A diagnosis of CCS could not be confirmed in any of the patients, and CCS was excluded as the reason for the patients' pain in the posteromedial part of the lower leg.

▶ These 2 papers present what appears to be a controversy with regard to the existence of CCS in the fifth compartment surrounding the posterior tibial muscle recently described by Davey et al. (1) using the slit catheter device. Based on this method, compartmental pressures in excess of 30–35 mm Hg in a normally perfused patient suggest the need for an open compartment fasciotomy. Melberg and Styf, on the other hand, using a Myopress catheter connected to an electromagnetic transducer and a multichannel recorder, although obtaining mean muscle exercise pressures of 45 mm Hg, reject the concept of the existence of CCS in the fifth compartment because the pressures return to normal immediately after exercise. Perhaps the case would be more convincing had they performed a prospective randomized study to determine the effect on symptomatology of patients with a history of posterior medial leg pain with exertion and elevated compartment pressures during exercise.—J.S. Torg, M.D.

Reference

1. Davey JR, et al: *Am J Sports Med* 12:391, 1984.

Achilles Tendon Rupture in Badminton
Kaalund S, Lass P, Høgsaa B, Nøhr M (Aalborg Hosp, Denmark)
Br J Sports Med 23:102–104, June 1989   10–120

Badminton is a frequent cause of Achilles tendon rupture. To investigate the mechanisms of injury, subsequent work and sport absences, and training and competition activity levels associated with Achilles tendon rupture, a 2½-year study was undertaken in 35 men and 4 women (mean age, 36 years) who were operated on for complete Achilles tendon ruptures. The injuries had occurred while the patients were playing badminton. All 39 patients were operated on within 48 hours by simple end-to-end suture. One patient also underwent plantaris tendon transposition. Postoperative treatment consisted of an above-knee plaster cast with the foot in the equinus position for 3 weeks, and a below-knee cast for an additional 3 weeks. A 3-cm heel lift was used for 3 months after cast removal. None of the patients had formal physical rehabilitation therapy. The mean follow-up period was 23 months.

One patient reruptured the Achilles tendon 2 months after operation. At follow-up, 2 patients had sural nerve damage. Twelve patients had loss of dorsiflexion of 5 to 10 degrees, 5 complained of pain in the tendon region when exercising, 3 had pain from the heeltabs of their shoes, 3 had a slight lack of subtalar movement, and 3 had scar adhesions. None of the patients had healing problems or wound infections.

Analysis of weekly badminton playing activity revealed that 51% played for less than 2 hours and 82% for less than 4 hours. Achilles tendon rupture had occurred at the start of the game in 10%, in the middle of the game in 23%, and at the end in 64% of the patients. Twenty-five patients reported limbering up before playing, including 2 of the 4 who sustained injuries early in the game. Rupture had occurred during a sudden forward movement in 34 cases. Thirty-two of the 39 players resumed the sport within 1 year, but 11 were unable to regain their former playing level. The other 7 did not return to any sport because of fear of injury. Eighteen players were able to resume badminton participation in less than 6 months after operation; 20 returned to work within 6 weeks.

▶ It is interesting to note that, although this injury resulted in a prolonged absence from vigorous physical activity for the majority of players, absence from work was not shortened. Half of the patients returned to work within 6 weeks and 87% within 3 months.—J.S. Torg, M.D.

Achilles Tendon Injuries: The Role of MR Imaging
Marcus DS, Reicher MA, Kellerhouse LE (Mercy Hosp and Med Ctr, San Diego)
J Comput Assist Tomogr 13:480–486, May–June 1989   10–121

Swelling may make the diagnosis of acute rupture of the Achilles tendon difficult based on physical examination alone. To correlate findings on magnetic resonance (MR) imaging with physical examination and

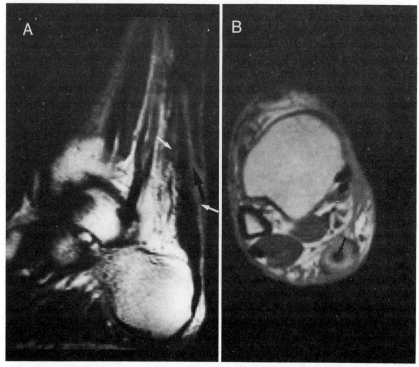

Fig 10–41.—**A,** sagittal scan reveals disruption of midportion of tendon *(black arrow)*. Moderate signal *(white arrows)*, presumed to represent hemorrhage and edema, surrounds region of tear (TR/TE 500/39). **B,** axial scan reveals remaining intact portion of tendon *(arrow)* surrounded by high-intensity hemorrhage (TR/TE 600/39). (Courtesy of Marcus DS, Reicher MA, Kellerhouse LE: *J Comput Assist Tomogr* 13:480–486, May–June 1989.)

clinical outcome, studies were made in 6 men and 1 woman with clinically suspected Achilles tendon injuries. The ankle was imaged in 30 patients without Achilles tendon injuries to establish the normal MR appearance of the tendon. Physical examination included assessment of plantar-flexion strength, recording of Thompson test results, and palpation of the tendon for defects.

The MR studies depicted the Achilles tendon in excellent detail and showed abnormalities with greater accuracy than physical examination. Five tendons were depicted as partially torn on MR (Fig 10–41); of these, only 1 had palpable tendinous defects, but 4 had plantar-flexion weakness. Surigcal findings and MR correlated precisely in 1 case.

Magnetic resonance has a role in the evaluation of clinically equivocal Achilles tendon tears. In the future, MR may be even more important as a research tool to determine optimal forms of treatment for specific Achilles tendon injuries.

▶ In the face of complete rupture of the Achilles tendon, the Thompson test is not only of comparable diagnostic value but is considerably more cost effective. When the diagnosis of partial Achilles tear was made, all of the patients were treated nonoperatively. Thus the merits of the MR imaging with regard to the decision-making process appear questionable.—J.S. Torg, M.D.

Surgical Treatment of Chronic Achilles Tendinitis
Nelen G, Martens M, Burssens A (Univ Hosp, Pellenberg, Belgium)
Am J Sports Med 17:754–759, November–December 1989   10–122

Achilles tendon lesions are the most common of the overuse syndromes of the lower leg, and conservative treatment does not always solve the problem. Between 1977 and 1985, 170 patients underwent operation in treatment of Achilles tendinitis. Of these, 78 males and 13 females aged 16–45 years with 143 involved tendons were available for follow-up.

Fifty-three patients had bilateral symptoms. Only patients whose lesions and symptoms were limited to the Achilles tendon segment 2–6 cm proximal of the insertion were included in this study. Patients with an insertion tendinopathy or a lesion at the musculotendinous junction were excluded. Eighteen patients were top-ranking athletes. The mean duration of preoperative symptoms was 18 months and ranged from 2 to 178 months. All patients had failed to respond to conservative treatment. The postoperative results were rated from excellent to poor, based on residual postoperative complaints and the patient's ability to return to sports.

Ninety-three tendons with evidence of pure peritendinitis were treated with a simple dorsal release of the fascia cruris and peritenon. The diseased tendon was resected in 50 tendons with tendinosis. In 26 of these the defect could be sutured side to side; the other 24 required reinforcement with a turned-down tendon flap because of extensive débridement.

The overall results were excellent in 81 tendons, good in 41, fair in 14, and poor in 7. Of the 93 tendons treated with only dorsal release, results were excellent in 54, good in 28, fair in 8, and poor in 3. Of the 26 tendons treated with side-to-side suture, results were excellent in 15, good in 4, fair in 4, and poor in 3. Of the 24 procedures in which a turned-down tendon flap procedure was required, the results were excellent in 12, good in 9, fair in 2, and poor in 1. Postoperative complications were rare, usually minor, and did not influence the end results. The surgical treatment of Achilles tendinitis caused by athletic overuse yields satisfactory results with low morbidity in a high percentage of cases.

▶ The postoperative results reported were based on residual complaints and the patient's ability to return to activities compared with the preinjury level. They were defined as follows: Excellent, no residual symptoms and unlimited performance; good, full return to same preoperative activity level with some stiffness after strenuous activities; fair, no complaints related to daily activity but stiffness and aching related to sports; and poor, no improvement. Apparently, postoperative complications were few and minor. The technique of reinforcing an extensive area of débridement with a trimmed-down tendon flap has not been reported previously for chronic tendinosis or for partial tear of the Achilles tendon.—J.S. Torg, M.D.

Reconstruction of Neglected Achilles Tendon Rupture With Marlex Mesh
Ozaki J, Fujiki J, Sugimoto K, Tamal S, Masuhara K (Nara Med Univ, Nara, Japan)
Clin Orthop 238:204–208, January 1989   10–123

There are several methods for surgical repair of neglected Achilles tendon rupture; however, some authors have reported unsatisfactory results, whereas others have used relatively complicated procedures. A previously unreported method of repair using polypropylene mesh may be successful. Six women had ruptured Achilles tendons resulting from fails during participation in sports. The principal symptoms were prolonged localized pain, weakness of plantar flexion power, limping, and calf swelling. Conservative measures were ineffective. The delay to surgery averaged 4.3 months.

Technique.—Scar tissue was resected to healthy tendinous tissue, and both ends were divided into 2 sections horizontally. Three layers of Marlex mesh were

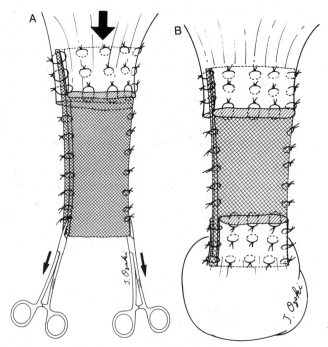

Fig 10–42.—Preparation of Marlex mesh. **A,** mesh is folded into 3 layers and fixed to proximal end of the tendon. The retracted gastrocnemius and soleus muscles are pulled distally to make the gap as narrow as possible. **B,** mesh is sandwiched with moderate tension to distal end in same fashion. (Courtesy of Ozaki J, Fujiki J, Sugimoto K, et al: *Clin Orthop* 238:204–208, January 1989.)

folded into an artificial tendon, sandwiched between the layers of natural tendon, and fixed at the proximal end (Fig 10–42). The retracted gastrocnemius and soleus muscles were pulled out to narrow the gap; using moderate tension, the mesh was sutured with the knee in 90 degrees of flexion and the ankle plantar in 60 degrees of flexion. After a long-leg cast was applied, the leg was immobilized for 6 weeks and was kept non-weight-bearing for 8 weeks.

The mean follow-up was 3 years. All patients had satisfactory function and were able to return to preinjury sports activities. There were minimal signs of foreign body reaction and little adhesion with adjacent tissues.

The procedure using Marlex mesh produces satisfactory results. The operative procedure is simple and does not require harvesting healthy tendon or fascia as donor material. Complications are minimal.

▶ My own experience in managing a neglected Achilles tendon rupture has been that if the patient is placed supine on the operating room table and the knee and hip are flexed and the ankle plantar flexed, opposition and repair can be achieved without autogenous or synthetic grafting. With regard to the use of polypropylene as described by the authors, it is interesting that they observed collagenous tissue in growth.—J.S. Torg, M.D.

Ankle Arthroscopy: Neurovascular and Arthroscopic Anatomy of Standard and Trans-Achilles Tendon Portal Placement
Voto SJ, Ewing JW, Fleissner PR Jr, Alfonso M, Kufel M (Akron City Hosp)
Arthroscopy 5:41–46, 1989   10–124

Because of the proximity of neurovascular and tendinous structures in the ankle, accurate arthroscopic portal placement is important. Ten fresh-frozen cadaver ankles were dissected after placing standard anterior and posterior arthroscopic portals. In addition, a trans-Achilles tendon approach was evaluated for portal use. This portal was placed through the central tendon fibers at the level of the joint line.

Analysis of the distances of neurovascular and tendinous structures from the lateral portals (Fig 10–43) indicated that arthroscopy can be performed safely by outlining the tendinous structures and keeping the knife blade parallel to them. Only the skin is penetrated with the knife. The use of anterocentral and posteromedial portals entails a potential risk to the respective neurovascular bundles. The trans-Achilles tendon approach appeared to be anatomically safe, and it offers an additional posterior portal. Distention of the ankle capsule did not significantly displace the superficial or deep structures. Intra-articular structures are best visualized when the arthroscope is on the same side of the structures to be assessed.

▶ This paper supplements previous descriptions of portals for ankle arthroscopy by Andrews et al. (1) and Parisien et al. (2). The authors emphasize caution in the use of anterocentral and posteromedial portals. However, no men-

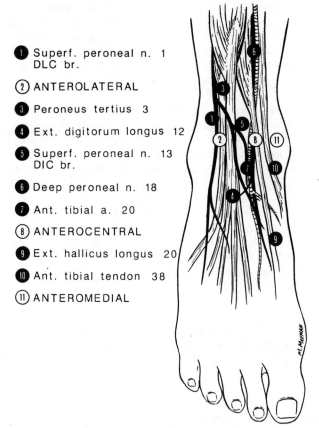

① Superf. peroneal n. 1
   DLC br.

② ANTEROLATERAL

③ Peroneus tertius 3

④ Ext. digitorum longus 12

⑤ Superf. peroneal n. 13
   DIC br.

⑥ Deep peroneal n. 18

⑦ Ant. tibial a. 20

⑧ ANTEROCENTRAL

⑨ Ext. hallicus longus 20

⑩ Ant. tibial tendon 38

⑪ ANTEROMEDIAL

Fig 10–43.—Mean distances of neurovascular and tendinous structures from the lateral portals. All distances are measured in millimeters based on the most laterally based portal (i.e., anterolateral or posterolateral). (Courtesy of Voto SJ, Ewing JW, Fleissner PR Jr, et al: *Arthroscopy* 5:41–46, 1989.)

tion is made of postoperative complications, real or imagined, resulting from this approach. It should be noted that, ". . . visualization of intraarticular structures was easiest when the arthroscope was placed on the same side of the structure."—J.S. Torg, M.D.

References

1. Andrews JR, et al: *J Foot Ankle* 6:29, 1985.
2. Parisien JS, et al: Clin Orthop 224:228, 1987.

Arthroscopic Treatment of Osteochondral Lesions of the Talar Dome
Frank A, Cohen P, Beaufils P, Lamare J (St-Germain-En-Laye Hosp Ctr; Versailles Hosp Ctr, Le Chesnay, France)
Arthroscopy 5:57–61, 1989

Arthroscopy was used to treat 9 osteochondral lesions of the talar dome, including 2 recent osteochondral fractures in a young patient with a free fragment detached in the joint; the loose body was ablated. In 4 men and 3 women, old lesions were associated with a partially loose osteocartilaginous body and necrosis of the underlying bone. These lesions were located posteromedially. The loose body was removed and the necrotic bone curetted. In some patients it was necessary to place the foot in talipes equinus to distract the joint and reach a posterior lesion.

All patients recovered some joint motion within 2 weeks but several had moderate pain on walking. After 6 months, 6 patients had no more than negligible pain; 2 others had moderate pain at the end of the day, and 1 patient had no relief. On follow-up for 10–24 months 6 patients were free of pain even while engaging in sports activities. Radiologic healing remained incomplete even after 1–2 years. The surface of the talar dome often was irregular. An area of necrosis persisted in the patient who had a poor clinical outcome.

Arthroscopy is a simple and satisfactory means of treating osteochondral lesions of the talar dome. The indications are the same as for open surgical treatment.

▶ The favorable clinical results reported by the authors in this series are similar to those reported by Parisien (1) and Pritsch et al. (2). The authors do admit to "technical difficulties . . . because of the posterior-medial positions of the lesions." This was apparently overcome by using a distractor placed between a transtibial and a transcalcaneous pin.—J.S. Torg, M.D.

References

1. Parisien JS: *Am J Sports Med* 14:211, 1986.
2. Pritsch M, et al: *J Bone Joint Surg* 86-A:862, 1986.

Entrapment of the Superficial Peroneal Nerve: Diagnosis and Results of Decompression
Styf J (Gothenburg Univ, Sweden)
J Bone Joint Surg 71-B:131–135, January 1989   10–126

Only a few reports of superficial peroneal nerve entrapment have appeared, but its incidence is probably higher than is suggested by the literature. The effects of decompression to relieve symptoms and nerve conduction velocity were assessed in 21 patients with chronic lateral compartment syndrome.

During a 5-year period, 21 patients aged 15–79 years underwent fasciotomy and neurolysis to relieve superficial peroneal nerve entrapment in 24 legs; 3 patients had bilateral symptoms. Conduction velocities in the superficial peroneal nerve were measured before and after operation, using surface electrodes from which electromyograms (EMGs) of both peroneal muscles and the anterior tibial muscles were recorded. Com-

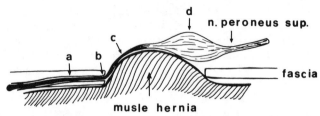

Fig 10−44.—Diagram of the superficial peroneal nerve showing findings at operation and some possible sites of entrapment. **a**, peroneus tunnel; **b**, impingement at the exit from the tunnel; **c**, compression by herniating muscle producing a waist on the nerve tissue; **d**, poststenotic swelling. (Courtesy of Styf J: *J Bone Joint Surg [Br]* 71-B:131−135, January 1989.)

partment pressure were recorded bilaterally in the lateral compartment in all patients and in the anterior compartment in 15. Nineteen patients were followed for a mean of 37 months.

At operation, clearly visible waisting of the superficial peroneal nerve was found in 12 legs (Fig 10−44). Associated poststenotic swelling was present in 5 legs. The superficial peroneal nerve had an anomalous course in 5 patients, and there were fascial defects over the lateral compartment in 11 patients.

Only 9 of the 19 patients were completely satisfied with the outcome, even though 13 had unlimited or increased physical ability. Physical ability was unchanged in the other 6. Of the 13 improved patients, 4 were not satisfied because they were athletes who could not attain the desired level of competitive activity. Only 1 patient required reoperation, during which the nerve was found to be trapped in scar tissue. All radiographs and all myograms were normal. Although conduction velocity in the superficial peroneal nerve was increased after operation, the increase was not significant. Decompression relieved the pain and sensory abnormalities of entrapment of the superficial peroneal nerve in 75% of the cases, but operation was less effective in athletes.

▶ Diagnostic criteria involved decreased sensibility and pain over the dorsum of the foot at rest or during an exercise test, as well as a positive response to at least 1 of 3 provocation tests. These were (1) nerve conduction velocity of less than 44 m/sec; (2) increased lateral compartment intermuscular pressure after exercise of more than 43−40 mm Hg; and (3) a positive exercise test. In the latter, a positive response was development of pain and diminished sensation to light touch over the dorsum of the foot.—J.S. Torg, M.D.

Early Postoperative Weight-Bearing and Muscle Activity in Patients Who Have a Fracture of the Ankle
Finsen V, Saetermo R, Kibsgaard L, Farram K, Engebretsen L, Bolz KD, Benum P (Trøndhiem Univ Hosp, Trøndheim, Norway)
J Bone Joint Surg 71-A:23−27, January 1989   10−127

Controversy exists regarding postoperative management after internal fixation of an ankle fracture. In a prospective study, 56 patients with displaced ankle fractures necessitating surgical fixation were randomly assigned to 1 of 3 postoperative treatment regimens; no plaster cast or weight-bearing, and active exercises of the ankle (18 patients); a non-weight-bearing plaster cast (19); or a plaster walking cast for the first 6 postoperative weeks (19). The duration of followup was approximately 2 years.

There were no consistent differences in the clinical results among the 3 groups. Specifically, the time lost from work and the proportion of excellent and good clinical results did not differ significantly among the 3 groups. Radiographs showed no significant differences among groups in the proportion of patients with widening of the ankle mortise. There were no adverse effects from weight-bearing with the syndesmosis screw in place.

None of the 3 postoperative regimens appears to be more advantageous than the others in a patient who has a stable osteosynthesis of an ankle fracture.

▶ Although the authors report no difference in the 3 postoperative regimens, they conclude that, "If stable osteosynthesis of a fracture of the ankle is achieved in a reliable patient, the surgeon and patient together can select any one of the postoperative regimens. For most patients, this will probably consist of weight-bearing with a plaster cast."—J.S. Torg, M.D.

Pressure Distribution in Morton's Foot Structure

Rodgers MM, Cavanagh PR (Wright State Univ, Dayton; Pennsylvania State Univ, University Park)
Med Sci Sports Exerc 21:23–28, February 1989   10–128

The Morton foot strucure (MFS) is a foot in which the head of the second metatarsal is more distally placed than the head of the first. The origin of this foot problem has been hypothesized to be an abnormal metatarsal head loading pattern found in the MFS. Plantar pressure distribution under the metatarsal head in 30 subjects with MFS was compared with that in 15 nonaffected controls.

Plantar pressure distributions during walking were collected using a 1,000-element piezoceramic pressure platform. The protrusion of the head of the second metatarsal beyond the first metatarsal was determined by palpation. Pressure distributions were collected from a mid-gait step onto the platform at a speed of 1.6 to 2 m/sec using a 15-m runway. Peak pressures and impulse values were determined for 3 forefoot regions.

The difference between the lengths of the first 2 metatarsals ranged from 0.8 to 2.8 cm in the MFS group. Peak loading in both groups occurred under the second metatarsal, but the magnitudes of second metatarsal peak pressures were significantly higher in the MFS group (Fig 10–45).

Although the loading pattern between the MFS and non-MFS foot

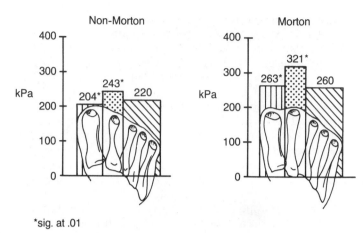

Non-Morton Morton

*sig. at .01

Fig 10–45.—Average peak pressures in kPa for the Morton and non-Morton groups. The first and second metatarsal head pressures were significantly different between groups. (Courtesy of Rodgers MM, Cavanagh PR: *Med Sci Sports Exerc* 21:23–28, February 1989.)

structures is similar, the significantly higher second metatarsal head peak pressure in the MFS may predispose this foot to problems associated with excessive localized pressure. This discrepancy in peak pressure may be related to a difference in dynamic function of the metatarsophalangeal joints during walking in which the more distally placed second metatarsal head serves as a pivot between 2 axes of motion and is rapidly loaded and unloaded.

▶ A major limitation of this study was the method in which metatarsal length was determined. Specifically, because radiologic evaluation apparently was not feasible, the examination was based on manual palpation of the first and second metatarsal heads. Apparently, "forensic footprints" were taken during walking and the difference in the metatarsal lengths was measured. I would question the accuracy of such a technique. Also, although an increased magnitude of pressure under the second metatarsal head in the MFS was demonstrated, the data do not support an association of this finding with the variety of foot problems that occur in the athlete.—J.S. Torg, M.D.

Turf Toe: Diagnosis and Treatment
Rodeo SA, O'Brien SJ, Warren RF, Barnes R, Wickiewicz TL (Cornell Univ; Hosp for Special Surgery, NY)
Physician Sports Med 17:132–147, April 1989   10–129

The installation of synthetic playing surfaces on football fields and the use of lightweight shoes on these surfaces have resulted in a dramatic increase in the incidence of metatarsophalangeal (MP) joint sprains of the great toe, a condition commonly known as turf toe.

Analysis of the mechanism of injury is necessary to understand the

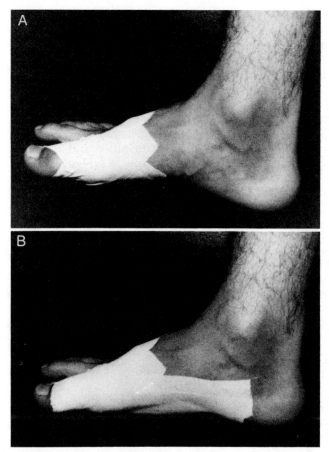

Fig 10–46.—Common taping technique used in turf toe: **A,** strips of 1-in. adhesive tape cross the metatarsophalangeal joint in a figure-8 strapping fashion. **B,** additional strips are applied from the tip of the toe to the middle of the longitudinal arch to serve as "checkreins." (Courtesy of Rodeo SA, O'Brien SJ, Warren RF, et al: *Physician Sports Med* 17:132–147, April 1989.)

joint pathology associated with the injury. The most common mechanism of a turf toe injury is hyperextension of the MP joint. Diastasis of the components of a tripartite medial sesamoid may result from disruption of the plantar capsular mechanism. Signs and symptoms include pain, hyperemia, and swelling around the joint. Roentgenograms show only generalized soft tissue swelling unless there is a concomitant fracture. The differential diagnosis includes metatarsal and phalangeal fracture, MP dislocation, and sesamoid stress fractures.

Initial treatment is conservative and includes ice application, compression, and elevation of the foot. Other treatment modalities are ultrasound, hot/cold contrast baths, and iontophoresis. The toe may be immobilized by taping, which consists of overlapping strips of 1-in. elastic tape around the great toe (Fig 10–46). These "checkreins" are secured by repeating the figure-8 strapping of 1-in. adhesive tape on top. Gradual weight-bearing is recommended until the full range of motion is pain free. During the return to activity, the shoe should be fitted with a splint to provide rigidity for the distal forefoot.

Prevention of turf toe injury should be recommended strongly to running backs, offensive linemen, and wide receivers. Rigid shoe inserts (e.g., those constructed of heat-sensitive plastic or a 0.51-mm spring steel splint) appear to be the most effective means of prevention. Appropriate shoe fit, such as those fitted both by length and width, is helpful. Artificial turf is also a predisposing factor to turf toe injury because it decreases shock absorption. The potential long-term sequelae of turf toe injury are undetermined, but separation of the medial and lateral sesamoid components, hallux rigidus, hallux valgus, and calcification have occurred.

▶ A soft shoe on an unforgiving artificial surface is an invitation to turf toe. It has been theorized that some players may be predisposed to this injury because of a loss of range of motion in the first MP joint. However, this study did not support that theory. We have tried various modalities, including nonsteroidal anti-inflammatory drugs and taping. We always fit the shoe with custom-molded plastic inserts to prevent recurrence of this injury. We recommend that the athlete use these inserts for the remainder of the season.—F.J. George, ATC, PT

Hazards of Long Distance Cycling
Desai KM, Gingell JC (Southmead Hosp, Bristol, England)
Br Med J 298:1072–1073, April 22, 1989   10–130

An unusual complication of long-distance cycling was reported in a young man who was not accustomed to riding more than a few kilometers.

Man, 27, complained of secondary erectile impotence. His sexual function was normal before he took part in a 2-day, 209-km bicycle race 5 months earlier. His bicycle had a hard, narrow leather saddle. During the race he experienced severe perineal pain and urgency of micturition. He stopped after about 32 km to void and noticed that his penis was completely shriveled and without any sensation. After a few minutes the pain stopped, and he continued the race. Despite recurrent perineal and gluteal pain, which caused him to make further brief stops, he finished the race. He then had total loss of erections for approximately 3 weeks. Although he improved gradually, his erections still lacked full rigidity and were sustained only briefly. Results of clinical examination and routine analysis of urine were normal, as were blood concentrations of glucose and serum concentrations of testosterone and prolactin. An intracavernosal injection of 15 mg of papaverine produced a fully rigid erection of almost 90 minutes' duration. There was no evidence of hemodynamic disturbance. Within 3 months his symptoms resolved completely.

This complication was probably caused by an ischemic neuropathy of the dorsal and cavernous nerves of the penis, which was induced by compression of the penile crura against the pubic bone by the bicycle seat. Short-term erectile impotence may be much more common in long-distance cyclists than has been appreciated previously.

▶ Another potential problem for male cyclists, who can also have painless gross hematuria after bumpy rides, presumably because of trauma to the perineum and posterior urethra. Bicycle-seat hematuria can be prevented by lowering the nose of the saddle, using a special seat cover, and rising off the saddle when railroad tracks and other bumps are encountered (1).—E.R. Eichner, M.D.

Reference

1. Salcedo JR: *N Engl J Med* 315:768, 1986 (letter).

Subject Index

Scintigraphy
thallium-201, after exercise and
coronary artery disease, 206
Self-esteem
exercise and, 126
Self-Motivation Inventory
predicting injury in cross country
runners with, 183
Semen
parameters in bodybuilders using
anabolic steroids, 198
Serotonergic
cells, tryptophan and 5-HT in, and
exercise, 84
Sex
differences
in heart response to supine exercise,
angiographic study, 30
in muscle cross-sectional area of
athletes, 32
Shift
test, dynamic posterior, in tibial
subluxation, 351
Shin
splints, compartment syndromes and
stress fractures, 281
Shoulder
arthroscopy (*see* Arthroscopy of
shoulder)
dislocation (*see* Dislocation, shoulder)
injuries
in archery, 299
athletic trainers evaluating, 250
in swimming, 319
instability
arthroscopic stapling repair, 322
rehabilitation, 320
pain
in throwing athlete, 330
and weakness, infraspinatus atrophy
causing, 336
Skating
pair, elite, injuries in, 300
speed skating simulator, ergometry of,
115
Skeletal
muscle (*see* Muscle, skeletal)
musculoskeletal (*see* Musculoskeletal)
Skiers
shoulder dislocations and Colles'
fractures, midazolam and diazepam
in, 321
women, working capacity, mental status
and menstrual cycle, 46
Skiing
downhill, injury risk in, 297
Skin
diving, ECG of, 158

Smoking
exercise after myocardial infarction and,
xvii
Snowboard
injuries, 298
Soccer
injuries
epidemiology and traumatology,
294
surface-related, 295
in women, menstrual cycle and oral
contraception in, 39
match, glucose polymer ingestion and
glycogen depletion during, 136
performance, effects of 100% oxygen
on, 147
women players, hematologic status of,
36
Somatomedin
C and muscle performance in aged, 9
Sonography (*see* Ultrasound)
Soreness
muscle
delayed, and postexercise static
stretching, 275
after high speed voluntary muscle
contractions, 274
from weight training, 10% trolamine
salicylate cream in, 275
in women, study of, 40
Spectroscopy, magnetic resonance
of wrist flexor muscles of elite rowers,
15
Spine
cervical, football-induced trauma, study
of, 293
fracture in winter sports, 308
lumbar, bone densities after physical
activity, 239
Splints
shin, compartment syndromes and stress
fractures, 281
Sports
eye injuries in, 303
nutrition, 133
winter, spine fracture in, 308
for women, medical problems of, 37
Sprain
knee lateral ligament compartment,
362
thumb, metacarpo-phalangeal, 343
Sprinting
hamstring injuries in, 272
Squash
players, competitive veteran, heart rate
and metabolic response of, 216
Squat
exercise and knee stability, 268

Author Index